RECENT ADVANCES IN
ANIMAL NUTRITION — 2012

Recent Advances in Animal Nutrition

2012

P.C. Garnsworthy, PhD
J. Wiseman, PhD
University of Nottingham

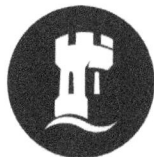

Nottingham
University Press

British Library Cataloguing in Publication Data
Recent Advances in Animal Nutrition — 2012:
University of Nottingham Feed Manufacturers
Conference (44th, 2012, Nottingham)
I. Garnsworthy, Philip C. II. Wiseman, J.

ISBN 9781789183016

Disclaimer

Every reasonable effort has been made to ensure that the material in this book is true, correct, complete and appropriate at the time of writing. Nevertheless the publishers, the editors and the authors do not accept responsibility for any omission or error, or for any injury, damage, loss or financial consequences arising from the use of the book.

Typeset by Nottingham University Press, Nottingham

EU GPSR Authorised Representative
LOGOS EUROPE, 9 rue Nicolas Poussin, 17000, LA ROCHELLE, France
E-mail: Contact@logoseurope.eu

PREFACE

The 44th University of Nottingham Feed Conference was held at the School of Biosciences, Sutton Bonington Campus, 27th – 28th June 2012. The Conference was divided into sessions that covered areas of topical interest to the animal feed industry. These sessions were Ruminants, Opportunities, Global Food and Farming, and Non-ruminants.

The Ruminant session started with a paper on monitoring the nutritional status of individual transition cows in order to improve reproduction and health of the whole herd. The second paper explained the relationships between feed intake and reproduction in cattle. The third paper reviewed the benefits of providing supplemental antioxidants in the diet to enhance fertility of dairy cows. The fourth paper provided a comprehensive review of rumen lipid metabolism and it various effects on the cow and milk composition.

The session on Opportunities comprised four papers that addressed issues of topical importance. The first paper explores the potential to formulate rations for lower environmental impact and the implications for overall feed costs. The second paper describes the animal feed industry in Germany. The third paper discusses the processes for obtaining EU registration of new feed additives. The fourth paper discusses the recent and likely future impacts of biofuels on the animal feed market.

The session on Global Food and Farming session contained two keynote papers addressing worldwide issues in food security. The first paper discusses the vital role of animal production, particularly from ruminants, in meeting global food requirements from a fixed area of land. The second paper complemented the first by exploring the potential for improving efficiency of animal production through advanced genetic techniques.

The non-ruminant session consisted of five papers concerned with aspects of nutrition, efficiency and environmental impact. The first paper considered how selection of poultry for digestive capacity impacts gut microflora and health. The second paper provided a progress report on the environmental road map used in the British pig industry. The third paper discussed the importance of methodology and definitions when considering amino acid digestibility of feeds for pigs. The fourth paper reviewed hormonal responses to nutrition in sows and implications for performance. The final paper provided an update on the role of phytase in diets for non-ruminants.

We would like to thank all speakers for their presentations and written papers, which have maintained the high standards and international standing of the Nottingham Feed Conference. We are grateful to all those members of the feed industry who provided suggestions and assistance in developing the conference programme. We would also like to acknowledge the input of those who helped us to chair sessions (Mike Wilkinson and Tim Parr) and the administrative (managed by Sue Golds), catering and support staff who ensure the smooth running of the conference. Finally we would like to thank the delegates who made valuable contributions both to the discussion sessions and the general atmosphere of the meeting.

P.C. Garnsworthy
J. Wiseman

CONTENTS

MONITORING NUTRITIONAL STATUS OF TRANSITION COWS TO IMPROVE HEALTH AND FERTILITY

R.L. COOPER AND J.A. HUSBAND

Evidence Based Veterinary Consultancy Ltd, Redhills Rural Enterprise, Penrith CA11 ODT, UK

Introduction

It is well recognised that how we choose to manage dairy cattle during their non-lactating period and in the few weeks following calving, can have extremely significant effects on their subsequent production, health and fertility. This period is often referred to as 'the transition period' and is commonly defined as the three weeks preceding calving and the three weeks after calving.

The main nutritional goals of transition cow management are:

• Prevention of excessive negative energy balance (NEB) and fat mobilisation, including subclinical or clinical ketosis and severe 'fatty liver'.

• Prevention of clinical and subclinical periparturient hypocalcaemia.

• Prevention of micronutrient deficiencies and additional supplementation of certain micronutrients where evidence suggests positive health benefits.

• Adaptation to the milking cow ration in a manner that encourages rumen health

Each of these has been robustly linked in scientific literature to the risk of other 'metabolic' diseases occurring, the probability of successful reproductive function or immune competency; a full review of the evidence is beyond the scope of this article and the authors instead would direct the reader to several good review articles (Overton and Waldron, 2004; Mulligan and Doherty, 2008; Santos, 2008)

Applying monitoring systems

BENEFITS OF MONITORING

It is commonly said that if something can be measured, it can be managed. This holds equally true in herd production medicine, particularly where many of the losses associated with poor transitioning are through subclinical disease or otherwise not immediately apparent. For the modern herd, data collection and analysis are vital in order to allow critical assessment of current management strategies and to provide early-warning systems to facilitate rapid intervention should problems occur. In addition, data are important in assessing management or interventions that have been applied, in order to assess whether the change has had a positive influence or been cost effective.

There are also benefits of monitoring on an individual animal basis. This particularly relates to subclinical (e.g. subclinical ketosis and hypocalcaemia) or inapparent disease (e.g. endometritis); by having a system in place for monitoring levels of that disease, there may potentially be opportunities available for early treatment. For example, McCart, Nydam and Oetzel (2012) tested cows six times from 3-16 days into lactation using a portable handheld ketone meter, and compared the effect of bolusing subclinically ketotic cows with propylene glycol against control cows. Treated animals were 1.6 times less likely to develop an abomasal displacement and 1.3 times more likely to conceive to first insemination. Clearly there are opportunities to be had through monitoring systems separate from herd level management interventions.

CHALLENGES TO MONITORING SYSTEMS

The goal of monitoring systems is to allow identification of an emerging problem within a timescale that allows interventions to circumvent or reduce the risks of a negative event occurring. Monitoring differs from herd performance analysis, which tends to focus on how the herd has performed over a longer time period in order to develop long-term intervention strategies, rather than how the herd is currently doing.

One of the difficulties of dairy monitoring systems is the small denominators (sample size) that end up being used in calculations of many performance indices. For example, if one out of two cows calving gets an abomasal displacement, does this necessarily indicate that the next one to calve has a 50% chance of getting one? When denominators are small, confidence intervals – the range over which we can be confident that the true mean lies – will be much greater for data that may still have the same mean and standard deviation.

The way to narrow confidence intervals and improve the 'robustness' of data is to increase the number of animals included in the denominators. In practical terms this means adding more historical performance to the dataset, e.g. moving from monitoring milk fever on a monthly incidence to a rolling three monthly incidence. The disadvantage of this approach is that while our confidence in the incidence figures generated improves, the 'momentum' of the rolling average also increases, and the longer it will take us to react when a problem arises.

There is a constant playoff between having confidence in the figures we use to make decisions, and how quickly we are able to respond to a potential problem; there is no 'one size fits all' approach and the decision over where the correct balance lies between the two must be made on both a herd and individual parameter basis i.e. in larger herds, it is probably appropriate to look at a disease incidence over a shorter time period.

Monitoring transition cow management in the UK is difficult, as herd size tends to be comparatively small. In an annual 2010 survey by DEFRA (DEFRA statistics, 2012), the average UK herd size was put at 113 cows. If we accept that the window of opportunity for monitoring transition cow management is approximately 42-63 days within a 420-day production cycle (Hudson, 2010), this infers an average denominator of 12-17 animals 'at risk' in a year-round calving herd. Set against a background of inherent environmental, nutritional and genetic variation, critical assessment and monitoring of transition cow systems is at best challenging.

MONITORING TECHNIQUES

Whatever technique is employed for monitoring, a relatively high sensitivity for initial screening tests ensures that herds with current or developing issues are readily identified and the undesirable outcome (compromise to the economic performance of the unit and animals' welfare) avoided. As such, these techniques should be cheap and easy to employ, but, due to the reciprocal relationship between sensitivity and specificity in most test characteristics, they should usually not be relied upon as diagnostic tools, especially where costly interventions are likely to follow due to the number of false positives that can typically be expected. Ideally, they should trigger further investigation using 'gold standard' techniques with a higher specificity and, hopefully, comparable sensitivity for conformation of diagnosis.

For example, if comparing the difference in body condition score (BCS) between dry stock and those 30-60 days into lactation demonstrated an average difference of >1.0 BCS units, then biochemical appraisal could be employed to make an assessment of fat mobilisation and ketosis. This would allow the advisor to differentiate between genuine BCS loss and the possibility of a cohort of lean animals following a cohort of over-conditioned animals around the production system – assuming that BCS data are not so historical that the opportunity for diagnosis has passed.

The way in which data are interpreted at a group level is an important part of monitoring systems. When examining data that have a uni-directional negative impact on cow health or are compared to threshold values, the proportion of animals above a threshold should be described, rather than just using the mean (Oetzel, 2004). For example, if animals are sampled for blood betahydroxybutyrate (BHB) concentrations, results should be expressed as the proportion of animals above the 1.2mmol/l cut-off, rather the mean BHB concentration for the group. For measurements that have a bi-directional negative effect on cow health (i.e. can be too high or low), then the mean or median may be more appropriate. For example, in a partial dietary cation anion balance (DCAB) system urine pH can be too acid (pH <6.5) or too alkali (pH >8.2), so a mean may be considered appropriate under some circumstances. BCS is frequently expressed as a mean and indeed may be considered bi-directional, but the authors contend that under most circumstances it is more appropriate to express it as a threshold value for a particular production group (e.g. proportion of cows with BCS >3.5). Means in particular may induce a false sense of confidence in data where equal proportions of too high and too low values exist.

Monitoring techniques can be broadly divided into direct or indirect measurements of the disease or fertility characteristic of interest; for example, direct measurement of subclinical ketosis could be blood biochemistry for the presence of a ketone body, while an indirect measurement would be milk fat:protein ratio (FPR) or the incidence of commonly associated diseases, such as abomasal displacement. Direct measurements are obviously the most robust approach from a diagnostic perspective, but may incur a time or labour cost that precludes or limits their application on-farm. In these circumstances, indirect measurements may be an acceptable compromise, provided their limitations are known, quantifiable and acknowledged.

Monitoring negative energy balance

DIRECT MEASUREMENTS

Biochemical appraisal

A wide variety of substrates, hormones and enzymes can be used to assess energy status of dairy cattle. Glucose, insulin, insulin-like growth factor (IGF), urea and aspartate aminotransferase (AST), amongst others, have all been shown to have varying associations with fertility or disease indices, and are potentially useful in building up a physiological profile at an individual animal level. However, due to difficulties in interpretation, commercial availability or expense, most of these are not widely used in practice for the purposes of monitoring; the two most commonly employed biochemical measurements of energy status for monitoring purposes are the ketone bodies (usually beta-hydroxybutyrate (BHB)) and non-esterified fatty acids (NEFA). Circulating concentrations of NEFA and BHB measure the success of adaptation to negative energy balance (NEB). NEFA reflects the magnitude of mobilization of fat from storage. BHB reflects the completeness of oxidization ("burning") of fat in the liver. Ketone bodies are the result of incomplete oxidation of fatty acids. As the supply of NEFA to the liver exceeds the ability of liver to completely oxidize the fatty acids to supply energy (Acetyl CoA for the TCA cycle), the amount of ketone production increases.

Following lipolysis and mobilisation of body fat reserves, fat is mobilised and NEFA are processed primarily by the liver. Blood concentration of NEFA is therefore a reliable measurement of the degree and rate of fat mobilisation in dairy cattle. Blood NEFA have been shown to be closely associated with liver triacyl-glycerol (TAG) content, increased risk of metabolic disease and decreased production, but moreover have been shown to have direct negative effects on fertility, including reducing oocyte competence (Bobe, Young and Beitz, 2004).

Ospina, Nydam, Stockol and Overton (2010) found that animals with blood NEFA concentrations ≥0.27mmol/l between 14 and 2 days prepartum had a reduced pregnancy risk of 19% and, if ≥0.33mmol/l, a 305-day milk yield reduced by 683 l. Post-partum cows (2-14 days in milk) with NEFA ≥0.72 mmol/l had a reduction in pregnancy risk of 16% and a reduction in 305-day milk yield of 393 l. The same group also identified associations between blood NEFA concentration and an increased incidence of metabolic disease in the individual animal (displaced abomasa, ketosis and metritis) if threshold concentrations of 0.29mmol/l pre-partum and 0.57mmol/l post-partum were exceeded.

Once NEFA reach the liver, their fate is either export as very low density lipoprotein (VLDL), storage as intrahepatic TAG, or oxidation. In situations of NEB, complete oxidation of NEFA is co-substrate limited, and partial oxidation pathways are employed, namely ketogenesis. Ketones bodies – acetoacetate, acetate and the carboxylic acid betahydroxybutyrate – are then exported and can be used as a source of energy by most body tissues.

Ketone testing forms the bulk of biochemical appraisal of energy status in cattle performed in the UK. It is possible to examine milk, urine and blood using both laboratory-based and cow-side assays, but the test characteristics of commercial available tests vary considerably.

Urine testing for the presence of ketone bodies essentially focuses on 'tablet' based systems that rely on a colour changing reaction between nitroprusside and acetoacetate and acetone, or semi-quantitative measurement of BHB via urine dip-strips. Although the nitroprusside-based tests are normally highly sensitive in urine, they have relatively poor specificity (Nielen, Aarts, Jonkers, Wensing, and Schukken, 1994; Carrier, Stewart, Godden, Fetrow and Rapniki, 2004), limiting their use to ruling out ketosis at the individual animal level. With this in mind, and given the time and labour involved in urine collection, it would appear unlikely that batch testing of urine for ketosis screening will ever become commonplace.

Milk testing for ketones has the obvious appeal of a non-invasive, low-labour method of assessing herd prevalence of subclinical ketosis. There have been various attempts to provide bulk laboratory testing through adaptation of methods normally used for serum assay, including fluorometric determination, gas liquid chromatography and Fourier transform infrared (FTIR) spectrometry (Larson and Neilson, 2005; Cook, Ward and Dobson, 2001; Eicher, 2004; Van Knegsel et al, 2010). Typically these have suffered from poor sensitivity, despite reasonable specificity, and have given relatively high numbers of false positives; the authors are unaware of any laboratories that are applying these techniques on a commercial basis.

Cow side milk testing has generally relied on nitroprusside-based tests that involve a colour change, as per the urine-based tests. These typically have high specificity in milk (>95%) but poor sensitivity (<45%) (Nielen et al, 2004; Carrier et al, 2004; Geishauser, Leslie, Ten Hag and Bashiri, 2000). A cow-side milk test, that semi-quantitatively measures BHB via formazin formation from nitrotetrazolium blue, exists under various names world-wide, including 'Ketolac'. This test has higher sensitivity in milk than the nitroprusside tests (73-95%) and reasonable specificity (69-96%) (Carrier et al, 2004; Oetzel, 2004; Osbourne, Leslie, Duffield, Petersson, Ten Hag and Okada, 2002; Geishauser et al, 2000). As this is a semi-quantitative test, different thresholds can be applied under different circumstances to alter test characteristics depending on the type of screening aimed for. As such, this test appears to represent the best non-invasive method of cow-side ketone testing available on the market at present.

In general, interpretation of milk tests is complicated by what 'gold standard' they are measured against and by the somewhat variable correlation between blood ketones and milk ketones. Although acetone concentrations appear to correlate well between blood and milk (r^2=0.96; Enjalbert, Nicot, Bayourthe and Moncoulon, 2001), BHB appears variable (r^2=0.00-0.87; Geishauser, Leslie, Kelton and Duffield, 1998) and acetoacetate apparently low (r^2=0.45; Enjalbert et al, 2001). Despite the limitations of milk testing, there is little doubt that they will be the focus of future commercial automated systems; there is currently a cooperative venture between Dansk Kvæg, DeLaval and FOSS being rolled out in Europe (Herd Navigator) that uses nitrotetrazolium blue-based dry-stick chemistry to measure milk BHB automatically. These results are then combined with other animal data in a statistical model to predict likelihood of subclinical ketosis. It is hoped that as the market for this type of screening develops, it will allow for refinement of milk ketone testing techniques and improved statistically-based interpretation systems.

At present, the 'gold standard' for metabolic appraisal of NEB remains blood biochemistry. Although options for ketone testing in milk and urine may be available, the techniques necessary for NEFA assay makes them the domain of commercial laboratory testing for the foreseeable future.

The disadvantages of blood-based biochemical appraisal are readily apparent. Firstly, these tests tend to be more expensive to run than milk and urine based tests (where they exist). This cost is related not only to the clinical biochemistry itself, but also the cost of labour in identifying and isolating animals for testing, and for either a qualified technician or veterinary surgeon's time in taking the samples. Secondly, blood sampling is generally regarded as an unpleasant experience, so there is an obvious animal welfare implication from using it as a routine monitoring tool.

To reduce these costs and the relative insult to cow welfare, statistical methods of sampling can be employed. Using hypergeometic distribution, it is possible to calculate the minimum number of samples required to identify one or more 'positive' animals at a defined prevalence and population at risk, and the probability that this threshold has been exceeded from the results of such sampling. In practical terms, 12 animals per group are generally required to make a well-informed decision about the likely prevalence of disease within a population. In sample sizes less than this number, there is an increasing likelihood that either insufficient animals will be available to reliably detect a problem, if present, or to allow meaningful interpretation of test results at a herd level.

Selecting the correct cohort of animals to sample is equally as important. Holtenius and Holtenius (1996) hypothesised that subclinical ketosis can be divided broadly into two types. Type 1 ketosis is largely a result of a mismatch between energy intake from feed and energy output (maintenance plus milk production requirements). This is typically thought to occur at around 25-45 days in milk when production is rapidly approaching peak but dry matter intake (DMI) is still rising slowly. Type 2 ketosis is thought to be largely a product of transition mismanagement and homeorrhetically-determined BCS loss (via uncoupling of the somatotrophic axis), resulting in accentuated insulin resistance and associated fat mobilisation. This is generally accepted to take place within the first two weeks post-calving.

It is suggested that the herd advisor selects animals on the basis of the problem most likely to be encountered. For example, a high-yielding TMR-fed herd feeding maize silage to their typically over-conditioned dry cows would be considered higher risk for Type 2 ketosis, and so may focus on NEFA and BHB testing in animals 2-15 days in milk. In contrast, a grass-based herd with minimal or no concentrate feeding would be considered higher risk for a Type 1 problem, so may choose to focus on BHB in cows 25-45 days into lactation. Although it is perfectly possible that either herd may have either both 'types' of ketosis present, or that they be the opposite way round to expected, it is suggested that appraisal of the clinical picture and relative risks for the management system can help to focus monitoring towards where it is more likely needed.

Fat mobilisation pre-calving, as shown by elevated NEFA, has been associated with subsequent increased risk of metabolic disease, including ketosis, as well as reduced production and decreased fertility. This fat mobilisation typically appears to be linked to the drop in DMI before calving, and in the authors' experience is greatest within the last seven days preceding parturition. Determination of blood NEFA concentrations in this group of animals is therefore a reasonable biochemical method of monitoring dry cow management.

Table 1. Suggested biochemical monitoring for dairy herds

	Target group relative to calving	*Biochemical substrate*	*No. animals to sample*
Pre-calving	-7 to -1 days	NEFA	12
Post calving			
'Type 2' ketosis	+1 to +15 days	BHB + NEFA	12
'Type 1' ketosis	+25 to +45 days	BHB +/- NEFA	12

There is now at least one cow-side test available for monitoring blood BHB. Originally used for diabetic monitoring in humans, these devices offer the benefit of rapid, affordable and relatively accurate diagnosis on-farm. Jeppesen, Enmark and Enevoldsen (2006) compared the devices to spectrophotometrically derived BHB concentrations and discovered a high correlation ($r^2=0.99$). When assessed as diagnostic devices for subclinical ketosis, at the 1.2mmol/l cut of point, sensitivity and specificity were found to be 85-88% and 94-96% respectively; at 1.4mmol/l cut-off this was raised to 90-96% and 97-98% respectively (Iwerson, Falkenberg, Voigtsberger, Forderung and Heuwieser, 2009; Voyvoda and Erdogan, 2010).

Body condition scoring

Body condition score is a widely used tool for determining changes in the body composition of dairy animals. Like mobility scoring, scales and definitions of BCS systems vary between countries but are essentially similar.

There is a strong evidence base that both BCS changes across the dry period and excessive BCS loss in early lactation are strongly and significantly associated with decreased performance, namely increased risk of disease and reduced fertility (Roche, Friggens, Kay, Fisher, Stafford and Berry, 2009). BCS loss could arguably be seen as an indirect measurement of excessive NEB, as mobilisation of tissue reserves (predominantly adipose) is a natural process and not necessarily a pathophysiological process in its own right. In practical terms, however, associations are so strong that changes over defined time periods and absolute values *per se* at particular points in the production cycle may be regarded as effective and practical monitoring method.

In practical terms, BCS scoring can be performed in two ways: the first relies on repeat measurements of individual cows at key points in their production cycle, allowing absolute changes to be identified on an individual and group basis. Provided that a well-defined method of scoring is employed, the number of operators kept to a minimum and regular cross checking between operators performed, this provides the best objective data on what is happening at a herd level. The main disadvantage is that the amount of labour involved in acquiring the data, and often poor feedback / utilisation of such data by farm advisors, means that all but the most dedicated units tend to lose enthusiasm. The other disadvantage in BCS scoring as a monitoring tool is that the lag from a problem emerging to the point at which it becomes apparent is relatively great. For example, if animals are scored at calving and 60 days into lactation, it may take a problem in dry cow management up to 3 months to be detected.

Another approach used by Caraviello, Weigel, Craven, Gianola, Cook, Nordlund, Fricke and Wiltbank (2006) is to examine cohorts of cattle in a single snapshot, looking at absolute prevalence rather than changes. Typically, this would focus on the proportion of animals in late lactation and late dry period BCS-UK >3. 5 or <2.0 and animals around peak lactation BCS-UK <1.75. This approach is well supported by scientific literature, in that many studies have identified risk associations with absolute body score condition values at key points in the production cycle (Roche et al 2009). It is also possible to compare average BCS between these cohorts to make a crude assessment of what the likely BCS loss or gain may be; this is no substitute for tracked individual cow data, but on farms where routine BCS is unable to be successfully implemented, it provides some limited information.

Modern parlours, particularly robotic systems currently apply repeat weight measurements as a proxy measurement of BCS. The difficulty of weight as a proxy for BCS is the ability to interpret absolute weight changes against individual and diurnal variations in frame size, gut fill, milk production (udder fill) and increasing feed intake across early lactation. There are some encouraging movements towards automated BC scoring by combining body weights with digital imaging of cows, but these systems require further refining before they are rolled out to commercial units.

INDIRECT MEASUREMENTS OF NEB

Milk constituents

Milk compositional data (MCD) at both a group and individual level are commonly employed as an indirect monitoring tool in the UK. The basic premise behind MCD is that during periods of excessive fat mobilisation, NEFA can be utilised by mammary epithelium in order to synthesise milk butterfat (BF). Animals mobilising a large degree of body-fat are more likely to have high BF than those in similar management conditions, not in excessive NEB. Similarly, there is a reasonably strong relationship between milk protein production and the energy intake of dairy cows (Coulon and Rémond, 1991), with animals in more positive energy balance having higher milk protein yield.

Bulk milk is a composite of all lactating animals, and therefore is inappropriate as a monitoring tool for energy status of early lactation animals in isolation. Nevertheless, it is common in the field for bulk milk composition, particularly protein, to be used as basic screening tool for herd energy status: typically, where bulk milk protein is below 3.1% in a year-round calving herd, advisors will often instigate further investigation. In this respect it remains a reasonable ancillary monitoring system: although tests characteristics are unknown, it can be assumed that sensitivity will be poor – due to concentration effects from peak and late lactation animals – but specificity moderate.

Monthly individual cow milk composition recording is relatively commonplace in the UK, and there promises to be an increasing move to parlour based composition measurements that can deliver daily testing of milk for BF and protein content. As such, this makes MCD an appealing monitoring tool, being readily available to farms and their advisors, and in the most part not attracting any additional testing costs.

The proportion of the herd with FPR >1.5 in the first 60 days in lactation, milk BF >5.5% and proportion of the herd with a total weight of milk protein <1.0 kg/d in the first 35 days into lactation feature in commercially available UK herd analysis software in the context of nutritional monitoring, (TotalVet, Sum-It), although with the exception of FPR none of the other parameters have a particularly good evidence base in peer-reviewed literature.

Unfortunately, although there is a strong statistical association between MCD and milk production, correlations with metabolic disease and fertility parameters are generally weak (Madouasse, Huxley, Browne, Bradley, Dryden and Green, 2010). In other words, excessive NEB (as measured by blood BHB and NEFA concentrations) accounts for only a small proportion of the variability seen in milk BF% and protein, whereas genetic factors, diet composition, age, season etc. account for the majority of the variability. The net effect is that at an individual cow, and probably herd level, MCD has poor sensitivity and specificity for detecting excessive NEB and is therefore inappropriate as a monitoring or diagnostic tool (Duffield, Kelton, Leslie, Lissemore, and Lumsden, 1997).

Although basic compositional data are unpromising in terms of diagnostic practicalities, there are currently efforts to determine the energy status of cows using mid-infrared spectrometry (MIR) to determine energy status of cows, primarily through the fatty acid profile of BF (McParland, Banos, Wall, Coffey, Soyeurt, Veerkamp and Berry, 2011). In the EU, this is being developed by a wide range of stakeholders from six countries in a joint project, OptiMIR, which runs through until 2015. Early data obtained though this and other international research appear to demonstrate better predictive power of NEB by milk NIR than FPR, but whether they will be a useful to diagnose NEB at an individual cow or herd level remains to be seen.

Methods for monitoring milk fever

The incidence of clinical milk fever is approximately 7 to 9% but varies considerably from farm to farm (Esslemont and Kossaibati, 1992). The incidence of subclinical disease is far higher (Jonsson, 1999) and in the authors' experience can be far in excess of 50% in the first 48 hours after calving (subclinical milk fever defined as blood calcium (Ca) concentration <2 mmol/l).

Where annual clinical incidence exceeds 7.5%, it is suggested that an investigation into the underlying causes followed by subsequent intervention strategies are appropriate. Due to the strong links between the occurrence of milk fever and the risk of other periparturient diseases (Curtis, Erb, Sniffen, Smith, Powers, Smith, White, Hillman and Pearson, 1983) it is also worthwhile assessing the prevalence of subclinical milk fever on a regular basis, especially in herds where there is a high incidence of other periparturient diseases.

Despite its economic impact on production, health, fertility and culling, clinical milk fever is poorly recorded on UK farms.

AETIOLOGY AND PREVENTION STRATEGIES

The aetiology of hypocalcaemia (milk fever) relates largely to the macro-mineral composition of the transition ration, but there is evidence that mobilisation of Ca from bone by parathyroid hormone (PTH) and calcitriol is possibly impaired under insulin resistance (Clemens and Karsenty, 2011). The risk of milk fever is most accurately assessed using the Dietary Cation Anion Balance or Difference (DCAB/D) of the transition pre-calving ration (Lean, DeGaris, McNeil and Block, 2006). The DCAB value of a ration or an individual feedstuff is calculated from the relative concentrations of sodium (Na) and potassium (K), the 'strong cations', relative to sulphur (present as SO_4) and chloride (Cl), the 'strong anions', and is measured in milliequivalents per kilogram dry matter (meq/kg DM). High DCAB value rations induce a metabolic alkalosis which decreases the efficiency of binding of PTH to its receptor and this reduces the activation of vitamin D_3. The role of vitamin D_3 is to increase Ca release from bone stores and increase Ca uptake from the gut.

Cows are usually metabolically alkalotic (urine pH in lactating cows is >8) due to the high K content of grass-based forages; virtually the only time strong metabolic alkalosis is a clinical problem is in the period prior to calving. The primary aim of the DCAB method of milk fever control is to reduce metabolic alkalosis. It is also important to ensure adequate magnesium (Mg) status as this is involved in the production, release and binding of PTH to its receptors (Horst, Goff and Reinhardt, 1994).

The partial DCAB approach is probably the most commonly used method of milk fever control and is based on selecting forages with low DCAB values (K concentration is the most important determinant of this) and ensuring an adequate Mg status. The full DCAB approach involves addition of anionic salts such as ammonium chloride, magnesium sulphate, calcium sulphate (gypsum) and calcium chloride. These have strongly negative DCAB values (an excess of Cl and S over Na and K) to induce a mild metabolic acidosis.

DIRECT MONITORING METHODS

Blood calcium measurements

Monitoring subclinical milk fever ideally focuses on the clinical output; sampling cohorts of cows for blood calcium. Evidence suggests that the window for diagnosis is relatively small for clinical milk fever, being up to 24 hours before calving, to a maximum of a week after. In the authors' practical experience, the window is substantially smaller, and animals should ideally be sampled within 48 hours after calving. No more than 30% of cows should have blood Ca below 2.00mmol/l in this cohort (Oetzel, 2004). Monitoring in this fashion attracts some logistical difficulties for UK herds. Firstly, due to small herd size it may take several weeks before a statistically robust number of animals have calved to estimate herd prevalence, and in that time diet and management may well have changed already. Secondly, in the UK it is illegal for technicians to sample animals for blood unless licensed to do so by DEFRA or the Home Office, and so the responsibility lies with the veterinary surgeon to either sample the animals themselves (this being possibly cost-prohibitive) or train the farmer – provided they are satisfied that it will be done in a responsible and safe manner - to blood sample their own cattle.

INDIRECT MEASUREMENTS

In practice monitoring is often best focused on either indirect biological measurements or on nutritional inputs.

Urinary monitoring

pH

In full DCAB systems, urinary pH is an acceptable method to assess acid-base status. Target ranges are oft-quoted as between pH 6 and 7 (Jardon, 1995) and provided that dietary Ca levels are kept sufficient to compensate for increased Ca mobilisation and excretion (typically 1.0-1.2% of dry matter), then this is considered adequate. The relationship between pH is the DCAB is not linear and in the partial DCAB range pH only falls slightly (and usually does not fall below 8.0) making urine pH monitoring unreliable. However, values >8.25 are considered to be high risk for milk fever (Seifi, Mohri and Zadeh, 2004). It is very important to note that pH meters need regular calibration to be accurate enough for this purpose.

Urinary macromineral testing

Urinary pH is less suitable for a partial DCAB system as described above. An alternative emerging method of assessment involves macromineral testing of urine. This allows appraisal of acidification of urine through measurement of Ca excretion, strong ion difference (SID) and TCO_2 (a measure of urine bicarbonate content and a proxy for blood bicarbonate), as well as providing ancillary information about Mg sufficiency and likely dietary intakes of K (often the cause of milk fever problems through high forage concentrations), Na and Cl.

Dietary macromineral assessment

Another indirect method of monitoring milk fever is simply regular evaluation of dietary components of the ration, principally the forages, for macromineral profile which must include Na, K, Cl, S (the components of the DCAB equation) and Mg. If a full DCAB prevention strategy is being used, it is important to know overall ration Ca concentration. Ca losses in the urine are normally low in the bovine, but at times of metabolic acidification they increase significantly (Husband, 2002) and there is a requirement for dietary Ca in excess of 1% of DM. As the mineral profile of forages may vary considerably between different cuts, growing areas and seasons, monitoring the risk of periparturient hypocalcaemia via frequent forage or TMR mineral analysis may be regarded as a reasonable ancillary monitoring strategy, despite the obvious limitations.

Table 2. Summary of prepartum urine analysis

Urine Parameter	Use
Calcium	Demonstrate Ca mobilization Demonstrate excessive demineralization with full DCAB.
pH	Demonstrate precalving metabolic acidification necessary for Ca mobilization
Magnesium	Demonstrate Mg status
SID (=Na+K-Cl)	Acid-base status, relates to DCAB (Roche et al., 2003)

Monitoring rumen health and adaptation

One of the goals of transition cow management is adaptation of the cow from the dry cow ration to the lactating ration without overt compromise to rumen health, and potentially

There is mixed evidence over whether provision of fermentable carbohydrates is necessary for rumen papillary development prior to calving (Reynolds, Durst, Lupoli, Humphries and Beever, 2004). As such, it seems unclear at the moment whether the greater risk for poor adaptation lies with changes in microbiological flora, anatomical considerations or rumen cell physiology.

Rumenocentesis is currently regarded as the gold standard for diagnosis and monitoring for subacute ruminal acidosis (SARA) (Enemark, 2007). The suggested guideline for herd-level diagnosis is that the prevalence of cows with a rumen pH ≤5.5 obtained by ventral sac rumenocentesis should not exceed a 25% prevalence. This diagnosis criterion should be applied with caution to UK herds: in the validation study the cut off of pH ≤5.5 was identified as the best discriminatory pH between a 'safe' ration fed to one group of cows and a 'SARA-inducing' ration fed to another. Both of these rations could have been considered high risk by UK standards, and it is arguably a false assumption to assume that there are no adverse effects on animal health from rumen pH reaching or remaining in the range of, for example, 5.7-6.1. It is advisable to consider rumen pH measurements in parallel with rumen fluid quality scoring; (Kleen, Hoojer, Rehageand Noordhuizen, 2004) composed a list of criteria that could be used to grade rumen fluid acquired during sampling and found that it highly correlated to presence of SARA.

Rumenocentesis is an invasive procedure that compromises cattle welfare, is expensive to apply on a routine basis and probably would be considered ethically unacceptable by the general public. As such, many alternative methods of monitoring have been suggested including animal-based observations, paper and physical assessment of the ration, and alternative methods of rumen fluid capture or assessment. Animal and ration based observations that have been advocated in popular literature can be found in Table 3.

Table 3. Methods of rumen health monitoring proposed in popular literature

Type of observation	Method
Animal-based	Proportion of awake, lying animals cudding 2-3 hours after feeding.
	Number of chews per cud
	Cleanliness scoring: especially flank & tail (Hughes, 2001)
	Presence or absence of 'dropped cuds'
Faecal-based	Faecal consistency scoring
	Presence or absence of fibre >1.25cm
	Presence or absence of undigested (processed) starch grains
	Presence or absence of fibrin casts
Ration based	Paper formulation (various formulation guidelines cited)
	Penn-state separator assessment (various guidelines cited)
	Ration water-flotation assessment
Substrate based	Proportion of the herd with low milk butterfat (<2.5%)
	Blood constituent changes: hypercalcaemia, hyperphosphataemia, low pH
	Urine constituent changes: increased phosphate excretion

Although these methods are widely employed in the field and many would argue their efficacy, peer-reviewed data relating to their validation are either scant or absent altogether; as such, the methods should be applied with healthy scepticism by the herd advisor, but certainly not dismissed outright.

There are a number of products currently available that are able to monitor rumen pH remotely via in-situ boluses (Mottram et al, 2008). These have been typically developed towards academic research, but are beginning to enter the commercial market. Although there have been some practical shortcomings relating to the lifetime and long-term accuracy of such boluses, it is understood that these shortcomings are being addressed, and such devices will hopefully be available as monitoring tools in the near future.

Monitoring micronutrient status

The most robust evidence with regard to influence of micronutrient status in cows relates mainly to those associated primarily with antioxidant function - Vitamin E, selenium and beta-carotene – or iodine (Underwood and Suttle, 1999; LeBlanc, Herdt, Seymor, Duffield and Leslie, 2004). Although the effects on cow and calf health of iodine relate largely to deficiency (via undersupply or antagonism), the 'antioxidants' have a more complicated relationship. Deficiency of these has been clearly shown to increase risk of metabolic disease and reduced immune competency, but several studies have demonstrated a benefit in health and performance from feeding supplementary levels.

At present the ability to monitor micronutrient status within a commercial setting is limited to the diagnosis of deficiency where clinical indicators suggest a problem; there is little or no capacity to assess whether dietary intake is sufficient to bring about additional health and performance benefits.

Summary

How we choose to manage dairy cattle during their non-lactating period and in the few weeks following calving (the transition period), can have extremely significant effects on their subsequent production, health and fertility. The aims of monitoring transition management are to see if goals are being achieved and to allow identification of an emerging problem within a timescale that allows interventions to circumvent or reduce the risks of a negative event occurring.

The main monitoring target is NEB in early lactation and there are direct and indirect methods available to do this, but it is important to know the limitations of the tests being used.

References

Bobe, G. J., Young, J.W. and Beitz, D.C. (2004) *Invited Review:* Pathology, Etiology, Prevention and Treatment of Fatty Liver in Dairy Cows. *J. Dairy Sci.* 87:3105–3124.

Carrier, J., Stewart, S., Godden,S., Fetrow, J., and Rapnicki, P. (2004). Evaluation and use of three cowside tests for detection of subclinical ketosis in early postpartum cows. *J. Dairy Sci.* 87:3725-3735.

Caraviello, D. Z., Weigel, K. A., Craven, M., Gianola, D., Cook, N. B. Nordlund, K. V., Fricke, P. M. and Wiltbank, M. C. (2006) Analysis of Reproductive Performance of Lactating Cows on Large Dairy Farms Using Machine Learning Algorithms. *J. Dairy Sci.* 89:4703–4722.

Clemens, T.L. and Karsenty, G. (2011) The Osteoblast: An Insulin Target Cell Controlling Glucose Homeostasis. *Journal of Bone and Mineral Research*, 26:4, 677–680.

Cook, N.B., Ward W.R. and Dobson, H. (2001) Concentrations of ketones in milk in early lactation, and reproductive performance of dairy cows. *Vet Rec*, 148: 769-772.

Coulon, J. B., and Rémond, B. (1991). Variations in milk output and milk protein content in response to the level of energy supply to the dairy cow: A review. *Livestock Production Science*, 29:31-47.

Curtis, E. R., Erb, H. N., Sniffen, G. J., Smith, R. D., Powers, P. A., Smith, M. C., White, M. E., Hillman, R. B. & Perason, E. J.(1983) Association of parturient hypocalcaemia with periparturient disorders in Holstein cows. *Journal of the American Veterinary Medical Association* 183, 559-561.

DEFRA Statistics (2012) http://www.defra.gov.uk/food-farm/food/food-industry/ milk-industry/ DEFRA, UK.

Duffield, T. F., Kelton, D. F., Leslie, K. E. , Lissemore, K. D. and Lumsden, J. H. (1997). Use of test day milk fat and milk protein to detect subclinical ketosis in dairy cattle in Ontario. *Canadian Veterinary Journal*, 38:713-718.

Eicher, R., (2004) Evaluation of the metabolic and nutritional situation in dairy herds: Diagnostic use of milk components. *23rd World Buiatrics Congress, Québec, Canada.*

Enemark, J.M.D. (2007) The monitoring, prevention and treatment of sub-acute ruminal acidosis (SARA): A review. *The Veterinary Journal* 176 32-43.

Enjalbert, F., Nicot, M.C., Bayourthe, C. and Moncoulon, R. (2001). Ketone bodies in milk and blood of dairy cows: Relationship between concentrations and utilization for detection of subclinical ketosis. *J Dairy Sci*, 84: 583-589.

Esslemont, R. & Kossaibati, M. (2002) Trends in fertility in 52 dairy herds over 11 seasons. *DAISY Research Report no. 5.* University of Reading.

Geishauser, T., Leslie, K. Kelton D. and Duffield, T. (1998). Evaluation of five cowside tests for use with milk to detect subclinical ketosis in dairy cows. *J Dairy Sci,* 81: 438-443.

Geishauser, T., Leslie, K., Ten Hag, J. and Bashiri, A. (2000). Evaluation of eight cow-side ketone tests in milk for detection of subclinical ketosis in dairy cows. *J. Dairy Sci.* 83:296-299.

Holtenius, P. and Holtenius, K. (1996) New aspects of ketone bodies in energy metabolism of dairy cows: A review. *J Vet Med A* 43:579.

Horst R L, Goff J P and Reinhardt T A. (1994) Calcium and vitamin D Metabolism in the dairy cow. Symposium: calcium metabolism and utilization. *J. Dairy Sci.* 77: 1936-1951.

Hudson, C.D., Breen, J.E., Bradley, A.J. and Green, M.J. (2010) Fertility In UK Dairy Herds: Preliminary Findings Of A Large-Scale Study. *Cattle Practice* 18:2 89-94.

Hughes (2001) A system for assessing cow cleanliness. *In Practice* 23:9 517-524.

Husband, J. A. (2002) The effect of feeding anionic salts on urine pH. *Cattle Practice* 10, 113-118.

Iwersen M, Falkenberg, U. Voigtsberger R., Forderung, D. and Heuwieser, W. (2009). Evaluation of an electronic cowside test to detect subclinical ketosis in dairy cows. *J Dairy Sci,* 92: 2618-2624.

Jardon, P. W. (1995) Using urine pH to monitor anionic salt programs. *Compendium on Continuing Education for the Practicing Veterinarian* 17, 860-862.

Jeppesen R, JMD Enemark and C Enevoldsen, (2006). Ketone body measurement in dairy cows. *Proc. 24th World Buiatrics Congress, Nice, France. World Assoc. Buiatrics, Vienna, Austria.*

Jonsson, N. N. (1999) The effects of subclinical hypocalcaemia on postpartum fertility. *Cattle Practice* 7, 255-260.

Kleen, J.L., Hooijer, G.A., Rehage, J. and Noordhuizen, J.P.T.M., (2004). Rumenocentesis (rumen puncture): a viable instrument in herd health diagnosis. *Deutsche Tierarztliche Wochenschrift* 111, 458–462.

Larsen T and N Nielsen, 2005. Fluorometric determination of β-hydroxybutyrate in milk and blood plasma. *J Dairy Sci,* 88: 2004-2009.

Lean, I.J., DeGaris, P.J., McNeil, D.M. and Block, E. (2006) Hypocalcemia in Dairy Cows: Meta-analysis and Dietary Cation Anion Difference Theory Revisited. *J. Dairy Sci.* 89:669–684.

LeBlanc, S. J., Herdt, T. H., Seymour, W. M. Duffield, T. F. and Leslie, K. E. (2004) Peripartum Serum Vitamin E, Retinol, and Beta-Carotene in Dairy Cattle and Their Associations with Disease. *J. Dairy Sci.* 87:609–619.

Madouasse, A, Huxley, J N, Browne, W J, Bradley, A J, Dryden, I L and Green, M J, (2010) Use of individual cow milk recording data at the start of lactation to predict the calving to conception interval. *J. Dairy Sci.* 93(10), 4677-90.

Madouasse, A, Huxley, J N, Browne, W J, Bradley, A J, Dryden, I L and Green, M J, (2010) Use of individual cow milk recording data at the start of lactation to predict the calving to conception interval. *J. Dairy Sci.* 93(10), 4677-90.

McArt J.A.A., Nydam, D.V. and Oetzel, G. R. (2012) A field trial on the effect of propylene glycol on displaced abomasum, removal from herd, and reproduction in fresh cows diagnosed with subclinical ketosis. *J Dairy Sci* 95:2505-2512.

McParland S., Banos, G., Wall, E., Coffey, M.P., Soyeurt, H., Veerkamp, R.F. and Berry, D.P. (2011) The use of mid-infrared spectrometry to predict body energy status of Holstein cows. *J Dairy Sci.* 94:7 3651-61.

Mottram, T., Lowe, J., McGowan, M., and Phillips, N. (2008) A wireless telemetric method of monitoring clinical acidosis in dairy cows. *Computers and Electronics in Agriculture* 64: 45-48.

Mulligan, F.J. and Doherty, M. L. (2008) Production diseases of the transition cow. *The Veterinary Journal* 176 3-9.

Nielen, M., Aarts, M. G. A., Jonkers, A. G. M., Wensing, T. and Schukken, Y. H. (1994). Evaluation of two cowside tests for the detection of subclinical ketosis in dairy cows. *Can. Vet. J.* 35:229-232.

Oetzel GR. (2004) Monitoring and testing dairy herds for metabolic disease. *Vet. Clin. North Amer: Food Animal Practice* 20:651-674.

Osborne, T.M., Leslie, K.E., Duffield, T., Petersson, C.S., Ten Hag, J. and Okada, Y. (2002) Evaluation of keto-test in urine and milk for the detection of subclinical ketosis in periparturient Holstein dairy cattle. *Proc. 35th Ann. AABP Conf.* 35:188.

Ospina P. A., Nydam, D. V., Stockol T. and Overton, T. R. (2010). Associations of elevated nonesterified fatty acids and β-hydroxybutyrate concentrations with early lactation reproductive performance and milk production in transition dairy cattle in the northeastern United States. *J Dairy Sci,* 93:1596-1603.

Overton, T.R. and Waldron, M. R. (2004) Nutritional Management of Transition Dairy Cows: Strategies to Optimize Metabolic Health. *J. Dairy Sci.* 87:(E. Suppl.):E105–E119.

Reynolds, C. K., Durst, B., Lupoli, B., Humphries, D. J. and Beever, D. E. (2004) Visceral Tissue Mass and Rumen Volume in Dairy Cows During the Transition from Late Gestation to Early Lactation. *J. Dairy Sci.* 87:961–971.

Roche, J. R., Friggens, N. C., Kay. J. K., Fisher, M. W. Stafford, K. J. and Berry, D. P. (2009) Body condition score and its association with dairy cow productivity, health, and welfare. *J. Dairy Sci.* 92:5769–5801.

Roche, J.R., Dalley, D., Moate, P., Grainger, C., Rath, M. and O'Mara, F. (2003) Dietary Cation-Anion Difference and the Health and Production of Pasture-Fed Dairy Cows 2. Non-lactating Periparturient Cows. *J. Dairy Sci.* 86:979–987.

Seifi, H., Mohri, M. and Zadeh, J. (2004) Use of prepartum urine pH to predict the risk of milk fever in dairy cows. *The Veterinary Journal*, 167:3 281-285.

Underwood, E.J. and Suttle, N.F. (1999) *The Mineral Nutrition of Livestock*, 3rd edn. CAB International, Wallingford, UK.

Van Knegsel, A.T.M., van der Drift, S.G.A., Horneman, M., de Roos, A.P.W., Kemp, B. and Graat, E.A.M. (2010). Ketone body concentration in milk determined by Fourier transform infrared spectroscopy: Value for the detection of hyperketonemia in dairy cows. *J Dairy Sci*, 93: 3065-3069.

Voyvoda H and H Erdogan, (2010) Use of a hand-held meter for detecting subclinical ketosis in dairy cows. *Res Vet Sci,* 89: 344-351

2

FEED INTAKE AND REPRODUCTION IN CATTLE

SARTORI, R., GUARDIEIRO, M.M., MOLLO, M.R. AND SURJUS, R.S.
Department of Animal Science, ESALQ, University of São Paulo (USP), Av. Pádua Dias, 11, Piracicaba, SP, Brazil 13418-900
E-mail: robertosartori@usp.br

Introduction

Nutrition has an important role in reproduction by directly affecting aspects of the reproductive physiology and performance in cattle. For example, several studies have linked nutrition to fertility problems, especially in dairy cows that have severe negative energy balance (NEB), evidenced by the decrease in body condition score (BCS) postpartum (Moreira *et al.*, 2000, López-Gatius, 2003) and furthermore, to the deleterious effects of high energy diets (Wiltbank *et al.*, 2006, Santos *et al.*, 2008a, Santos *et al.*, 2008b), the toxic effects of nitrogen compounds (Butler, 1998, Dawuda *et al.*, 2002, Rhoads *et al.*, 2006), and vitamin and/or mineral deficiencies (Ingraham *et al.*, 1987, Aréchiga *et al.*, 1994, Aréchiga *et al.*, 1998). Moreover, there is still much controversy about the effects of nutritional "flushing" or increase in dry matter intake (DMI) on fertility and embryo production in ruminants (Diskin and Morris, 2008, Santos *et al.*, 2008b, Leroy *et al.*, 2008). On the other hand, some but not all studies have found positive results on the reproductive efficiency in cattle using fat supplementation.

Due to the vast amount of information on this subject, we will be focusing mainly in this chapter, on data related to feed intake and reproduction, emphasizing studies developed by our group that have not been published elsewhere. Data from published studies from other groups will be either described in less detail or summarized in tables.

Influence of feed intake on ovarian structures and hormone concentrations

Several studies have shown that dry matter intake affects several aspects of reproductive physiology in cattle. Most of these observations were by indirect comparisons, such as comparing heifers vs. lactating dairy cows. There were, however, experiments that were specifically designed to evaluate the effects of nutrition on reproduction in animals of the same category, differing only in feed supply. These studies reported many effects of feed intake on reproduction such as: changes in number and size of ovarian structures; changes in circulating hormone concentrations; and alteration in the duration of oestrus, and will be described below.

INFLUENCE OF FEED INTAKE ON NUMBER OF OVARIAN ANTRAL FOLLICLES

Some researchers described greater superovulatory responses to ovarian superstimulation in cattle overfed previously (Gong *et al.*, 2002, Singh *et al.*, 2004, Ireland *et al.*, 2007, Surjus *et al.*, 2012). Similarly, treatment with recombinant bovine somatotrophin (rBST) improved antral follicle population in cattle (Gong *et al.*, 1991, Buratini *et al.*, 2000). It is likely that the mechanisms involved in the follicle number improvement due to high feed intake are related to circulating insulin and IGF-I concentrations, being augmented especially by increased propionate concentrations. Additionally, increase of insulin concentrations induced by high feed intake decreased IGF binding proteins (IGFBP) expression, increasing the bioavailability of IGF-I (Armstrong *et al.*, 2001, Gong *et al.*, 2002). Both insulin and IGF-I act as potent stimulators of granulosa cell proliferation and steroidogenesis in cattle (Webb *et al.*, 2004). IGF-I acts in synergism with FSH on steroidogenesis by increasing the P450 aromatase activity (Echternkamp *et al.*, 1994). Silva and Price (2002) showed that in vitro culture of bovine granulosa cells with ~100 ng/ml of insulin stimulated mRNA expression and P450 aromatase activity, and increased oestradiol secretion by these cells. Recently, Mani *et al.* (2010) cultured bovine granulosa cells with different concentrations of IGF-I (1, 50 and 100 ng/ml) in a serum-free system without insulin. These authors found that culture with IGF-I (50 or 100 ng/ml) significantly increased: 17β-oestradiol production, cell number, mRNA expression of genes related to steroidogenesis (CYP11A1, HSD3B1, and CYP19A1), and expression of genes that encode receptors for IGF-I and FSH (FSHR and IGF-IR) as compared to granulosa cells cultured only with FSH. Furthermore, because the corpus luteum (CL) also has

IGF-I receptors, it may respond to an IGF-I stimulus with increase in gonadotrophin activity and progesterone synthesis. Data from a recent study from our lab also suggest a relationship between circulating IGF-I and insulin and ovarian function in cattle. By directly comparing *Bos indicus* vs. *Bos taurus* non-lactating cows, fed on maintenance diets, Bastos *et al.* (2010) observed that *Bos indicus* cows had higher number of follicles (42.7 ± 5.9) than *Bos taurus* cows (19.7 ± 3.2; p < 0.05), as well as higher circulating insulin (9.9 ± 1.5 vs. 3.0 ± 0.7 µIU/ml) and higher circulating IGF-I concentrations (245.5 ± 12.0 vs. 198.3 ± 10.3 ng/ml; p < 0.05). Moreover, despite having smaller ovarian structures (ovulatory follicle and CL), *Bos indicus* cows had higher circulating oestradiol and progesterone concentrations.

Although, as discussed above, there are studies that have shown a positive relationship between high feed intake and number of antral follicles, results from other authors, including data from studies performed in our lab, either have found no effect or have described a negative relationship. Below, we present the results of two experiments in which there was no relationship or there was a negative relationship between feed intake and follicle number. Interestingly, in both studies, the animal model used was *Bos indicus* heifers.

It has been shown that the BCS at the beginning of a nutritional "flushing" treatment may influence embryo production in *Bos taurus* cattle (Adamiak *et al.*, 2005). Based on this assumption, we developed a study to investigate if differences in BCS associated or not with nutritional flushing influence the superovulatory response in Nelore (*Bos indicus*) heifers (Bastos *et al.*, 2007). Thirty six pubertal heifers with lower (2.7 ± 0.1; n = 18) or higher (3.7 ± 0.1; n = 18) BCS (scale from 1 to 5) were assigned to two groups and each group was subdivided into Maintenance (M; fed at nutritional requirements for maintenance) or Flushing (F; 1.8 x M). Therefore, there were four subgroups: <BCS + maintenance (<M), <BCS + flushing (<F), >BCS + maintenance (>M), and >BCS + flushing (>F). Nutritional flushing occurred throughout the 14 d prior to the first FSH injection of the superovulation treatment, after which heifers returned to the maintenance diet. Heifers were superovulated with a total of 150 IU of FSHp. Twelve h after the last FSH treatment, GnRH was injected i.m. and all heifers were inseminated 12 and 24 h later using the same sire. Seven d after GnRH, embryos were collected and evaluated. Each heifer was superovulated twice and the interval between embryo collections was 35 d. Heifers that had received F at the first superovulation were kept on M at the second superovulation, and vice-versa. Ovarian ultrasonography was performed to evaluate follicular population at the time of the first and last FSH injection. Moreover, ultrasound examination was also done 2 and 7 d after the GnRH injection in order to estimate the number of ovulated follicles. The number of follicles ≥ 3mm at the time of the first FSH did not differ (p > 0.10) among groups >M (56.4 ± 6.0), >F (55.1 ± 4.5), <M (54.3 ± 6.9), and <F (48.2 ± 4.8).

One of the studies showing a negative relationship between feed intake and follicle population used 39 *Bos indicus* heifers that were fed on a diet with 40.8% coast-cross hay, 51.9% corn silage, 7.3% energy/protein-urea/mineral/vitamin supplement for 9 weeks (Mollo *et al.*, 2007a). Heifers were divided in two groups according to dietary maintenance levels: Group H = 1.7 x M and Group L = 0.7 x M. At the end of the 7th week of nutritional treatments, heifers underwent superovulatory treatments. In spite of Group H heifers having higher BCS, body weight (BW; Figure 1) and serum insulin concentrations (14.3 ± 1.7 vs. 3.0 ± 0.8 µIU/ml) than Group L heifers, Group L had a greater number of follicles ≥ 3 mm at the time of the first FSH treatment (42.6 ± 6.6 vs. 32.6 ± 2.5; P = 0.10). Superovulatory responses and embryo production data of the above experiments will be presented in a later section below.

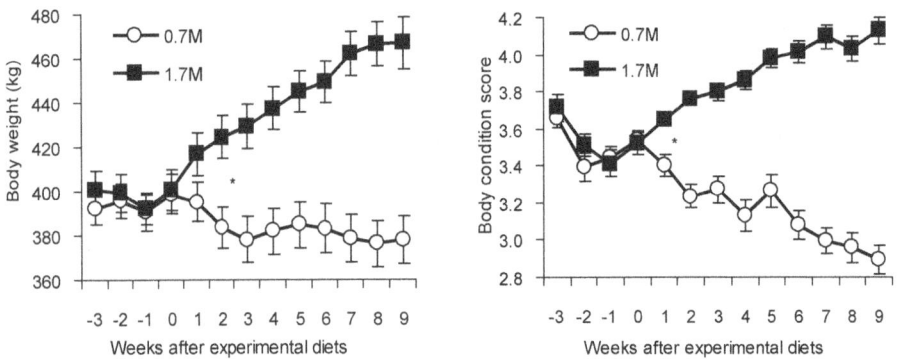

Figure 1. Body weight and body condition score of *Bos indicus* heifers under low (0.7 x M; n = 19) or high (1.7 x M; n = 20) feed intake.

Data from studies that evaluated the relationship between feed intake and follicle population are summarized in Table 1.

INFLUENCE OF FEED INTAKE ON NUMBER OF FOLLICULAR WAVES

Although a previous study in *Bos taurus* heifers had suggested there was an effect of feed intake on number of follicle waves in cattle (Murphy *et al.*, 1991), another study performed by our group in *Bos indicus* heifers did not see this effect (Mollo *et al.*, 2007b). In the study of Murphy *et al.* (1991), heifers receiving 0.7 of maintenance diets (0.7 x M) tended to have more oestrous cycles with three waves (5/7) than heifers receiving 1.8 x M (1/5). In our research using 39 Nelore heifers described above, there was no effect of feed intake on number of follicle

Table 1. Studies performed in Bos taurus, *Bos indicus* or crossbred cattle showing the influence of feed intake on antral follicle population before ovum pick up or superovulation. Experimental animals were fed maintenance (1 x M) or below maintenance (< M) diets vs. above maintenance (> M) diets throughout different supplementation periods of time.

Reference	N	Genetic group	Category	Supple-mentation period	1 x M or < M	> M	Difference	P
Gutierrez *et al*. (1997)	**28**	***Bos taurus***	**Heifers**	**30**	**18.0**	**25.0**	**+38.9**	**<0.05**
Nolan *et al*. (1998)	33	*Bos taurus*	Heifers	17	6.7	6.7	0.0	>0.10
Mackey *et al*. (2000)	**11**	***Bos taurus***	**Heifers**	**14**	**5.9**	**9.2**	**+55.9**	**0.10**
Armstrong *et al*. (2001)	**24**	***Bos taurus***	**Heifers**	**12**	**8.1**	**11.0**	**+35.8**	**<0.05**
Gong *et al*. (2002)	**24**	***Bos taurus***	**Heifers**	**16**	**8.7**	**14.5**	**+66.7**	**<0.05**
Adamiak *et al*. (2005)	48	*Bos taurus*	Heifers	70	12.6	13.0	+3.2	>0.10
Bastos *et al*. (2009)	28	*Taurus* x *Indicus*	Crossbred dry cows	7	19.5	16.4	-15.9	>0.10
Sales *et al*. (2011)	28	*Taurus* OR *Indicus*	Dry cows	42	25.2	24.5	-2.8	>0.10
Martins *et al*. (2006)	**20**	***Bos indicus***	**Dry cows**	**35**	**14.8**	**17.1**	**+15.5**	**<0.05**
Bastos *et al*. (2007)	72	*Bos indicus*	Heifers	7	54.4	51.6	-5.1	>0.1
Mollo *et al*. (2007a)	39	*Bos indicus*	Heifers	63	42.6	32.6	-23.5	0.10
Surjus *et al*. (2012)	**66**	***Bos indicus***	**Dry cows**	**32**	**11.1**	**12.8**	**+15.3**	**<0.05**

*Data in bold represent studies having positive effects of high feed intake on number of follicles before superovulation or ovum pick up.

waves (Figure 2). The percentage of cycles with two, three, or four waves was 25.0, 50.0 and 18.0%, respectively for Group L (0.7 x M) and 27.8, 55.6 and 16.6%, respectively for Group H (1.7 x M). When comparing lactating dairy cows to heifers, which have very different feed intakes, other studies also did not detect differences in number of waves during an oestrous cycle (Sartori *et al.*, 2004, Wolfenson *et al.*, 2004).

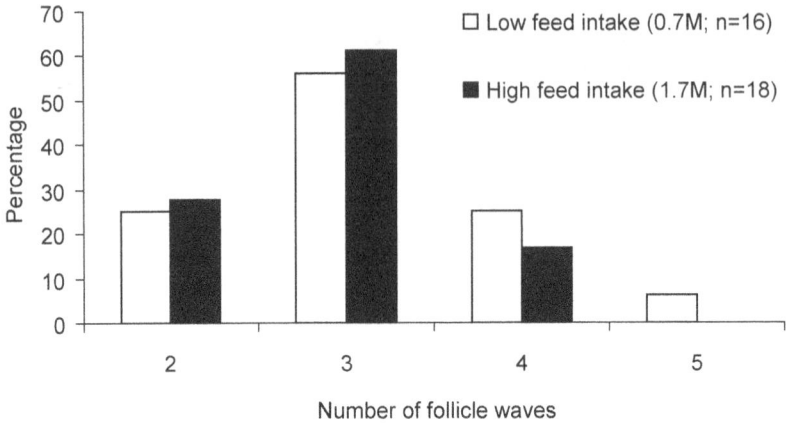

Figure 2. Percentage of *Bos indicus* heifers with two to five follicle waves during an oestrous cycle in relation to feed intake.

INFLUENCE OF FEED INTAKE ON SIZE OF OVARIAN STRUCTURES AND CIRCULATING HORMONES

In lactating dairy cows there is a high and positive correlation (r = 0.88) between dry matter intake and milk production (Harrison *et al.*, 1990). High feed intake can alter ovarian physiology and hormone concentrations. In fact, high producing cows have greater follicle sizes; however steroid concentrations in blood are lower compared to heifers and dry cows (Sartori *et al.*, 2002, Wolfenson *et al.*, 2004). Sartori *et al.* (2004) compared ovarian function of pubertal heifers (n = 27) and lactating dairy cows (n = 14) with a mean milk yield of 45.7 ± 1.3 kg/d, during one complete oestrous cycle. Similarly, Mollo *et al.* (2007b) followed one complete oestrous cycle of pubertal Nelore heifers under high (H; 1.7 x M) or low (L; 0.7 x M) feed intake. For the sake of making an indirect comparison, we grouped data from both studies in the same table (Table 2) and discussed the influence of feed intake on reproductive variables of *Bos indicus* beef and *Bos taurus* dairy cattle.

Despite differences between breeds in size of ovarian structures and circulating hormones, as reported elsewhere (Sartori *et al.*, 2010), there was a clear effect of feed intake on reproductive variables in both breeds. Likewise, in another study of our laboratory, we observed greater (P < 0.03) serum oestradiol concentrations in non-lactating Zebu cows with restricted feeding (0.7 x M) as compared to overfed cows (1.7 x M; 17.2 ± 2.5, n = 7 vs. 9.8 ± 1.2 pg/ml, n = 6; Martins *et al.*, 2006).

Table 2. Mean (± SE) serum hormone concentrations and size of ovarian structures in heifers and lactating cows. Study 1 used 39 Nelore heifers under low (0.7 x M) or high (1.7 x M) feed intake [adapted from Mollo *et al.* (2007b)]. Study 2 compared lactating dairy cows milking 45.7 ± 1.3 kg/d to pubertal heifers (Sartori *et al.*, 2004).

	Study 1 (Nelore heifers)			Study 2 (Holstein cattle)		
	Low intake (n = 19)	High intake (n = 20)	P	Heifers (n = 27)	Cows (n = 14)	P
Oestrus duration (h)	17.1 ± 2.5	10.7 ± 2.2	0.07	-	-	-
Mounts during oestrus	29.8 ± 5.1	8.9 ± 1.9	<0.01			
Codominant follicles during first wave; %	-	-	-	3.7	35.7	0.01
Multiple ovulation rate; %[1]	-	-	-	1.9	17.9	0.02
Maximum size of ovulatory follicle (mm)[1]	11.8 ± 0.2	14.0 ± 0.2	<0.01	15.0 ± 0.2	17.2 ± 0.5	<0.01
Serum oestradiol peak preceding ovulation (pg/ml)	14.3 ± 1.5	12.8 ± 0.6	0.35	11.3 ± 0.6	7.9 ± 0.8	<0.01
Growth rate of ovulatory follicle (mm/d)[1]	0.9 ± 0.1	1.2 ± 0.1	<0.01	1.2 ± 0.1	1.2 ± 0.1	0.97
Days between luteolysis and ovulation (n)	6.9 ± 0.5	5.2 ± 0.3	<0.01	4.6 ± 0.1	5.2 ± 0.2	0.01
Corpus luteum volume (mm³)	4096 ± 174	5199 ± 376	<0.01	7303 ± 308	11120 ± 678	<0.01
Maximal serum progesterone (ng/ml)	5.2 ± 0.6	5.6 ± 0.4	0.50	7.3 ± 0.4	5.6 ± 0.5	<0.01
Serum total IGF-I (ng/ml)	588.9 ± 23.2	569.8 ± 22.5	0.56	-	-	-
Serum insulin (µIU/ml)	11.8 ± 0.2	14.3 ± 1.8	0.02	-	-	-

[1]Results include ovulatory follicles that initiated and ended the evaluated cycle of each heifer.
*For both studies, only data from animals with typical cycles and single ovulation were used.

There was, however, no difference in the size of ovulatory follicles between groups. Working with prepubertal ewes, we observed higher concentrations of progesterone in restricted than *ad libitum* ewes supplemented with an intravaginal progesterone releasing device (4.4 ± 0.3 vs. 2.5 ± 0.2 ng/ml; P < 0.0001; Mattos *et al.*, 2010).

It is well known that size of the ovulatory follicle has a positive and high correlation with size of CL (Vasconcelos *et al.*, 2001, Sartori *et al.*, 2002) and consequently may reflect circulating progesterone concentrations. However, despite lactating dairy cows having bigger CL, their circulating progesterone concentrations are lower as compared to heifers and dry cows (Sartori *et al.*, 2002, Sartori *et al.*, 2004, Wolfenson *et al.*, 2004). Comparing studies in which cattle underwent different feed intake regimens (Mollo *et al.*, 2007b), similar results were obtained. Nelore heifers under high feed intake had larger CL, but there was no difference in serum progesterone concentration (Table 2). In another study (Bastos and Sartori, unpublished), Nelore and Holstein non-lactating cows were submitted to high or low feed intake. Independent of breed, overfed cows had greater CL (5146 ± 287 vs. 3964 ± 306 mm3; P < 0.01), and lower concentrations of progesterone (2.3 ± 0.2 vs. 3.0 ± 0.2 ng/ml; P = 0.03) than those in low feed intake. Lower circulating progesterone associated or not with heat stress has also been related to increased codominance and double ovulation rates observed in lactating cows, but not in heifers. Increasing blood progesterone by manipulating the oestrous cycle with exogenous hormonal treatments has reduced the incidence of multiple ovulations in dairy cows (Wiltbank *et al.*, 2012).

The lower circulating steroid concentrations in ruminants under high nutritional plane may be due to two causes. The first is related to lower steroidogenesis in follicles or CL of animals fed on high energy diets than those in restricted feeding. However, no study has adequately measured production of ovarian steroids. Thus, the most reliable explanation is that overfed cattle have higher liver blood flow, due to increased feed intake (Sangsritavong *et al.*, 2002, Vasconcelos *et al.*, 2003), and consequently, steroid hormones are metabolized at a faster rate, resulting in decreased circulating concentrations. Lactating dairy cows, compared with dry cows, have twice the hepatic blood flow and metabolize much more progesterone and oestradiol (Sangsritavong *et al.*, 2002).

Due to lower blood oestradiol concentrations, the follicles of lactating dairy cows need to grow for a longer period of time to achieve a GnRH/LH peak than those of heifers. Confirming these findings, Sartori *et al.* (2004) reported that high producing dairy cattle have a longer time between luteolysis and ovulation than heifers (Table 2). Surprisingly, underfed Nelore heifers took longer to ovulate than overfed heifers (Table 2). Besides metabolism of steroid hormones, circulating insulin may also play an important role in follicle development, especially in Zebu cattle that have much higher circulating insulin than *Bos taurus* cattle (Sartori *et al.*, 2010). Differences in LH pulse frequency between *Bos indicus* and *Bos taurus* may also be associated with differences in follicle growth.

A longer time between luteolysis and ovulation, or a longer period of follicle dominance may affect embryo quality. Cerri *et al.* (2009) reported that almost 80% of embryos were viable in cows with a 5.5 to 6.0 d period of follicle dominance, whereas only 45% of embryos were considered viable in cows with a period of dominance lasting 8.5 to 11.5 d. Moreover, a negative correlation (r = -0.22) has been reported between period of follicle dominance and conception rate (Bleach *et al.*, 2004). Furthermore, differences in size of follicles may be associated with alterations in their growth rate, which also can be affected by dietary energy level. The growth rate per day of follicles was increased in heifers that were offered an *ad libitum* diet in comparison to heifers fed on restricted diets (1.58 mm/d vs. 1.11 mm/d; P < 0.05; Mackey *et al.*, 2000).

Blood oestradiol concentration has a strong positive correlation with standing heat and intensity of oestrus (0.57). Moreover, there is a strong negative correlation between milk production and oestrus duration (-0.45; Lopez *et al.*, 2004). Thus, lactating dairy cows have shorter oestrus duration than heifers (7.3 vs. 10.7 h; P < 0.05; Nebel *et al.*, 1997). Corroborating these data, Mollo *et al.* (2007b) observed shorter oestrus duration in heifers fed *ad libitum* compared with a restricted feed intake diet (Table 2). Likewise, Lopez *et al.* (2004) reported reductions in oestrus duration (6.2 ± 0.5 vs. 10.9 ± 0.7 h; P < 0.001) and intensity (6.3 ± 0.4 vs. 8.8 ± 0.6 mounts; P < 0.01) in cows with higher (46.4 kg/d) compared with lower (33.5 kg/d) milk yield.

Influence of dry matter or energy intake on in vivo and in vitro embryo production/quality

The general aspects of the influence of dry matter intake on embryo production have been discussed recently by us in the Cattle Practice journal (Sartori *et al.*, 2012). Most of the researchers that have studied the effect of feed intake on embryo production, reported negative results on reproductive function of overfed cattle in comparison to those fed restricted diets (Sartori *et al.*, 2012). The causes of compromised embryo production linked to feed intake are still not well elucidated, however, changes in liver blood flow, in local and circulating metabolites (glucose, IGF-I) and hormones (insulin and steroids) concentrations, as well as the predominant volatile fatty acid source, may be involved in this process. Furthermore, we hypothesized that the effect of feed intake on embryo quality may be different between *Bos taurus* and *Bos indicus* breeds, which consistently have different circulating insulin, IGF-I and steroid hormone concentrations (Sartori *et al.*, 2010). As shown below, it is tempting to speculate that Zebu cattle may be more resistant to the effects of changes in feed intake on embryo production and quality.

Alterations in blood steroids concentrations can affect patterns of follicular development, oocyte quality, fertilization or transport of embryo/ovum and early embryonic development (Folman *et al.*, 1973, Fonseca *et al.*, 1983, King *et al.*, 1994, Mann *et al.*, 1998, Inskeep, 2004), resulting in reduced fertility. Amount of diet also may markedly change IGF-I and insulin concentrations. These hormones/metabolites affect production of steroids by follicles, number of follicles (Gutiérrez *et al.*, 1997, Armstrong *et al.*, 2002, Gong *et al.*, 2002) and sensitivity of follicles to reproductive hormones (FSH and LH; Webb *et al.*, 2004). On the other hand, hyperinsulinaemia and increased plasma and intrafollicular IGF-I concentrations impair oocyte quality and subsequent embryo development (Armstrong *et al.*, 2001, Adamiak *et al.*, 2005). Due to these relevant and interesting observations reported in the literature, mainly in *Bos taurus* cattle, a series of experiments was performed to investigate the influence of dry matter intake on embryo production in *Bos indicus* cattle.

In our studies we investigated if and how dry matter or/energy intake affects *in vivo* and *in vitro* embryo production in Nelore cattle.

In the study by Mollo *et al.* (2007a), after feeding treatment diets for 9 weeks, overfed heifers (1.7 x M, n = 20) surprisingly presented lower superstimulatory (24.0 ± 1.1 vs. 48.4 ± 1.6 follicles ≥ 6 mm; P < 0.001) and superovulatory (15.7 ± 0.9 vs. 33.6 ± 1.4 CL; P < 0.0001) responses in comparison to those fed on a restricted diet (0.7 x M, n = 19). Moreover, the numbers of recovered embryos/ova (6.7 ± 0.9 vs. 10.5 ± 0.6; P = 0.0003) and transferable embryos (3.8 ± 0.4 vs. 5.7 ± 0.6; P = 0.01) were also lower for the high feed intake heifers. The superstimulatory and superovulatory responses and the number of total and transferable embryos seemed to be compromised by higher circulating insulin concentrations at the first day of FSH treatment (14.3 ± 1.7 vs. 3.0 ± 0.8 μIU/ml; P < 0.001). Therefore, high feed intake negatively affected follicle development before and throughout the superstimulatory treatment. In contrast, it did not affect oocyte/embryo quality, as seen by the similar percentage of viable embryos recovered in both groups (~62%; P > 0.10).

Bastos *et al.* (2007) did not detect any effect on superovulatory response, embryo production, or embryo quality in heifers (n = 36) with higher or lower BCS fed on maintenance (1 x M) or flushing (1.8 x M) diets for 14 d before a superovulation treatment. Little variation of the superestimulatory response (14.6 ± 1.6[a] vs. 12.6 ± 1.4[b] vs. 13.6 ± 1.5[ab] number of follicles > 6 mm; P < 0.05) also was reported in non-lactating cows (n = 32) fed on maintenance (M, 1.2% of DM/kg of BW), 0.7 x M (0.84% of DM/kg of BW) or 1.5 x M (1.8% of DM/kg of BW) diets after 42 d of feeding, in a cross-over design (Surjus *et al.*, 2012). In this study, there was no difference in the superovulatory response (11.0 ± 1.4 vs. 9.8 ± 1.3 vs. 10.2 ± 1.3 CL; P > 0.10), fertilization rate (P = 0.71) or percentage of viable embryos (P

= 0.98) among experimental groups (Surjus *et al.*, 2012).

Guardieiro *et al.* (2010) supplied to 40 heifers concentrates with or without rumen-protected fat (Megalac-E, rich in linoleic acid) starting 50 d before superovulation, in a cross-over experimental design. The embryos recovered were cryopreserved and subsequently evaluated for *in vitro* embryo development. The superstimulatory response, total number of embryos/ova, viable embryos, degenerate embryos, or unfertilized oocytes recovered were similar between groups. Although, beyond the energy effect, there was a negative effect of unsaturated fatty acids on the superovulatory response (15.7 ± 1.2 vs. 18.0 ± 1.3 CL; P = 0.06), hatching rate at 48 h (17.3 ± 3.3%; n = 137 vs. 33.1 ± 4.0%, n = 148, P = 0.009) and at 72 h (30.9 ± 4.0%, n = 137 vs. 44.3 ± 4.2%; n = 148, P = 0.04) of *in vitro* culture.

Our group also performed two studies to investigate the effects of feed intake on *in vitro* embryo production (Martins *et al.*, 2006; Prata *et al.*, 2011). At the first study, overfed cows (1.7 x M, n = 10) in comparison to those under low feed intake (0.7 x M, n = 10), had a discrete but significant increase in number of follicles ≥ 3 mm in diameter at the time of ovum pick up (OPU) and, associated with this finding, there was a higher circulating concentration of insulin in the 1.7 x M group (5.6 ± 0.8 vs. 3.5 ± 0.7 µIU/ml, P = 0.06, unpublished). Moreover, the diet with higher energy content tended to reduce the percentage of viable oocytes (44.0%, n = 732 vs. 48.6%, n = 623; P = 0.08). Despite similar numbers of cleaved oocytes and blastocysts between groups, there was a higher expression of the BAX gene and global expression of all evaluated genes in embryos from the lower feed intake group, which may be related to better embryo quality (Martins *et al.*, 2006).

Our most recent research was performed in a cross-over design (Prata *et al.*, 2011). Increases in total number of oocytes (20.2 ± 2.0[b], 23.0 ± 2.3[a], and 21.5 ± 2.2[ab]; P = 0.02) and viable oocytes (14.4 ± 1.6[b], 17.0 ± 1.9[a], and 15.7 ± 1.7[ab]; P = 0.006) were observed for non-lactating cows fed on a 0.7 x M diet compared with a 1.0 x M diet (experimental diets were offered for 30 d before OPU). Surprisingly, cows receiving a 1.5 x M diet did not differ from the other groups. Although the number of cleaved oocytes was also higher in 0.7 x M cows than in 1.0 x M cows (10.7 ± 1.4[b], 13.4 ± 1,7[a], and 12.6 ± 1.6[ab] for 1.0, 0.7, and 1.5 x M; P = 0.04), we did not detect an influence of diet on the number (5.4 ± 0.8, 6.9 ± 0.9, and 5.9 ± 0.8; P = 0.15) or percentage of blastocysts produced *in vitro* (31.9, 30.6, and 31.1%; P = 0.67).

Acknowledgments

The authors would like to acknowledge the support from EMBRAPA, FAPESP, CNPq and CAPES of Brazil.

References

Adamiak, S.J., Mackie, K., Watt, R.G., Webb, R. and Sinclair, K.D. (2005) Impact of nutrition on oocyte quality: cumulative effects of body composition and diet leading to hyperinsulinemia in cattle. *Biology of Reproduction*, **73**, 918-926.

Armstrong, D., Gong, J., Gardner, J., Baxter, G., Hogg, C. and Webb, R. (2002) Steroidogenesis in bovine granulosa cells: the effect of short-term changes in dietary intake. *Reproduction*, **123**, 371-378.

Armstrong, D.G., McEvoy, T.G., Baxter, G., Robinson, J.J., Hogg, C.O., Woad, K.J., Webb, R. and Sinclair, K.D. (2001) Effect of dietary energy and protein on bovine follicular dynamics and embryo production in vitro: associations with the ovarian insulin-like growth factor system. *Biology of Reproduction*, **64**, 1624-1632.

Aréchiga, C.F., Ortíz, O. and Hansen, P.J. (1994) Effect of prepartum injection of vitamin E and selenium on postpartum reproductive function of dairy cattle. *Theriogenology*, **41**, 1251-1258.

Aréchiga, C.F., Vázquez-Flores, S., Ortíz, O., Hernández-Cerón, J., Porras, A., McDowell, L.R. and Hansen, P.J. (1998) Effect of injection of beta-carotene or vitamin E and selenium on fertility of lactating dairy cows. *Theriogenology*, **50**, 65-76.

Bastos, M.R., Martins, A.C., Melo, L., Carrijo, L.H.D., Rumpf, R. and Sartori, R. (2007) Effect of body condition score and feed intake on the superovulatory response and embryo production in Nelore heifers. *Acta Scientiae Veterinariae*, **35** Suppl 3, 1242 (abstract).

Bastos, M.R., Mattos, M.C.C., Meschiatti, M.A.P., Surjus, R.S., Guardieiro, M.M., Ferreira, J.C.P., Mourão, G.B., Pires, A.V., Biehl, M.V., Pedroso, A.M., Santos, F.A.P. and Sartori, R. (2010) Ovarian function and circulating hormones in nonlactating Nelore versus Holstein cows. *Acta Scientiae Veterinariae*, **38** Suppl 2, 776 (abstract).

Bastos, M.R., Ramos, A.F., Driessen, K., Martins, A.C., Rumpf, R., Sartori, R. (2009) Influence of high dry matter intake on the superovulatory response of crossbred cows. *Ciência Animal Brasileira*, **10**, 1066-1073.

Bleach, E.C., Glencross, R.G. and Knight, P.G. (2004) Association between ovarian follicle development and pregnancy rates in dairy cows undergoing spontaneous oestrous cycles. *Reproduction*, **127**, 621-629.

Buratini, J., Price, C., Visintin, J. and Bo, G. (2000) Effects of dominant follicle aspiration and treatment with recombinant bovine somatotropin (BST) on ovarian follicular development in Nelore (*Bos indicus*) heifers. *Theriogenology*, **54**, 421-431.

Butler, W.R. (1998) Review: effect of protein nutrition on ovarian and uterine physiology in dairy cattle. *Journal of Dairy Science*, **81**, 2533-2539.

Cerri, R.L., Rutigliano, H.M., Chebel, R.C. and Santos, J.E. (2009) Period of dominance of the ovulatory follicle influences embryo quality in lactating dairy cows. *Reproduction*, **137**, 813-823.

Dawuda, P.M., Scaramuzzi, R.J., Leese, H.J., Hall, C.J., Peters, A.R., Drew, S.B. and Wathes, D.C. (2002) Effect of timing of urea feeding on the yield and quality of embryos in lactating dairy cows. *Theriogenology*, **58**, 1443-1455.

Diskin, M.G. and Morris, D.G. (2008) Embryonic and early foetal losses in cattle and other ruminants. *Reproduction in Domestic Animals*, **43** Suppl 2, 260-267.

Echternkamp, S.E., Howard, H.J., Roberts, A.J., Grizzle, J. and Wise, T. (1994) Relationships among concentrations of steroids, insulin-like growth factor-I, and insulin-like growth factor binding proteins in ovarian follicular fluid of beef cattle. *Biology of Reproduction*, **51**, 971-981.

Folman, Y., Rosenberg, M., Herz, Z. and Davidson, M. (1973) The relationship between plasma progesterone concentration and conception in post-partum dairy cows maintained on two levels of nutrition. *Journal of Reproduction and Fertility*, **34**, 267-278.

Fonseca, F.A., Britt, J.H., McDaniel, B.T., Wilk, J.C. and Rakes, A.H. (1983) Reproductive traits of Holsteins and Jerseys. Effects of age, milk yield, and clinical abnormalities on involution of cervix and uterus, ovulation, estrous cycles, detection of estrus, conception rate, and days open. *Journal of Dairy Science*, **66**, 1128-1147.

Gong, J., Bramley, T. and Webb, R. (1991) The effect of recombinant bovine somatotropin on ovarian-function in heifers - follicular populations and peripheral hormones. *Biology of Reproduction*, **45**, 941-949.

Gong, J.G., Armstrong, D.G., Baxter, G., Hogg, C.O., Garnsworthy, P.C. and Webb, R. 2002. The effect of increased dietary intake on superovulatory response to FSH in heifers. *Theriogenology*, **57**, 1591-1602.

Guardieiro, M.M., Machado, G.M., Bastos, M.R., Mourão, G.B., Carrijo, L.H.D., Dode, M.A.N. and Sartori, R. (2010) Postcryopreservation viability of embryos from Nellore heifers supplemented with rumen-protected fat. *Reproduction, Fertility and Development*, **22**, 205-206 (abstract).

Gutiérrez, C.G., Oldham, J., Bramley, T.A., Gong, J.G., Campbell, B.K. and Webb, R. (1997) The recruitment of ovarian follicles is enhanced by increased dietary intake in heifers. *Journal of Animal Science*, **75**, 1876-1884.

Ingraham, R.H., Kappel, L.C., Morgan, E.B. and Srikandakumar, A. (1987) Correction of subnormal fertility with copper and magnesium supplementation. *Journal of Dairy Science*, **70**, 167-180.

Inskeep, E.K. (2004) Preovulatory, postovulatory, and postmaternal recognition effects of concentrations of progesterone on embryonic survival in the cow. *Journal of Animal Science*, **82** E-Suppl, E24-39.

Ireland, J., Ward, F., Jimenez-Krassel, F., Ireland, J., Smith, G., Lonergan, P. and Evans, A. (2007) Follicle numbers are highly repeatable within individual animals but are inversely correlated with FSH concentrations and the proportion of good-quality embryos after ovarian stimulation in cattle. *Human Reproduction*, **22**, 1687-1695.

King, R.S., Anderson, S.H. and Killian, G.J. (1994) Effect of bovine oviductal estrus-associated protein on the ability of sperm to capacitate and fertilize oocytes. *Journal of Andrology*, **15**, 468-478.

Leroy, J.L., Opsomer, G., Van Soom, A., Goovaerts, I.G. & Bols, P.E. (2008) Reduced fertility in high-yielding dairy cows: are the oocyte and embryo in danger? Part I. The importance of negative energy balance and altered corpus luteum function to the reduction of oocyte and embryo quality in high-yielding dairy cows. *Reproduction in Domestic Animals*, **43**, 612-622.

Lopez, H., Satter, L.D. and Wiltbank, M.C. (2004) Relationship between level of milk production and estrous behavior of lactating dairy cows. *Animal Reproduction Science*, **81**, 209-223.

López-Gatius, F. (2003) Is fertility declining in dairy cattle? A retrospective study in northeastern Spain. *Theriogenology*, **60**, 89-99.

Mackey, D.R., Wylie, A.R., Sreenan, J.M., Roche, J.F. and Diskin, M.G. (2000) The effect of acute nutritional change on follicle wave turnover, gonadotropin, and steroid concentration in beef heifers. *Journal of Animal Science*, **78**, 429-442.

Mann, G.E., Lamming, G.E. and Payne, J.H. (1998) Role of early luteal phase progesterone in control of the timing of the luteolytic signal in cows. *Journal of Reproduction and Fertility*, **113**, 47-51.

Martins, A.C., Ramos, A.F., Mollo, M.R., Pivato, I., Camara, J.L., Carrijo, L.H.D., Driessen, K., Rumpf, R. and Sartori, R. (2006) Influence of high or low feed intake on in vitro embryo production in cattle. *Acta Scientiae Veterinariae*, **34** Suppl 1, 290 (abstract).

Mattos, F.C.S.Z., Bastos, M.R., Lemes, A., Mattos, M.C., Guardieiro, M.M., Marques-Filho, W., Canavessi, A., Susin, I., Mourão, G.B. and Sartori, R. (2010) Influence of high or low feed intake on circulating insulin and progesterone concentrations in prepubertal ewes. *Acta Scientiae Veterinariae* **38**, s784 (abstract).

Mollo, M.R, Rumpf, R., Martins, A.C., Carrijo, L.H.D., Saueressig, M. and Sartori, R. 2007a. Embryo production in superovulated Nelore heifers under low or high feed intake. Acta Scientiae Veterinariae **35** Suppl, 1241 (abstract).

Mollo, M.R., Rumpf, R., Martins, A.C., Mattos, M.C.C., Lopes Jr, G., Carrijo, L.H.D. and Sartori, R. (2007b) Ovarian function in Nelore heifers under low or high feed intake. *Acta Scientiae Veterinariae*, **35**, 958 (abstract).

Moreira, F., Risco, C., Pires, M.F., Ambrose, J.D., Drost, M., DeLorenzo, M. and Thatcher, W.W. (2000) Effect of body condition on reproductive efficiency of lactating dairy cows receiving a timed insemination. *Theriogenology*, **53**, 1305-1319.

Murphy, M.G., Enright, W.J., Crowe, M.A., McConnell, K., Spicer, L.J., Boland, M.P. and Roche, J.F. (1991) Effect of dietary intake on pattern of growth of dominant follicles during the oestrous cycle in beef heifers. *Journal of Reproduction and Fertility*, **92**, 333-338.

Nebel, R., Jobst, S., Dransfield, M., Pandolfi, S. and Bailey, T. (1997) Use of radiofrequency data communication system, Heat Watch, to describe behavioral estrus in dairy cattle. *Journal of Dairy Science*, **80**, 151 (abstract).

Prata, A.B., Surjus, R., Borsato, M., Martins da Silveira, M., Mattos, M.C., Mourão, G.B., Santos, F.A.P., Basso, A., Pontes, J.H. and Sartori, R. (2011) Influence of high or low intake of dry matter/energy on *in vitro* production of bovine embryos. Cumbuco, Brazil: Proceedings of the XXI Annual Meeting of the Brazilian Society of Embryo Technology, **1**, 332 (abstract).

Rhoads, M.L., Rhoads, R.P., Gilbert, R.O., Toole, R. and Butler, W.R. 2006. Detrimental effects of high plasma urea nitrogen levels on viability of embryos from lactating dairy cows. *Animal Reproduction Science*, **91**, 1-10.

Sales, J.N., Iguma, L., Quintão, C., Gama, M., Freitas, C., Pereira, M., Camargo, L.S., Viana, J.H.M. and Baruselli, P.S. (2011). Effect of high energy diet on metabolic, endocrine and reproductive parameters in *Bos indicus* and *Bos taurus* cows. Cumbuco, Brazil: Proceedings of the XXI Annual Meeting of the Brazilian Society of Embryo Technology, **1**, 395 (abstract).

Sangsritavong, S., Combs, D.K., Sartori, R., Armentano, L.E. and Wiltbank, M.C. (2002) High feed intake increases liver blood flow and metabolism of progesterone and estradiol-17beta in dairy cattle. *Journal of Dairy Science*, **85**, 2831-2842.

Santos, J.E., Bilby, T.R., Thatcher, W.W., Staples, C.R. and Silvestre, F.T. (2008a) Long chain fatty acids of diet as factors influencing reproduction in cattle. *Reproduction in Domestic Animals*, **43** Suppl 2, 23-30.

Santos, J.E., Cerri, R.L. and Sartori, R. (2008b) Nutritional management of the donor cow. *Theriogenology*, **69**, 88-97.

Sartori, R., Guardieiro, M.M. and Surjus, R. (2012) Effects of dry matter or energy intake on embryo quality in cattle. Cattle Practice [In Press].

Sartori, R., Bastos, M.R., Baruselli, P.S., Gimenes, L.U., Ereno, R.L. and Barros, C.M. (2010) Physiological differences and implications to reproductive management of *Bos taurus* and *Bos indicus* cattle in a tropical environment. In: M.C. Lucy, J.L. Pate, M.F. Smith and T.E. Spencer. (Org.). *Reproduction in Domestic Ruminants VII*. 1 ed. Nottingham: Nottingham University Press **1**, 357-375.

Sartori, R., Haughian, J.M., Shaver, R.D., Rosa, G.J. and Wiltbank, M.C. (2004) Comparison of ovarian function and circulating steroids in estrous cycles of Holstein heifers and lactating cows. *Journal of Dairy Science*, **87**, 905-920.

Sartori, R., Rosa, G.J. and Wiltbank, M.C. (2002) Ovarian structures and circulating steroids in heifers and lactating cows in summer and lactating and dry cows in winter. *Journal of Dairy Science*, **85**, 2813-2822.

Silva, J.M. and Price, C.A. (2002) Insulin and IGF-I are necessary for FSH-induced cytochrome P450 aromatase but not cytochrome P450 side-chain cleavage gene expression in oestrogenic bovine granulosa cells in vitro. *Journal of Endocrinology*, **174**, 499-507.

Singh, J., Dominguez, M., Jaiswal, R. and Adams, G. (2004) A simple ultrasound test to predict the superstimulatory response in cattle. *Theriogenology*, **62**, 227-243.

Surjus, R.S., Prata, A.B., Borsato, M., Martins da Silveira, M., Mattos, M.C., Mattos, F.C.S.Z., Monteiro Jr, P.L., Mourão, G.B., Santos, F.A.P. and Sartori, R. (2012) Influence of high or low intake of dry matter and energy on *in vivo* production of bovine embryos. *Reproduction, Fertility and Development*, **24**: 227 (abstract).

Vasconcelos, J.L., Sangsritavong, S., Tsai, S.J. and Wiltbank, M.C. (2003) Acute reduction in serum progesterone concentrations after feed intake in dairy cows. *Theriogenology*, **60**, 795-807.

Vasconcelos, J.L., Sartori, R., Oliveira, H.N., Guenther, J.G. and Wiltbank, M.C. (2001) Reduction in size of the ovulatory follicle reduces subsequent luteal size and pregnancy rate. *Theriogenology*, **56**, 307-314.

Webb, R., Garnsworthy, P.C., Gong, J.G. and Armstrong, D.G. (2004) Control of follicular growth: local interactions and nutritional influences. *Journal of Animal Science*, **82** E-Suppl, E63-74.

Wiltbank, M., Lopez, H., Sartori, R., Sangsritavong, S. and Gümen, A. (2006) Changes in reproductive physiology of lactating dairy cows due to elevated steroid metabolism. *Theriogenology*, **65**, 17-29.

Wiltbank, M.C., Souza, A.H., Carvalho, P.D., Bender, R.W. and Nascimento, A.B. (2012) Improving fertility to timed artificial insemination by manipulation of circulating progesterone concentrations in lactating dairy cattle. *Reproduction, Fertility and Development*, **24**, 238-243.

Wolfenson, D., Inbar, G., Roth, Z., Kaim, M., Bloch, A. and Braw-Tal, R. (2004) Follicular dynamics and concentrations of steroids and gonadotropins in lactating cows and nulliparous heifers. *Theriogenology*, **62**, 1042-1055.

3

SUPPLEMENTAL ANTIOXIDANTS TO IMPROVE REPRODUCTION IN DAIRY CATTLE – WHY, WHEN AND HOW EFFECTIVE ARE THEY?

PETER J. HANSEN

Department of Animal Sciences, University of Florida, Gainesville FL 32611-0910, USA

Worldwide, many tons of vitamin E have been consumed by the public with little or no beneficial effects to their health and even a suggestion of harm..... Perhaps the best we can hope for, as a result of this, is that the excreted vitamin E may have helped to decrease corrosion in our sewage systems, especially those using plastic piping...

Gutteridge and Halliwell (2010)

Introduction

The choice to begin this review with the piquant quote from the free radical biologists, John M.C. Gutteridge and Barry Halliwell, was made so as to inject a note of caution into the discussion as to whether the reproductive process of lactating dairy cows can be enhanced by providing antioxidants. As Gutteridge and Halliwell (2010) point out, using nutrition to scavenge reactive oxygen species is not always easy or even desirable. Many molecules classified as antioxidants can promote free radical formation in certain situations, many pro-oxidants can act as antioxidants, and it is likely that a variety of molecules with antioxidant activity in vitro are not effective in vivo. Gutteridge and Halliwell (2010) also point out that reactive oxygen species play important roles in many biochemical processes and that supplemental administration of antioxidants could lead to unintended consequences that, among other things, aggravate damage associated with microbial infection.

Another quote, this time from the Roman dramatist Terence, illuminates a principle pertinent to free radical biology - "Moderation in all things (*Ne quid nimis*)". Indeed, an antioxidant regimen that has no benefit when organisms can regulate reactive oxygen metabolism could provide important benefits when the balance of oxidation and reduction tips towards oxidation.

37

The transition dairy cow is potentially at that tipping point. Feed consumption decreases about 3 to 4 weeks before parturition and then increases gradually thereafter (Rastani *et al.*, 2005). As a result, dietary consumption of antioxidants is reduced in the transition period. Neutrophils, which are very active at producing reactive oxygen species (Robinson, 2009), are probably involved in the parturition process (Kimura *et al.*, 2002) and are certainly activated as part of the inflammatory reaction in the uterus in the early postpartum period (Sheldon *et al.*, 2009). Moreover, lactation causes a large increase in oxygen demand and, as a necessary result, increased production of reactive oxygen products. Cows with higher milk yields have been reported to have higher concentrations of lipid hydroperoxides in serum (Löhrke *et al.*, 2005).

Despite the apparent risks that the transition cow faces with respect to free radical damage, the responses to antioxidant supplementation have been modest and variable. Indeed, as illustrated in Figure 1, biochemical evidence for an increase in the net production of reactive oxygen species after parturition has often been observed (Bernabucci *et al.*, 2005; Castillo *et al.*, 2005; Mudron and Konvicná, 2006; Tanaka *et al.*, 2011; Wullepit *et al.*, 2012), although not always (Bernabucci *et al.*, 2002; Turk *et al.*, 2008).

As will be delineated in this chapter, the most consistent benefit to antioxidant supplementation for dairy cow reproduction is a reduction in the incidence of retained placenta. This is an important effect of antioxidants because occurrence of retained placenta is associated with subsequent endometritis, metritis, and reduced fertility (Beagley *et al.*, 2010). In contrast to the effects of antioxidants on reducing the incidence of retained placenta, benefits of antioxidant supplementation on uterine health, resumption of cyclicity, and fertility have been variable. Some of this variation probably reflects differences in chemical structure, route, and dosage of the antioxidant tested. To the extent this is true, it may be possible to develop antioxidant treatments that are more effective at reducing excess free radical production than currently available treatments. It is likely, however, that much of the variation in effectiveness of antioxidant treatments reflects variation in the antioxidant status of unsupplemented cows. Depending on diet and physiological and immune status, innate antioxidant defences of the cow are probably sufficient in many cases to protect cells involved in reproductive processes from the oxidizing actions of reactive oxygen species. In those cows, like the humans taking vitamin E alluded to by Gutteridge and Halliwell (2010), additional antioxidants are not required.

Production of reactive oxygen species

Production of incompletely reduced oxygen species is a requisite of aerobic life. During oxidative phosphorylation, molecular oxygen is usually reduced by the

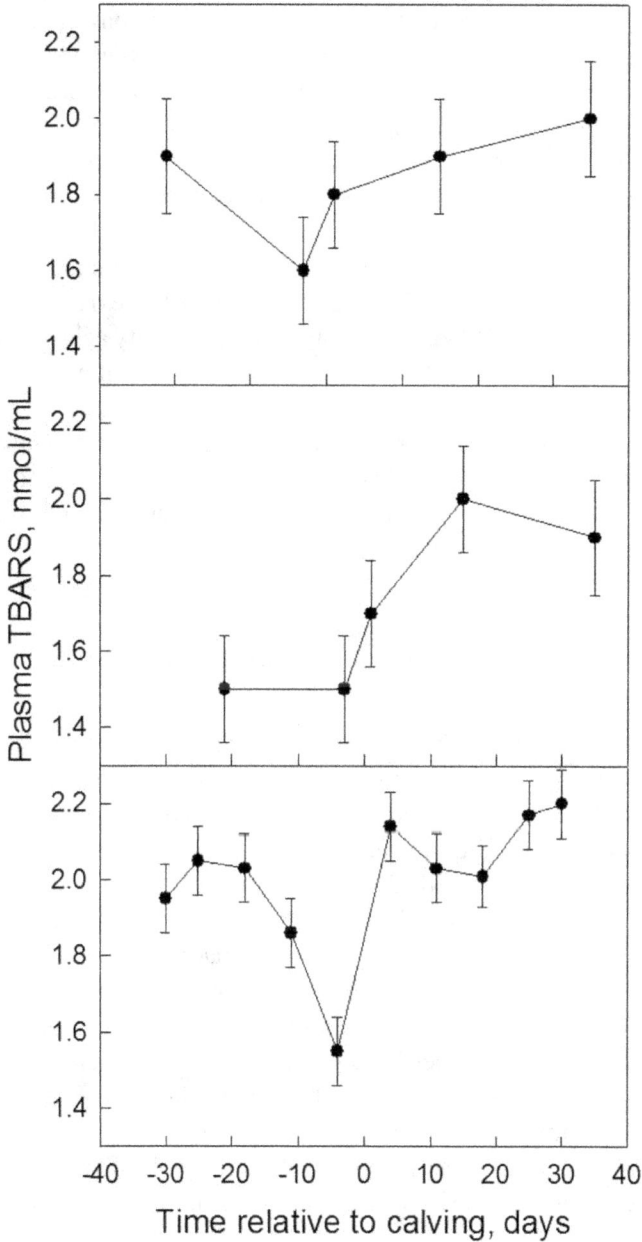

Figure 1. Plasma concentrations of thiobarbituric acid reactive substances (TBARS) in dairy cows during the transition period. Formed as a result of lipid peroxidation, TBARS are used to assess oxidative status. Data in the top and middle panel are from Bernabucci *et al.* (2002); data in the bottom panel are from Bernabucci *et al.* (2005). Season of calving was spring (top panel), summer (middle panel), or was not described (bottom panel).

addition of four electrons to produce two molecules of water (Figure 2). However, some of the oxygen metabolized in the cell is not completely reduced. For example, about 2% of the oxygen consumed by mitochondria is converted to hydrogen peroxide (Chance, Sies, and Boveris, 1979). Reactive oxygen species are also generated by a variety of enzymes in the peroxisome, microsomes and cytosol.

Often, reaction of reactive oxygen species with other molecules leads to generation of additional reactive oxygen species. A chain reaction that consumes polyunsaturated fatty acids in membranes can ensue when oxidation of polyunsaturated fatty acids by reactive oxygen species in the presence of iron generates lipid peroxides (Spiteller, 2011). The aldehydes generated as a result are measured in the TBARS (thiobarbiric acid reactive substances) assay to assess the degree of oxidative stress. Provision of polyunsaturated fatty acids in the diet may increase production of reactive oxygen species in cattle (Wullepit *et al.*, 2012).

Inflammation leads to an increase in production of reactive oxygen species because of their production during prostaglandin and nitric oxide synthesis and by neutrophils (Robinson, 2009; Cho, Seo, and Kim, 2011; Hou *et al.*, 2011). There is little direct evidence that inflammation increases oxidative stress in dairy cattle, with the exception of abdominal surgery (Mudron *et al.*, 2007).

Common antioxidants administered to dairy cattle

There are two systems for eliminating reactive oxygen species in the body (Figure 2). The first consists of enzymes that facilitate electron donation to reactive oxygen species. These enzymes, which include superoxide dismutase, glutathione peroxidase, and catalase, require metal cofactors for enzymatic activity. For example, there are two superoxide dismutases, one requiring copper and zinc and the other requiring manganese. Glutathione peroxidase requires selenium and catalase requires iron. One commonly used approach to improving antioxidant status in dairy cattle has been to increase administration of these metal cofactors by increasing dietary content or, for selenium, by injection. Most efforts have focused on selenium and copper because there are deficiencies in amounts of these metals in many soils (Steinnes, 2009). Bioavailability of selenium can be improved by providing an organic form incorporated into methionine through yeast fermentation. In one experiment, the organic form of selenium improved neutrophil function and uterine health as compared to inorganic selenium (Thatcher *et al.*, 2010).

There are a second group of antioxidants that directly react with reactive oxygen species and cause their elimination (Figure 2). These molecules, which include vitamin E (a-tocopherol and other tocopherols) and β-carotene in the lipophilic

$$O_2 \xrightarrow{e^-} O_2^{\bullet-} \xrightarrow{e^-} H_2O_2 \xrightarrow{e^-} OH\bullet \xrightarrow{e^-} H_2O$$

Scavenging Enzymes — CuZn superoxide dismustase (Cu Zn)
Mn superoxide dismutase (Mn)
Catalase (Fe)
GSH peroxidase (Se)

Free Radical Sinks ——————————————→
Aqueous (glutathione and ascorbic acid) and lipophilic (vitamin E, β-carotene)

Reduction of hydrogen peroxide by glutathione peroxidase

2 GSH + H_2O_2

↓ *GSH peroxidase*

GSSG + $2H_2O$

NADPH + H^+ ↓ *GSH reductase*

2 GSH + $NADP^+$

SH
|
γ-glu-cys-gly   *Reduced glutathione*

Reduction of peroxy radicals by β-carotene

ROO•

Double bonds susceptible to oxidation

ROO• + CAR ⟶ ROO-CAR•
ROO-CAR• ⟶ ROO^- + CAR•
CAR• + AscH ⟶ CAR + $Asc^{-\bullet}$
$Asc^{-\bullet}$ + H^+ ⟶ $AscH^-$

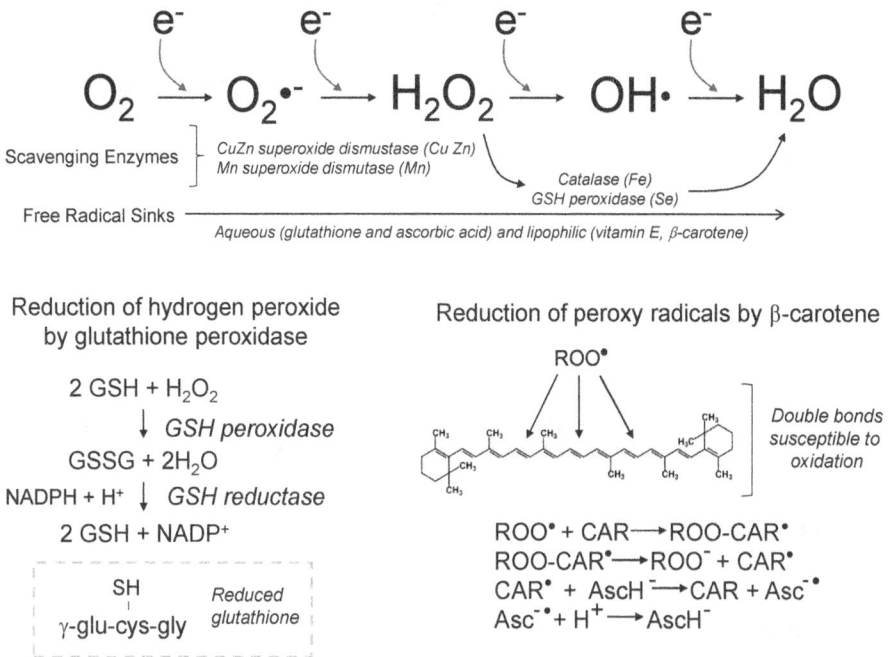

Figure 2. Role of antioxidants commonly fed to dairy cattle in removal of reactive oxygen species. Reactive oxygen species are formed from the incomplete reduction of oxygen, as shown at the top of the figure for reduction of oxygen to water. Other molecules can also give rise to reactive oxygen species, most notably unsaturated fatty acids (not shown). There are two main mechanisms for the removal of free radicals. First, a variety of enzymes reduce reactive oxygen species. For example, superoxide dismutase reduces singlet oxygen to peroxide, and peroxidase and catalase reduce peroxides to water. These enzymes require metal cofactors that are derived from the diet. An example of how one enzyme, glutathione peroxidase, functions is shown. In particular, GSH peroxidase uses the hydrogen on the sulphydryl group of reduced glutathione (GSH) to reduce peroxide to water. Subsequently oxidized glutathione is reduced by glutathione reductase. Antioxidants of the second type are scavenging molecules that are readily oxidized by reactive oxygen species. Present in high concentrations, these molecules act as free radical sinks to cause elimination of reactive oxygen species. Many free radical sinks are derived from the diet, including vitamin E (tocopherol) and β-carotene in the hydrophobic portion of cells, and ascorbic acid in the aqueous portion of cells. An example of how one of these free radical sinks can react with reactive oxygen species is the reduction of peroxy radicals by β-carotene. The double bonds of β-carotene can react with peroxyl radicals to produce a carotene radical. Subsequently, the caretonoid molecule (CAR) is reduced by a hydrogen donated by ascorbic acid (AscH). Ascorbic acid in turn is returned to the reduced state by addition of a hydrogen. Note that components of antioxidant systems that are provided directly through the diet are indicated in red. Chemical reactions between reactive oxygen species and antioxidants are taken from Krinsky and Yeum (2003), Namitha and Negi (2010) and Lubos, Loscalzo and Handy (2011).

compartment of cells and glutathione and ascorbic acid (vitamin C) in the aqueous compartment, act as scavenging molecules to reduce reactive oxygen molecules. Existing in high concentration, these molecules can be thought of as free radical sinks that provide a source of electrons for reduction of molecules with unpaired electrons. There are biochemical interactions between several of these scavenging molecules. For example, free radicals of β-carotene formed by reduction of peroxyl molecules can be in turn reduced by either vitamin E or ascorbic acid (Krinsky and Yeum, 2003). Thus, altering the concentration of one scavenging molecule could affect the concentrations of other such molecules. The most important scavenging molecules for dairy cattle nutrition have been vitamin E and β-carotene. These have been fed as supplements or provided through injection. There are also commercial products that combine vitamin E with selenium.

Consequences of antioxidant therapy for reproduction

RETAINED PLACENTA

The most consistent benefit of antioxidants in dairy cattle is a reduction in incidence of retained placenta. This action of antioxidants is probably caused by an improvement in neutrophil function. Occurrence of retained placenta has been associated with defects in function of neutrophils (Kimura *et al.*, 2002) and function of neutrophils can be enhanced by vitamin E (Politis *et al.*, 1995, 2004) and β-carotene (Michal *et al.*, 1994). Among the antioxidant regimens administered before or at calving that have reduced incidence of retained placenta are injections of vitamin E (Erskine *et al.*, 1997), selenium (Eger *et al.*, 1985), vitamin E and selenium in combination (Eger *et al.*, 1985; Aréchiga *et al.*, 1994; Bourne *et al.*, 2008), and feeding of supplemental β-carotene (Michal *et al.*, 1994). Representative results are shown in Table 1. In a meta-analysis of 44 studies examining effectiveness of vitamin E, alone or in combination with selenium, Bourne *et al.*, (2007) reported that beneficial results were obtained in 20 studies (45%), adverse effects in 3 studies (7%) and no effect in 21 studies (48%). Some of the experiments in which no effect was observed had little statistical power. In other cases in which no effect was seen, it is likely that control cows received adequate amounts of antioxidants so that no benefit of antioxidant supplementation would occur.

UTERINE HEALTH

Despite the fact that antioxidant therapy can improve neutrophil, macrophage and lymphocyte function (Spears and Weiss, 2008; Sordillo and Aitken, 2009), and the reduction in incidence of retained placenta, which predisposes cows to uterine infections (Le Blanc, 2008), improvements in uterine health during the

Table 1. Representative results from experiments evaluating antioxidant supplementation in the prepartum period on incidence of retained placenta and uterine infections, and on interval from calving to conception

Study	Location	Number of animals	Antioxidant treatment	Incidence of retained foetal membranes	Incidence of uterine infections	Interval, calving to conception (days)
Aréchiga et al., 1994	Mexico	99	No treatment	10.1%		141 ± 7.7[a]
		99	500 mg vitamin E & 50 mg Se, i.m., 3 wk before expected calving	3.0%		121 ± 7.6†
Michal et al., 1994	Washington, United States	14	No supplement	41%	18%[b]	
		14	300 mg β-carotene/d, dietaryl, beginning 14 d before expected calving	33% †	7%*	
		14	600 mg β-carotene/d	25%**	8%*	
Erskine et al., 1997	Michigan, United States	216	Untreated	12.5%	8.8%[b]	
		204	3000 mg vitamin E, i.m., 8-14 d before expected calving	6.4%	3.9%	
Le Blanc et al., 2002	Ontario, Canada	568	Placebo	14.4%	14.0[c]	
		574	3000 IU, vitamin E, s.c., 1 wk before expected calving	15.0%	16.3	
Cook and Green, 2007	United Kingdom	223	No treatment	10.3%	N.S.[cd]	N.S.[d]

Table 1. Contd.

Study	Location	Number of animals	Antioxidant treatment	Incidence of retained foetal membranes	Incidence of uterine infections	Interval, calving to conception (days)
		202	6800 mg I, 1000 mg selenium, 70 mg Co, intraruminal, dry off	4.4%		
Bourne et al., 2008	Essex, England	277	No treatment	6.5% †	12.6%	140
		271	2100 IU Vitamin E &7 mg Se, i.m., d -14 and 0 before calving	3%	17.7%	154

[a] Percent pregnant at first service was 25% for untreated and 41% for treated (P<0.05); [b] Metritis; [c] Endometritis; [d] Data not reported

Differences from control: † P<0.10 * P<0.05, ** P<0.01

postpartum period have been inconsistently reported. As shown in Table 1, the incidence of metritis was reduced by intramuscular injection of 3000 mg vitamin E at 8-14 d before calving (Erskine *et al.*, 1997) or by feeding 300 or 600 mg/d β-carotene for 8 wk beginning 4 wk before expected calving (Michal *et al.*, 1994). There was, however, no alteration in endometritis caused by an intrauminal bolus containing iodine, cobalt and selenium at dry off (Cook and Green, 2007) or a single injection of vitamin E at 1 wk before expected calving (Le Blanc *et al.*, 2002). Similarly, injections of vitamin E and selenium at 2 wk before expected calving and at within 24 h of parturition did not affect incidence of abnormal discharge from the vulva (Bourne *et al.* 2008).

Perhaps, antioxidants affect development of metritis to a greater extent than development of endometritis. More likely, however, is that the effectiveness of antioxidant treatments depend upon availability of antioxidants and pro-oxidants in the diet as well as physiological characteristics of cows. For instance, Thatcher *et al.* (2010), working in Florida, found that feeding of organic selenium before and after calving improved neutrophil function and antibody response to an injected immunogen (ovalbumin), reduced incidence of fever in the first ten days postpartum, and reduced the proportion of cows with a mucopurulent discharge at Days 5 and 10 postpartum. The effect of selenium source was different for multiparous cows than for multiparous cows. As an example, incidence of fever was reduced by organic selenium in multiparous cows (13% vs 25%) but not in primiparous cows (average of 41%). Using a very similar design, Rutigliano *et al.* (2008), working in California, saw no effect of selenium source. Importantly, serum concentrations of selenium were higher in the California study than in the Florida study so source of selenium may have been less important in the former.

FERTILITY

Reactive oxygen species can damage the spermatozoa, oocyte and preimplantation embryo (Moss, Pontes, and Hansen, 2009; Hendricks and Hansen, 2010; Bain, Madan, and Betts, 2011), so increasing the antioxidant status of the reproductive tract could potentially improve fertilization rate or development of the resulting embryo. Antioxidants could also theoretically enhance fertility by reducing the incidence of retained placenta or uterine infections because the probability of pregnancy following insemination is reduced when these disorders have occurred (Kim and Kang, 2003; López-Gatius *et al.*, 2006; McDougall, Macauley, and Compton, 2007; Gilbert, 2011).

In general, however, fertility has not been improved by antioxidant supplementation, regardless of whether treatments were administered prepartum

Table 2. Summary of selected experiments evaluating antioxidant supplementation in the postpartum period on fertility.

Study	Location	Number of animals	Antioxidant treatment	Pregnancy rate at first service	Pregnancy rate at second service	Interval, calving to conception (days)	Services per conception
Aréchiga et al., 1998a	Mexico	89	No treatment	46%	52	98.1 ± 4.5	2.0
		97	500 mg vitamin E & 50 mg Se, i.m., 30 d postpartum	45%	70†	84.6 ± 4.3*	1.7*
Aréchiga et al., 1998b	Florida, United States	100	No treatment	17%			
		91	400 mg β-carotene/d, beginning 15-30 d after calving	13%			
Paula Lopes et al., 2003	Florida, United States	125	Saline, i.m.	31	31%		
		122	500 mg vitamin E & 50 mg Se, i.m., 21 d before calving and 30 and 80 d after calving	33%	27%		

Differences from control: † $P<0.10$ * $P<0.05$

or postpartum. Results from selected studies are shown in Table 1 (prepartum administration) and Table 2 (postpartum administration). Among the treatments ineffective at altering fertility were injection of vitamin E with or without selenium (Ealy *et al.*, 1994; Paula-Lopes *et al.*, 2003; Bourne *et al.*, 2008), feeding of vitamin E (Persson Waller *et al*), replacing inorganic selenium with organic selenium (Rutigliano *et al.*, 2008) and injection (Gossen, Feldmann, and Hoedemaker, 2004; Aréchiga *et al.*, 1998b) or feeding of β-carotene (Aréchiga *et al.*, 1998a). In contrast, there was one study in which prepartum injection with vitamin E and selenium improved pregnancy rate at first service (Aréchiga, Ortíz and Hansen, 1994). Also, a single injection of vitamin E and selenium at 30 days postpartum had no effect on pregnancy rate at first service but did improve pregnancy rate to second service (Aréchiga *et al.*, 1998b). Similarly, pregnancy rate to second service was higher for cows fed organic selenium than for those fed inorganic selenium even though pregnancy rate at first service was not different between groups (Thatcher *et al.*, 2010). It is possible that antioxidants are more beneficial for the subset of cows that do not get pregnant to first insemination because these cows are more likely to be experiencing oxidative stress. Rizzo *et al.* (2007) reported that reactive oxygen metabolites were higher in repeat-breeder cows than in other cows.

It may also be that the treatments devised to alter antioxidant status are not sufficient to do so in the reproductive tract where fertilization and embryonic development take place.

Where do we go from here?

The situation revealed by the literature is one where effects of administration of supplemental antioxidants are beneficial but inconsistent. When effective, provision of antioxidants through the diet or injection can reduce the incidence of retained placenta, improve uterine health and increase fertility. A result that is just as likely, however, if not more so, is the inability to improve cow performance through antioxidant supplementation. What seems true is that there are cows that experience oxidative stress of sufficient magnitude that provision of antioxidants improves physiological and immune function of the cow. When these cows are numerous in a herd, effects of antioxidant supplementation are detected as treatment effects. When these cows are not numerous, antioxidant supplementation tends not to have a significant effect on physiological function on average, even if the few cows experiencing oxidative stress benefit from additional antioxidants. Thus, there was a benefit of organic selenium on second service pregnancy rate when blood selenium concentrations were low (Thatcher *et al.*, 2010), but not when they were high (Rutagliano *et al.*, 2008).

One way to improve the efficacy of antioxidant supplementation for the dairy cow is to assess which cows are at risk for oxidative stress and whether the incidence of these cows in the herd is sufficiently high to warrant intervention with supplemental antioxidants. Analysis of feed composition to determine levels of vitamins and minerals involved in antioxidant defence can be one tool for assessing risk for oxidative stress. It is also likely that blood metabolites can be used to assess the oxidative status of individual cows and groups of cows. To date, there are insufficient data to establish benchmark values of key metabolites that predict cow response to antioxidant supplementation. However, establishing such benchmarks can be useful in identifying cows or herds that respond to antioxidant supplementation. Le Blanc *et al.* (2002), for example, found that the mass ratio of a-tocopherol:cholesterol in serum before treatment was predictive of the effect of 3000 IU vitamin E injection, s.c., one week before calving on incidence of retained placenta.   For cows with a mass ratio of 2.5×10^{-3} or less, the odds ratio of incidence of retained placenta for treated cows as compared to control cows was 0.27 for primiparous cows and 0.47 for multiparous cows. For cows with higher mass ratios, the odds ratio was 0.71 and 1.46 for primiparous and multiparous cows, respectively.

There are also opportunities to develop new antioxidant supplements. Indeed, it may be that the antioxidants used most often to date (vitamin E, selenium, and β-carotene) are not the best antioxidants to escape the rumen, become distributed to reproductive tissues and react with reactive oxygen species. The literature is rich with descriptions of molecules with antioxidant properties, and many of these are natural products that could conceivably be fed to dairy cattle. One of these is the polyamine resveratrol found in grape skin that has been reported to increase sperm output in rats (Juan *et al.*, 2005). Another is the class of molecules called anthocyanins that are found in purple sweet potato and which have been reported to reduce effects of elevated temperature on embryo survival in vitro (Sakatani *et al.*, 2007).

References

Aréchiga, C.F., Ortíz, O., and Hansen, P.J. (1994) Effect of prepartum injection of vitamin E and selenium on postpartum reproductive function of dairy cattle. *Theriogenology* **41**, 1251-1258.

Aréchiga, C.F., Staples, C.R., McDowell, L.R., and Hansen, P.J. (1998b) Effects of timed insemination and supplemental β-carotene on reproduction and milk yield of dairy cows under heat stress. *Journal of Dairy Science* **81**, 390-402.

Aréchiga, C.F., Vázquez-Flores, S., Ortíz, O., Hernández-Cerón, J., Porras,

A., McDowell, L.R., and Hansen, P.J. (1998a) Effect of injection of β-carotene or vitamin E and selenium on fertility of lactating dairy cows. *Theriogenology* **50**, 65-76.

Bain, N.T., Madan, P., and Betts, D.H. (2011) The early embryo response to intracellular reactive oxygen species is developmentally regulated. *Reproduction Fertility and Development* **23**, 561-575.

Beagley, J.C., Whitman, K.J., Baptiste, K.E., and Scherzer, J. (2010) Physiology and treatment of retained fetal membranes in cattle. *Journal of Veterinary Internal Medicine* **24**, 261-268.

Bernabucci, U., Ronchi, B., Lacetera, N., and Nardone, A. (2002) Markers of oxidative status in plasma and erythrocytes of transition dairy cows during hot season. *Journal of Dairy Science* **85**, 2173-2179.

Bernabucci, U., Ronchi, B., Lacetera, N., and Nardone, A. (2005) Influence of body condition score on relationships between metabolic status and oxidative stress in periparturient dairy cows. *Journal of Dairy Science* **88**, 2017-2026.

Bourne, N., Laven, R., Wathes, D.C., Martinez, T., and McGowan, M. (2007) A meta-analysis of the effects of Vitamin E supplementation on the incidence of retained foetal membranes in dairy cows. *Theriogenology* **67**, 494-501.

Bourne, N., Wathes, D.C., Lawrence, K.E., McGowan, M., and Laven, R.A. (2008) The effect of parenteral supplementation of vitamin E with selenium on the health and productivity of dairy cattle in the UK. *Veterinary Journal* **177**, 381-387.

Castillo C, Hernandez J, Bravo A, Lopez-Alonso M, Pereira V, Benedito JL. (2005) Oxidative status during late pregnancy and early lactation in dairy cows. *Veterinary Journal* **169**, 286-292.

Chance, B., Sies, H., and Boveris, A. (1976) Hydroperoxide metabolism in mammalian organs. *Physiological Reviews* **59**, 529-605.

Cho, K.J., Seo, J.M., and Kim, J.H. (2011) Bioactive lipoxygenase metabolites stimulation of NADPH oxidases and reactive oxygen species. *Molecules and Cells* **32**, 1-5.

Cook, J.G., and Green, M.J. (2007) Reduced incidence of retained fetal membranes in dairy herds supplemented with iodine, selenium and cobalt. *Veterinary Record* **161**, 625-626.

Eger, S., Drori, D., Kadoori, I., Miller, N., and Schindler, H. (1985) Effects of selenium and vitamin E on incidence of retained placenta. *Journal of Dairy Science* **68**, 2119-2122.

Erskine, R.J., Bartlett, P.C., Herdt, T., and Gaston, P. (1997) Effects of parenteral administration of vitamin E on health of periparturient dairy cows. Journal of the American Veterinary Medical Association **211**, 466-469.

Gilbert, R.O. (2011) The effects of endometritis on the establishment of pregnancy in cattle. *Reproduction Fertility and Development* 2011 **24**, 252-257.

Gossen, N., Feldmann, M., and Hoedemaker, M. (2004) Einfluss einer parenteralen Supplementierung mit beta-Karotin in Form einer Injektionslösung (Carofertin®) auf die Fruchtbarkeitsleistung von Milchkühen. *Deutsche Tierarztliche Wochenschrifte* **111**, 14-21.

Gutteridge, J.M., and Halliwell, B. (2010) Antioxidants: Molecules, medicines, and myths. *Biochemical and Biophysical Research Communications* **393**, 561-564.

Hendricks, K.E., and Hansen, P.J. (2010)Consequences for the bovine embryo of being derived from a spermatozoon subjected to oxidative stress. *Australian Veterinary Journal*;**88**, 307-310.

Hou, C.C., Lin, H., Chang, C.P., Huang, W.T., and Lin, M.T. (2011) Oxidative stress and pyrogenic fever pathogenesis. *European Journal of Pharmacology* **667**, 6-12.

Juan, M.E., González-Pons, E., Munuera, T., Ballester, J., Rodríguez-Gil, J.E., and Planas, J.M. (2005) trans-Resveratrol, a natural antioxidant from grapes, increases sperm output in healthy rats. *Journal of Nutrition* **135**, 757-760.

Kim, I.H., and Kang, H.G. (2003) Risk factors for postpartum endometritis and the effect of endometritis on reproductive performance in dairy cows in Korea. *Journal of Reproduction and Development* **49**, 485-491.

Kimura, K., Goff, J.P., Kehrli, M.E. Jr., and Reinhardt, T.A. (2002) Decreased neutrophil function as a cause of retained placenta in dairy cattle. *Journal of Dairy Science* **85**, 544-550.

Krinsky, N.I., and Yeum, K.J. (2003) Carotenoid-radical interactions. *Biochemical and Biophysical Research Communications* **305**, 754-760.

LeBlanc, S.J., Duffield, T.F., Leslie, K.E., Bateman, K.G., TenHag, J., Walton, J.S., and Johnson, W.H. (2002) The effect of prepartum injection of vitamin E on health in transition dairy cows. *Journal of Dairy Science* **85**, 1416-1426.

LeBlanc, S.J. (2008) Postpartum uterine disease and dairy herd reproductive performance: a review. *Veterinary Journal* **176**, 102-114.

Löhrke, B., Viergutz, T., Kanitz, W., Losand, B., Weiss, D.G., and Simko, M. (2005) Short communication: hydroperoxides in circulating lipids from dairy cows: implications for bioactivity of endogenous-oxidized lipids. *Journal of Dairy Science* **88**, 1708-1710.

López-Gatius, F., García-Ispierto, I., Santolaria, P., Yániz, J., Nogareda, C., and López-Béjar, M. (2006) Screening for high fertility in high-producing dairy cows. *Theriogenology* **65**, 1678-1689.

Lubos, E, Loscalzo, J., and Handy, D.E. (2011) Glutathione peroxidase-1 in health and disease: from molecular mechanisms to therapeutic opportunities. Antioxidant and Redox Signaling **15**, 1957-1997.

McDougall, S., Macaulay, R., and Compton, C. (2007) Association between endometritis diagnosis using a novel intravaginal device and reproductive performance in dairy cattle. *Animal Reproduction Science* **99**, 9-23.

Michal, J.J., Heirman, L.R., Wong, T.S., Chew, B.P., Frigg, M., and Volker, L. (1994) Modulatory effects of dietary β-carotene on blood and mammary leukocyte function in periparturient dairy cows. *Journal of Dairy Science* **77**, 1408-1421.

Moss, J.I., Pontes, E., and Hansen, P.J. (2009) Insulin-like growth factor-1 protects preimplantation embryos from anti-developmental actions of menadione. *Archives of Toxicology* **83**, 1001-1007.

Mudron, P., and Konvicná, J. (2006) Thiobarbituric acid reactive substances and plasma antioxidative capacity in dairy cows at different lactation stages. *Deutsche Tierarztliche Wochenschrifte* **113**, 189-191.

Mudron, P., Herzog, K., Höltershinken, M., and Rehage, J. (2007) Effects of abdominal surgery on thiobarbituric acid reactive substances and plasma anti-oxidative capacity in dairy cows. *Journal of Veterinary Medicine Series A Physiology, Pathology and Clinical Medicine* **54**, 441-444.

Namitha, K.K. and Negi, P.S. (2010) Chemistry and biotechnology of carotenoids. *Critical Reviews in Food Science and Nutrition* **50**, 728-760.

Paula-Lopes, F.F., Al-Katanani, Y.M., Majewski, A.C., McDowell, L.R., and Hansen, P.J. (2003) Manipulation of antioxidant status fails to improve fertility of lactating cows or survival of heat-shocked embryos. *Journal of Dairy Science* **86**, 2343-2351.

Persson Waller, K., Hallén Sandgren, C., Emanuelson, U., and Jensen, S.K. (2007) Supplementation of RRR-alpha-tocopheryl acetate to periparturient dairy cows in commercial herds with high mastitis incidence. *Journal of Dairy Science* **90**, 3640 3646.

Politis, I., Hidiroglou, M., Batra, T.R., Gilmore, J.A., Gorewit, R.C., and Scherf, H. (1995) Effects of vitamin E on immune function of dairy cows. *American Journal of Veterinary Research* **56**, 179-184.

Politis, I., Bizelis, I., Tsiaras, A., and Baldi, A. (2004) Effect of vitamin E supplementation on neutrophil function, milk composition and plasmin activity in dairy cows in a commercial herd. *Journal of Dairy Research* **71**, 273-278.

Rastani, R.R., Grummer, R.R., Bertics, S.J., Gümen, A., Wiltbank, M.C., Mashek, D.G., and Schwab, M.C. (2005) Reducing dry period length to simplify feeding transition cows: milk production, energy balance, and metabolic profiles. *Journal of Dairy Science* **88**, 1004-1014.

Rizzo, A., Minoia, G., Trisolini, C., Manca, R., and Sciorsci, R.L. (2007) Concentrations of free radicals and beta-endorphins in repeat breeder cows. *Animal Reproduction Science* **100**, 257-263.

Robinson, J.M. (2009) Phagocytic leukocytes and reactive oxygen species. *Histochemistry and Cell Biology* **131**, 465-469.

Rutigliano, H.M., Lima, F.S., Cerri, R.L., Greco, L.F., Vilela, J.M., Magalhães, V., Silvestre, F.T., Thatcher, W.W., and Santos, J.E. (2008) Effects of method of presynchronization and source of selenium on uterine health and reproduction in dairy cows. *Journal of Dairy Science* **91**, 3323-3336.

Sakatani, M., Suda, I., Oki, T., Kobayashi, S., Kobayashi S, and Takahashi, M. (2007) Effects of purple sweet potato anthocyanins on development and intracellular redox status of bovine preimplantation embryos exposed to heat shock. *Journal of Reproduction and Development* **53**, 605-614.

Sheldon, I.M., Cronin, J., Goetze, L., Donofrio, G., and Schuberth, H.J. (2009) Defining postpartum uterine disease and the mechanisms of infection and immunity in the female reproductive tract in cattle. *Biology of Reproduction* **81**, 1025-1032.

Sordillo, L.M., and Aitken, S.L. (2009) Impact of oxidative stress on the health and immune function of dairy cattle. *Veterinary Immunology and Immunopathology* **128**, 104-109.

Spears, J.W., and Weiss, W.P. (2008) Role of antioxidants and trace elements in health and immunity of transition dairy cows. *Veterinary Journal* **176**, 70-76.

Spiteller, G (2010). Is lipid peroxidation of polyunsaturated acids the only source of free radicals that induce aging and age-related diseases? *Rejuvenation Research* **13**, 91-103.

Steinnes, E. (2009) Soils and geomedicine. *Environmental and Geochemical Health* **31**, 523-535.

Tanaka, M., Kamiya, Y., Suzuki, T., and Nakai, Y. (2011). Changes in oxidative status in periparturient dairy cows in hot conditions. *Animal Science Journal* **82**, 320-324.

Thatcher, W.W., Santos, J.E.P., Silvestre, F.T., Kim, I.H., and Staples, C.R. (2010) Perspective on physiological/endocrine and nutritional factors influencing fertility in post-partum dairy cows. *Reprodution in Domestic Animals* **45** (Suppl. 3), 2-14.

Turk R, Juretić D, Geres D, Svetina A, Turk N, Flegar-Mestrić Z. (2008) Influence of oxidative stress and metabolic adaptation on PON1 activity and MDA level in transition dairy cows. *Animal Reproduction Science* **108**, 98-106.

Wilde, D. (2006) Influence of macro and micro minerals in the peri-parturient period on fertility in dairy cattle. *Animal Reproduction Science* **96**, 240-249.

Wullepit, N., Hostens, M., Ginneberge, C., Fievez, V., Opsomer, G., Fremaut, D., De Smet, S. (2012) Influence of a marine algae supplementation on the oxidative status of plasma in dairy cows during the periparturient period. *Preventative Veterinary Medicine* **103**, 298-303.

4

RUMEN LIPID METABOLISM AND ITS IMPACTS ON MILK PRODUCTION AND QUALITY

K.J. SHINGFIELD[1] AND P.C. GARNSWORTHY[2]
[1]*MTT Agrifood Research, Animal Production Research, FI-31600, Jokioinen, Finland*
[2]*University of Nottingham, Sutton Bonington Campus, Loughborough, Leics LE12 5RD, UK*

Introduction

Ruminants have evolved an efficient compartmentalised digestive system enabling them to utilise fibrous feedstuffs. More than 900 g/kg of neutral detergent fibre digestion occurs in the rumino-reticulum due to the activity of numerous species of bacteria, protozoa and fungi. Digestion of dietary carbohydrate and protein in the rumen and reticulum results in production of volatile fatty acid fermentation products (principally acetate, propionate and butyrate), microbial protein and ammonia. Ruminant diets contain relatively low amounts of fat. However, lipids in forages, cereal grains and seed oils are rich in unsaturated fatty acids that are toxic to many rumen bacteria, particularly those that are involved in fibre digestion. Specific populations of bacteria, and to a lesser extent protozoa and fungi in the rumen, are capable of biohydrogenation, a process which converts unsaturated to saturated fatty acids (SFA). Fat supplements are often used to increase dietary energy content, but a major concern is the potential adverse effects on rumen function. Negative effects on ruminal digestion can be minimized when fats are fed as calcium soaps or encapsulated within a matrix of saturated fat or formaldehyde-treated protein, but the amount of protection from biohydrogenation varies depending on the technologies used. In addition to increasing energy intake, supplementing the diet with specific fat sources can be used as a means to lower rumen ammonia concentrations, modify rumen fermentation, decrease enteric methane production, alter milk and milk fat composition, improve fertility and enhance immune competence in lactating cows. In the following chapter, the effects of dietary fat supplements, specifically seed oils, fish oil and marine algae on rumen function, milk production and milk fatty acid composition are considered.

Lipids in the ruminant diet

Ruminant diets are variable in composition and can contain different forage species of variable quality (pasture, maize silage, grass or legume hay, or mixed grass and legume hay, and hay silage) and varying combinations of forage, cereals and protein supplements. Numerous by-products of the food industry may also be included. A general characteristic of ruminant diets is the relatively high fibre content (> 300 g cell wall constituents/kg dry matter (DM)) and low amounts of lipid (< 50 g/kg DM).

Lipid in cereal grains, plant oils, oilseeds, fish oil and byproducts are predominantly in the form of triacylglycerides (TAG) in which three fatty acid molecules are esterfied to a single glycerol molecule (Figure 1). Glycolipids are the major lipid class in forages with galactolipids being the most common. These differ from TAG in that one or more sugar molecules are linked to one position of the glycerol backbone (Figure 1). Forages and oilseeds also contain phospholipids present as structural components of cell membranes. Most phospholipids contain a diacylglyceride covalently bonded to a phosphate group, which is often esterified to a simple organic molecule such as choline (Figure 1). In general, both fatty acid molecules bound to glycerol in glycoglycerolipids or phospholipids are unsaturated. Free fatty acids are minor components of most ruminant feeds, but are the major lipid class in some proprietary fat supplements, including calcium soaps.

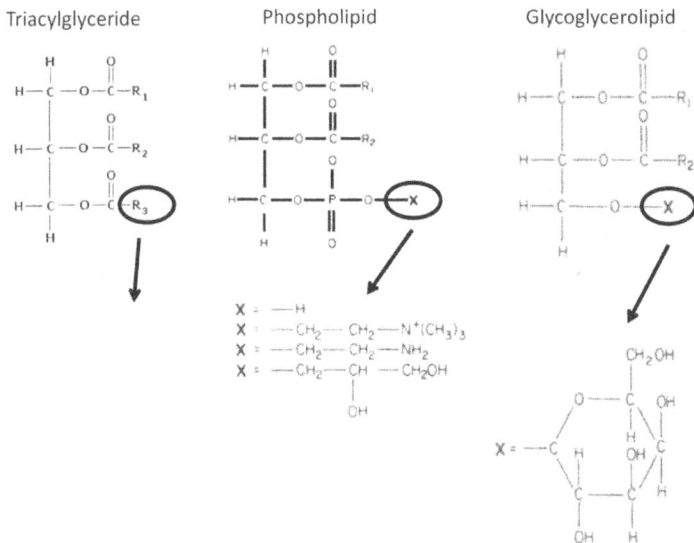

R1, R2 and R3 are unbranched hydrocarbon chains of 12 carbon atoms or longer that may not identical

Figure 1. Chemical structure of lipids in the ruminant diet.

The amount and composition of fatty acids in typical ruminant feed ingredients differs (Table 1). Fatty acid content of grass and legume forages is generally lower than 50 g/kg DM with 18:3n-3 (α-linolenic acid) as the major fatty acid (> 50 g/100 g fatty acids). In contrast, 18:2n-6 (linoleic acid) is the predominant fatty acid in forage maize, whole crop silages and cereal grains (Table 1). Rapeseeds are a rich source of *cis*-9 18:1 (oleic acid), safflower, soyabeans and sunflowerseeds are abundant in 18:2n-6, whereas linseeds and camelina contain high proportions of 18:3n-3 (Table 1). Fish oil and marine algae are the major sources of 20:5n-3 (eicospentaenoic acid) and 22:6n-3 (docosahexaenoic acid) for use in ruminant diets.

Ruminal lipid metabolism

Ruminants rely on microbial digestion of forages and supplementary feeds in the rumen to provide nutrients that would otherwise be unavailable to the host animal. Even though ruminant diets contain relatively low amounts of fat, a high proportion of the fatty acids are unsaturated. Unsaturated fatty acids are toxic to many species of rumen bacteria, particularly those that are involved in fibre digestion. Effects on rumen bacteria are related to the degree of unsaturation with the highly unsaturated fatty acids 18:3n-3 and 20:5n-3 being more toxic than *cis*-9 18:1 or 18:2n-6 (Maia, Chaudhary, Figueres and Wallace, 2007). In contrast to the digestion of carbohydrates and protein in the rumen, metabolism of dietary lipid does not provide rumen microbes with a source of energy, but rather represents a survival mechanism for sustaining the microbial community and rumen function, i.e. minimise the toxic effects of dietary unsaturated fatty acids on bacterial growth (Lourenço, Ramos-Morales and Wallace, 2010).

Lipolysis

Upon ingestion, plant lipids are liberated from the surrounding matrices through the action of mastication and digestion enabling ester linkages in dietary TAG, phospholipids and glycolipids to be hydrolysed by the action of bacterial lipases causing the release of non-esterified fatty acids (NEFA) and glycerol into the rumen. Lipolysis represents the first step in the complete metabolism of esterified dietary lipids and is thought to be rate limiting for the biohydrogenation of unsaturated fatty acids (Harfoot and Hazlewood, 1988). Typically more than 85% of esterified lipid is hydrolysed in the rumen (Palmquist, Lock, Shingfield and

Table 1 Typical lipid content and fatty acid composition of forages, oilseeds, fish oil and marine algae

Ingredient	Oil (g/kg DM)	16:0	18:0	cis-9 18:1	18:2n-6	18:3n-3	20:5n-3	22:6n-3	Reference
				Fatty acid composition (g/100 g fatty acids)					
Grass									
3-week growth	25.0	16.1	1.4	1.94	10.9	67.3	-	-	Dewhurst et al., 2001
6-week growth	15.2	19.4	2.0	2.40	11.9	60.7	-	-	
Early cut	33.2	15.1	2.3	4.4	18.2	49.9	-	-	Vanhatalo et al., 2007
Late cut	28.2	14.5	2.2	6.5	28.8	37.6	-	-	
Wilted	20.5	19.0	0.3	1.09	3.7	18.0	-	-	Shingfield et al., 2005a
Red clover									
Early cut	33.3	21.5	7.1	4.2	17.3	35.6	-	-	Vanhatalo et al., 2007
Late cut	30.2	19.5	3.8	3.5	21.4	38.8	-	-	
Silage									
Grass	18.5	17.9	0.3	1.40	4.0	17.0	-	-	Shingfield et al., 2005a
Grass	19.8	20.1	2.1	2.5	14.2	50.4	-	-	Shingfield et al., 2005b
Maize	25.3	17.4	2.2	20.3	44.8	6.6	-	-	
Red clover	30.4	20.6	6.5	3.4	17.4	40.0	-	-	Vanhatalo et al., 2007
Whole crop wheat	21.0	17.3	1.02	12.2	40.9	23.2	-	-	Noci et al., 2005
Grass hay	8.1	35.0	0.6	2.59	5.4	15.6	-	-	Shingfield et al., 2005a
Rape									
Oil	963	6.0	2.3	48.1	27.4	10.3	-	-	Givens et al., 2009
Whole seeds	408	4.8	2.0	56.8	19.3	8.3	-	-	

Table 1. Contd

Ingredient	Oil (g/kg DM)	Fatty acid composition (g/100 g fatty acids)							Reference
		16:0	18:0	cis-9 18:1	18:2n-6	18:3n-3	20:5n-3	22:6n-3	
Sunflower									
Oil	962	6.1	3.6	26.5	60.4	0.1	-	-	Shingfield *et al.*, 2008a
Whole seeds	400	5.1	4.3	21.6	66.8	0.2	-	-	Woods and Fearon, 2009
Linseed									
Oil	953	4.2	2.7	16.5	15.8	57.8	-	-	Shingfield *et al.*, 2011
Whole seeds	360	6.1	3.4	18.8	16.3	54.4	-	-	Woods and Fearon, 2009
Fish oil	950	15.0	2.6	11.0	1.2	0.9	16.5	10.5	Shingfield *et al.*, 2011
Marine algae, Schizochytrium sp.	581	26.3	0.9	1.1	0.3	0.2	<0.1	37.8	Boeckaert *et al.*, 2008

Bauman, 2005). Lipolysis of TAG in the rumen involves sequential hydrolysis of tri-, di- and mono-acylglycerides to liberate NEFA. Several factors are thought to influence the rate and extent of lipolysis in the rumen including dietary protein and fibre content, forage maturity and rumen pH (Palmquist *et al.*, 2005; Jenkins, Wallace, Moate and Mosley, 2008). The rate of lipolysis of TAG in oilseeds is related to melting point; also, fish oils are thought to be hydrolyzed more slowly, possibly due to stearic hindrance of the ester bonds (Palmquist *et al.*, 2005). Even though lipolysis is known to be a prerequisite for further metabolism of unsaturated fatty acids in the rumen, most of what is known about ruminal lipolysis is based on investigations in vitro (Palmquist *et al.*, 2005; Jenkins *et al.*, 2008).

Biohydrogenation

Following lipolysis, the predominantly unsaturated NEFA are released into the rumen, adsorbed onto feed particles and hydrogenated or incorporated directly into bacterial lipids. Bacteria are thought to be primarily responsible (Harfoot and Hazlewood, 1988; Jenkins *et al.*, 2008; Lourenço *et al.*, 2010). Mixed rumen protozoa have been found capable of isomerising 18:2n-6 to a mixture of conjugated linoleic acid (CLA) isomers (Or-Rashid, **Wright and McBride**, 2009), while fungi isolated from the rumen can hydrogenate 18:2n-6 to 18:0, albeit at much lower rates compared with mixed ruminal bacteria (Nam and Garnsworthy, 2007).

Biohydrogenation of 18:2n-6 and 18:3n-3 in the rumen has for many years been described as a process involving at least two distinct populations of ruminal bacteria with the first committed step proceeding via the isomerisation of the *cis*-12 double bond leading to the formation of conjugated 18:2 or 18:3, respectively (Harfoot and Hazlewood, 1988; Figure 2). Conjugated intermediates are transient and reduced sequentially to yield 18:0 as the final end product via *trans*-11 18:1 as a common intermediate. The final reduction step is considered to be rate limiting and therefore *trans* 18:1 intermediates accumulate. Fewer studies have examined the fate of *cis*-9 18:1 in the rumen. Incubations with mixed or pure cultures of rumen bacteria demonstrated that *cis*-9 18:1 can be biohydrogenated to 18:0 or isomerised to yield numerous *trans*-18:1 intermediates with double bonds at positions $\Delta6$-$\Delta16$ (Jenkins *et al.*, 2008; McKain, Shingfield and Wallace, 2010; Shingfield, Bernard, Leroux and Chilliard, 2010a; Figure 2).

Further investigations indicate that the biochemical pathways responsible for the transformations of NEFA in the rumen are much more complicated and result in the formation of numerous minor biohydrogenation intermediates. For example, incubations of 18:2n-6 with ruminal fluid and pure cultures of several

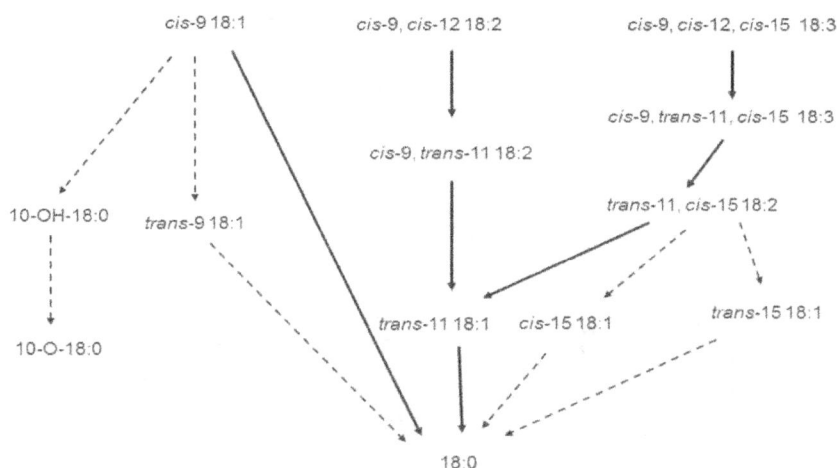

Figure 2. Major metabolic pathways of oleic acid, linoleic and linolenic acid biohydrogenation in the rumen (adapted from Shingfield *et al.*, 2010a).

ruminal bacteria was shown to yield geometric isomers of 9,11 conjugated linoleic acid (CLA) and 10,12 CLA formed via different mechanisms (Wallace, McKain, Shingfield and Devillard, 2007). Incubations with rumen contents or pure strains of ruminal bacteria also demonstrated that 18-carbon unsaturated fatty acids can also be hydrated (Jenkins *et al.*, 2008; McKain *et al.*, 2010). Recent investigations on the fate of [13]C 18:3n-3 during incubations with bovine rumen contents have provided the first evidence that biohydrogenation of 18:3n-3 results in formation of several isomers of non-conjugated 18:3 and *cis*-9, *trans*-11 CLA 18:2 as transient intermediates (Lee and Jenkins, 2011).

For typical ruminant diets, ruminal biohydrogenation varies between 58 and 87 g/100 g for *cis*-9 18:1, between 70 and 95 g/100 g for 18:2n-6, and between 85 and 100g/100 g for 18:3n-3 (Jenkins and Bridges, 2007; Glasser, Schmidely, Sauvant and Doreau, 2008; Shingfield *et al.*, 2010a), indicating that, with the exception of diets containing fish oil or marine algae, 18:0 is the major fatty acid leaving the rumen (Table 2). In general, the extent of ruminal biohydrogenation of 18-carbon unsaturated fatty acids tends to increase linearly in response to dietary intake, with little evidence that processed oilseeds offer substantial protection compared with plant oils (Chilliard, Glasser, Ferlay, Bernard, Rouel and Doreau, 2007; Jenkins and Bridges, 2007; Schmidely, Glasser, Doreau and Sauvant, 2008). Although biohydrogenation of 18-carbon unsaturated fatty acids in the rumen is extensive, conversion of 18-carbon unsaturated fatty acids to 18:0 is incomplete. Therefore, inclusion of plant-based lipids in the diet can alter the supply of fatty acids available for absorption in the small intestine, not only in terms of the amount of fatty acids in the supplement escaping the rumen, but also with respect to the

Table 2 Effect of dietary lipid supplements on flow of fatty acids at the omasum or duodenum in dry or lactating cows

Lipid Supplement	Oil (g/d)	Site[a]	Flow (g/d)								Reference
			16:0	18:0	cis-9 18:1	trans 18:1	18:2n-6	CLA	trans 18:2	18:3n-3	
Control	-	D	58.7	175	45.6	11.5	13.5	<0.1	NR	3.86	Chelikani et al., 2004
Rapeseed oil	1000		104	441	242	53.8	16.9	3.1	NR	2.32	
Control	-	O	58	293	10.8	41	8.0	3.9	4.7	4.3	Shingfield et al., unpublished
Whole rapeseeds	990		100	787	87.8	86	26.2	5.2	6.5	14.4	
Milled rapeseeds	930		103	1020	44.6	103	10.6	5.7	7.5	6.7	
Rapeseed oil	910		111	963	28.3	162	8.1	5.9	9.6	5.6	
Control	-	O	46.5	237.0	7.2	30.3	3.0	3.0	46.5	1.5	Shingfield et al., 2008a
Sunflower oil	250		59.8	408.0	12.7	67.2	6.3	2.5	59.8	1.2	
Sunflower oil	500		68.3	514.0	17.0	118.0	11.4	2.3	68.3	1.0	
Sunflower oil	750		94.2	672.0	26.4	226.0	15.3	2.7	94.2	0.9	
Control[b]	-	D	72.2	196.5	24.0	37.1	2.2	21.8	4.2	8.9	Loor et al., 2004
Linseed oil[b]	588		96.9	454.7	21.6	144.6	3.6	20.2	13.8	12.9	
Control[c]	-		73.5	201.7	47.1	80.7	1.7	36.5	6.5	8.8	
Linseed oil[c]	612		113.6	313.7	54.9	303.9	4.7	42.8	78.0	29.6	
Control	-	D	49.0	168.8	10.7	32.1	1.0	10.6	2.1	2.1	Doreau et al., 2009b
Rolled linseeds	235		53.5	252.3	11.4	56.1	1.7	7.9	5.9	5.9	
Extruded linseeds	235		55.0	228.9	15.5	82.4	2.7	12.1	13.6	7.8	
Linseed oil	235		56.3	227.9	14.7	93.3	3.0	12.0	15.3	4.7	

Table 2. Contd

Lipid Supplement	Oil (g/d)	Site[a]	16:0	18:0	cis-9 18:1	trans 18:1	18:2n-6	CLA	trans 18:2	18:3n-3	Reference
						Flow (g/d)					
Control	-	O	64.6	339	17.6	53.6	6.48	4.44	5.74	1.85	Shingfield et al., 2012
Fish oil	75		80.7	313	15.4	80.7	4.59	5.13	8.63	1.34	
Fish oil	150		90.4	169.0	16.1	149.0	3.87	4.92	14.54	1.07	
Fish oil	300		111	87.8	19.6	168.0	6.84	3.82	45.16	1.41	

[a]Fatty acid flows measured at the duodenum (D) or omasum (O).
[b]Grass hay based diet 65:35 forage:concentrate ratio on a dry matter basis.
[c]Grass hay based diet 35:65 forage:concentrate ratio on a dry matter basis.
NR, not reported.

amount and profile of biohydrogenation end products and intermediates (Table 2). As a result, increases in the amount of 18:0 leaving the rumen following addition of plant oils and oilseeds to the diet are accompanied by increases in *trans* 18:1, *trans* 18:2 and CLA, depending on the amount, type and form of lipid supplement, and also composition of the basal diet (Table 2). Typically, accumulation of biohydrogenation intermediates in animals fed on diets containing plant lipids tends to be higher for high concentrate diets compared with high forage diets.

Studies in cattle indicate that hydrogenation in the rumen is extensive for both 20:5n-3 (49 to 97 g/100 g) and 22:6n-3 (74 to 96 g/100 g) (Shingfield, Lee, Humphries, Scollan, Toivonen, Reynolds and Beever 2010b). Biochemical pathways of 20:5n-3 and 22:6n-3 biohydrogenation in the rumen are not known. Recent investigations have shown, however, that dietary fish oil supplements result in formation of several unique 20- and 22-carbon fatty acids containing at least one *trans* double bond (Toral, Shingfield, Hervás, Toivonen and Frutos, 2010; Kairenius, Toivonen and Shingfield, 2011; Shingfield, Kairenius, Ärölä, Paillard, Muetzel, Ahvenjärvi, Vanhatalo, Huhtanen, Toivonen, Griinari and Wallace, 2012).

Even though fish oil and marine algae contain relatively low amounts of 18-carbon unsaturated fatty acids (Table 1), supplementing the diet with marine lipids modifies 18-carbon fatty acid metabolism in the rumen (Table 2). It is thought that 20:5n-3 and 22:6n-3 in fish oil are responsible for inhibition of complete biohydrogenation of 18-carbon unsaturated fatty acids to 18:0, causing *trans* 18:1 and *trans* 18:2 intermediates to accumulate in the rumen (Jenkins *et al.*, 2008). Fish oil has no major effect on accumulation of CLA isomers or on extent of ruminal *cis*-9 18:1, 18:2n-6 and 18:3n-3 biohydrogenation (Shingfield, Ahvenjärvi, Toivonen, Ärölä, Nurmela, Huhtanen and Griinari, 2003; Shingfield *et al.*, 2010b, 2012).

Microbial lipid synthesis

Fatty acids available for absorption in the small intestine are derived also from rumen microbes, primarily in the form of structural membrane lipids. Bacterial and protozoal lipids originate from both biohydrogenation and utilization of dietary fatty acids, and fatty acids synthesis *de novo* (Harfoot and Hazlewood, 1988; Vlaeminck, Fievez, Cabrita, Fonseca and Dewhurst, 2006). In ruminants fed on diets containing less than 20 g fatty acids/kg DM, microbial lipid accounts for more than 600 g/kg of total fatty acid flow at the duodenum, but this contribution decreases to less than 500 g/kg for diets containing more than 40 g fatty acids/kg DM (Schmidely *et al.*, 2008). Evaluation of data from 95 experiments in sheep and cattle involving comparisons of 303 dietary treatments estimated that the amount of fatty acids at the duodenum of microbial origin is on average 10.8 g/ kg DM intake (Schmidely *et al.*, 2008).

Effect of dietary lipid supplements on rumen function

RUMINAL CARBOHYDRATE AND NITROGEN METABOLISM

A major concern with including fat in the diet is the potential to adversely affect nutrient digestion in the rumen. Several experiments in the 1980s reported negative effects of linseed oil (50 to 70 g/kg DM) on ruminal digestion in sheep fed at maintenance (Doreau and Ferlay, 1994). However, more recent experiments in dairy cows have demonstrated that plant and marine fat supplements can be fed at rates of between 20 and 30 g additional oil/kg DM without lowering NDF digestion, but higher amounts (> 50 g/kg DM) may lower ruminal and total tract organic matter and neutral detergent fibre digestibility coefficients (Table 3). Plant lipid supplements tend to have a more adverse effect on ruminal carbohydrate digestion when fed as free oil compared with whole or cracked seeds, possibly due to slower release of fatty acids into the rumen. Extrusion, which is often used to improve the nutritive value of protein in seeds, may give intermediate results since it disrupts most cells leading to increased oil release compared to whole or rolled seeds (Table 3). Overall, the amount and form of supplemental fat are the major factors influencing ruminal carbohydrate digestion.

For many years a number of technologies or experimental approaches have been investigated to protect unsaturated fatty acids from biohydrogenation and minimise potential disruption of nutrient digestion. Approaches to protect lipids include encapsulation of oil in a matrix of formaldehyde-treated soya and casein or SFA, xylose-treated protein or whey protein gel, saponification of fatty acids with calcium, or chemical conversion to fatty acyl amides (Jenkins and Bridges, 2007). Meta-analysis of measurements of fatty acid flow at the duodenum in cattle fed on diets containing oils, oilseeds or rumen protected lipids confirmed that in most cases, the technologies evaluated thus far do not afford significant protection of 18-carbon unsaturated fatty acids from ruminal biohydrogenation (Jenkins and Bridges, 2007). Nevertheless, despite the inconsistent and often limited degree of protection, rumen-protect fat supplements may have additional value over unprotected fats by minimising effects on rumen function and ease of handling (Jenkins and Bridges, 2007).

During microbial digestion of neutral detergent fibre, sugars and starches in the rumen, volatile fatty acids (VFA) are produced that can meet between 50 and 80% of ruminant energy requirements. Absorption of VFA via the rumen

Table 3 Effect of dietary lipid supplements on ruminal and total tract nutrient digestibility coefficients in dry or lactating cows

Lipid Supplement	Oil (g/d)	DMI (kg/d)	Ruminal		Total tract			Reference
			OM	NDF	OM	NDF	N	
Control	-	14.0	0.454	0.433	0.669	0.494	0.668	Chelikani et al., 2004
Rapeseed oil	1000	14.5	0.485	0.507	0.628	0.448	0.691	
Control	-	19.5	0.464	0.621	0.756	0.678	0.690	Shingfield et al., Unpublished
Whole rapeseeds	990	19.8	0.419	0.598	0.711	0.650	0.654	
Milled rapeseeds	930	18.6	0.470	0.594	0.742	0.653	0.714	
Rapeseed oil	910	18.2	0.428	0.586	0.730	0.628	0.704	
Control	-	15.1	0.507	0.562	0.714	0.650	0.634	Shingfield et al., 2008a
Sunflower oil	250	15.0	0.494	0.549	0.722	0.658	0.627	
Sunflower oil	500	14.7	0.527	0.582	0.725	0.651	0.640	
Sunflower oil	750	14.9	0.459	0.496	0.711	0.621	0.626	
Control[a]	-	20.4	0.572	0.427	0.685	0.614	0.675	Ueda et al., 2003
Linseed oil[a]	588	19.6	0.608	0.582	0.700	0.633	0.722	
Control[b]	-	20.5	0.618	0.443	0.700	0.510	0.673	
Linseed oil[b]	612	20.4	0.572	0.342	0.733	0.540	0.730	
Control	-	10.5	0.533	0.400	0.718	0.527	0.687	Doreau et al., 2009a
Rolled linseeds	235	10.0	0.598	0.476	0.720	0.558	0.685	
Extruded linseeds	235	9.9	0.518	0.456	0.718	0.541	0.702	
Linseed oil	235	9.9	0.517	0.419	0.724	0.525	0.695	
Control	-	18.7	0.397	0.565	0.712	0.628	0.666	Shingfield et al., 2012

Table 3. Contd

Lipid Supplement	Oil (g/d)	DMI (kg/d)	Ruminal				Total tract			Reference
			OM	NDF	OM	NDF	N			
Fish oil	75	18.8	0.463	0.619	0.731	0.654	0.684			
Fish oil	150	17.8	0.479	0.622	0.745	0.665	0.703			
Fish oil	300	15.6	0.440	0.582	0.740	0.647	0.686			

[a]Grass hay based diet 65:35 forage:concentrate ratio on a dry matter basis.
[b]Grass hay based diet 35:65 forage:concentrate ratio on a dry matter basis.
DMI, dry matter intake; N, nitrogen; NDF, neutral detergent fibre; OM, organic matter.

epithelium is the primary form in which energy yielding substrates enter the blood in ruminants. Fat supplements do not generally alter rumen pH, unless DM intake is substantially decreased, but often modify rumen fermentation characteristics (Table 4). Depending on the composition of the basal diet, plant oils and oilseeds may increase molar proportions of propionate at the expense of acetate and/or butyrate (Table 4), effects that have often been attributed to an inhibition of the activity and growth of ruminal fibrolytic species (Steward, Flint and Bryant, 1997). Fish oil or marine algae supplements often increase molar butyrate proportion and decrease that of acetate, and when fed in high amounts, may increase the ratio of glucogenic:lipogenic precursors in the rumen (Table 4).

Given that dietary fats are potent modifiers of ruminal fermentation, there has been interest in their use to lower protozoal predation and intraruminal recycling of bacterial protein, and thereby improve the efficiency of dietary protein utilization and decrease N losses into the environment (Hristov and Jouany, 2005). However, although lipid supplements often lower ruminal ammonia-N concentration (Table 4), no consistent improvement in the energetic efficiency of microbial protein synthesis can be expected unless ruminal protozoal numbers are decreased (Doreau and Ferlay, 1995). Fatty acids in coconut oil and linseed oil are known to have potent defaunating properties in the rumen (Machmüller, 2006; Hristov, Vander Pol, Agle, Zaman, Schneider, Ndegwa, Vaddella, Johnson, Shingfield and Karnati, 2009).

Ruminal methane production

Due to the concerns of increases in greenhouse gas emissions into the environment and potential effects on global warming, there has been renewed interest in the potential role of lipid supplements to decrease enteric methane (CH_4) production in ruminants. Enteric CH_4 is produced by archaea within the rumen. These microorganisms combine carbon dioxide with metabolic hydrogen released by bacteria during fermentation of cellulose to acetate. As a consequence, CH_4 production is strongly linked to the amount of neutral detergent fibre digested within the rumen. Thus far, the only long-term successful strategies to lower enteric CH_4 involve decreasing the reliance on fibre digestion through increasing either the proportion of starch or fat in the diet.

Supplementing diets with lipids is arguably one of the most practical and effective strategies to lower enteric CH_4 emissions in ruminants. Depending on the amount and composition, fat supplements may lower CH_4 production via several mechanisms; 1) increase energy intake and lower forage requirements, 2) lower neutral detergent fibre digestibility and intake, thereby decreasing total

Table 4 Effect of dietary lipid supplements on rumen fermentation characteristics in dry or lactating cows

Lipid Supplement	Oil (g/d)	pH	Ammonia-N mmol/l	Total VFA mmol/l	Molar proportions (mmol/mol)			Reference
					Acetate	Propionate	Butyrate	
Control	-	6.21	8.40	94.2	601	220	125	Hristov et al., 2009
Coconut oil	530	6.37	6.51	84.9	609	230	105	
Control	-	6.29	8.94	107	657	238	124	Chelikani et al., 2004
Rapeseed oil	1000	6.23	9.65	105	656	206	140	
Control	-	6.25	5.18	125	747	295	156	Hristov et al., 2011
Canola meal	609	6.34	4.19	121	688	318	144	
Rapeseed meal	648	6.25	5.35	120	695	297	148	
Control	-	6.50	5.89	104	670	164	132	Shingfield et al., 2008
Sunflower oil	250	6.39	6.07	102	670	165	132	
Sunflower oil	500	6.40	5.98	103	667	167	134	
Sunflower oil	750	6.54	4.63	98.1	660	190	129	
Control[a]	-	6.34	5.68	95.7	660	201	105	Ueda et al., 2003
Linseed oil[a]	588	6.44	7.80	94.8	658	207	97	
Control[b]	-	6.31	2.81	91.3	611	220	112	
Linseed oil[b]	612	6.44	4.80	91.3	598	247	94	
Control	-	NR	2.68	109	652	190	104	Doreau et al., 2009a
Rolled linseeds	235	NR	2.84	105	670	188	102	
Extruded linseeds	235	NR	2.63	99.0	667	183	104	
Linseed oil	235	NR	2.54	102	664	188	105	

Table 4. Contd

Lipid Supplement	Oil (g/d)	pH	Ammonia-N mmol/l	Total VFA mmol/l	Molar proportions (mmol/mol)			Reference
					Acetate	Propionate	Butyrate	
Control	-	6.47	6.62	115	659	174	131	Shingfield et al., 2012
Fish oil	75	6.59	6.21	111	657	176	131	
Fish oil	150	6.63	6.85	110	644	179	141	
Fish oil	300	6.62	5.29	105	611	208	146	
Control	-	6.01	NR	151	626	216	123	Boeckaert et al., 2008
Marine algae, Schizochytrium sp.	114	6.28	NR	124	605	209	145	

[a]Grass hay based diet 65:35 forage:concentrate ratio on a dry matter basis.
[b]Grass hay based diet 35:65 forage:concentrate ratio on a dry matter basis.
NR, not reported.

production of acetate and as a consequence hydrogen and CH_4 formation, 3) inhibit the growth of archaea, protozoa and cellulolytic bacteria and lower ruminal hydrogen production and 4) remove metabolic hydrogen in the rumen during biohydrogenation of unsaturated fatty acids. The importance of biohydrogenation as an alternative hydrogen sink to CH_4 in the rumen is quantitatively minor.

Long-chain polyunsaturated fatty acids (PUFA) are known to decrease methanogenesis through a toxic effect on microorganisms involved in fibre digestion and hydrogen production by protozoa (Doreau and Ferlay, 1995). Such effects, observed for all 18-carbon unsaturated fatty acids, are thought to be mediated via fatty acid effects on gram-positive rumen bacteria. Studies in vitro have demonstrated that 18:3n-3 inhibits growth of the cellulolytic bacteria, *Fibrobacter succinogenes, Ruminococcus albus*, and *Ruminococcus flavefaciens)* due to disruption of cell integrity (Maia, Chaudhary, Figueres and Wallace, 2007). Medium-chain saturated fatty acids, such as 12:0 (lauric acid) and 14:9 (myristic acid), also modify ruminal fermentation due to their potent antiprotozoal properties and, by association, reduce CH_4 production (Machmüller, 2006). Suppression of ruminal CH_4 production by 12:0 and 14:0, or by coconut oil, palm kernel oil and genetically modified rapeseed oil as a source of these medium chain fatty acids, is known to be mediated via a decrease in ruminal protozoal numbers and also through direct inhibition of rumen methanogens (Machmüller, 2006; Hristov *et al.*, 2009).

Meta-analysis of 37 dietary treatments fed to lactating cows revealed a significant negative relationship between DM intake and CH_4 emissions per kg DM intake (Giger-Reverdin, Morand-Fehr and Tran, 2003). Addition of terms for 18:3n-3 and longer chain (> 20 carbon atoms) fatty acids significantly improved accuracy of prediction. Similarly, a review of 17 studies of CH_4 emissions by beef cattle, dairy cows and lambs, reported that CH_4 (g/kg DMI) was decreased by 5.6 percentage units per 10 g/kg DM addition of supplemental fat, with no evidence that 18:3n-3 was more potent in lowering CH_4 compared with other PUFA (Beauchemin, Kreuzer, Mara and McAllister, 2008). In a more recent evaluation based on 67 treatment comparisons in cows, growing cattle and sheep, lipid supplements were found to decrease enteric CH_4 output on average by 3.8 percentage units per 10 g/kg DM addition of supplemental fat (Martin, Morgavi and Doreau, 2010).

Direct comparisons of linseed fatty acids in the form of meal, whole linseed, extruded linseed and linseed oil revealed that daily CH_4 emissions in lactating cows decreased from 418 g/d to 369, 258 and 149 g/d, respectively (Martin, Rouel, Jouany, Doreau and Chilliard, 2008). Part of the decrease in CH_4 was related to lowered digestibility and intake of successive diets, such that when expressed per kg digested NDF or per kg milk yield, only linseed oil significantly lowered CH_4, with no difference between other treatments. However, most studies reporting decreases in CH_4 due to dietary lipid supplements have been relatively short in duration, and there are few data on the efficacy over an extended period (Martin *et al.*, 2010). It remains unclear if the inhibitory effects of fatty acids on rumen methanogenesis persist for long periods, or whether microbial communities in the rumen adapt over time. Nevertheless, dietary fat addition results in the most consistent decreases in CH_4, compared with changes in the forage:concentrate ratio of the diet or other feed additives, which when fed in moderate amounts can lower greenhouse gas emissions without compromising the performance of growing or lactating cattle (Grainger and Beauchemin, 2011).

Effect of dietary lipid supplements on milk production and composition

The gross energy of fat is about double that of grass and cereals; metabolisable energy is about three times as high; and net energy about four times (Garnsworthy, 1997). Dietary fat supplements are often used to increase the energy concentration of the diet to support higher milk yields. Provided that there are no excessive decreases in DM intake, fat supplements increase energy intake with expected benefits on milk production, energy balance, body condition and fertility (Garnsworthy, 1997; Lock and Shingfield, 2004; Sinclair and Garnsworthy, 2010).

MILK YIELD

Although supplemental fat often increases milk yield, the response varies and is often difficult to predict (Table 5). Changes in milk yield depend on the amount of fat included in the diet, fatty acid composition, degree of protection from lipolysis and biohydrogenation in the rumen, composition of the basal diet, overall feeding level, and the stage of lactation and genetic merit of the cow (Garnsworthty, 1997). In most cases, milk yield responses to fat supplements can be explained by the increase in total net energy intake. Much lower than expected increases in milk production can occur when additional lipid disrupts rumen function and lowers both DM intake and nutrient digestion. Stage of lactation and genetic merit are also important determinants; cows in early lactation, and those of higher genetic merit, partition more energy towards the mammary gland for milk production at the expense of body fat reserves. Cows normally lose 0.5-1.0 kg of body weight each day for the first eight weeks of lactation, most of which is due to the mobilisation of lipid stored in adipose. Therefore increased energy intake at this stage of lactation may stimulate further increases in milk yield if the genetic potential of the cow has not been reached, or lower body fat depletion. In established lactation, when DM intakes are higher and milk yield less, energy tends to be partitioned more towards body reserves, so increased energy supply results in higher fat deposition in body reserves. Cows that have a high level of body fat reserves respond to high-fat diets by lowering fat mobilisation, whereas cows with a low level of body reserves generally respond by increasing milk yield (Garnsworthy, 1997). Cows of lower genetic merit have a greater propensity for fat deposition and will partition a greater proportion of surplus energy towards body tissues (Garnsworthy, 1997).

MILK PROTEIN CONTENT

It is generally accepted that energy intake is the major attribute of the diet influencing milk protein content. However, the relationship between increases in metabolisable energy and milk protein only holds true for non-lipid sources (Lock and Shingfield, 2004). Depending on inclusion rate, dietary lipid supplements typically result in a 1 to 4 g/kg decrease in milk protein concentration (Table 5). Often the decrease has been attributed to increases in milk yield rather than lowered milk protein output, but there is evidence to indicate that the decrease in milk protein content is not simply due to dilution, but reflect true physiological responses to fat supplements (Wu and Huber, 1994; Garnsworthy, 1997). Possible mechanisms underlying changes in milk protein content in response to fat supplements have been attributed to deficiencies in glucose supply, insulin resistance, improved energetic efficiency of milk production or reduced somatotrophin production (Wu and Huber, 1994). Of these, limitations in glucose supply appears to be the most plausible. It has been argued that glucose could become more limiting due to decreases in propionate production and microbial protein synthesis when fat replaces starch in the diet, or due to increased glucose requirements for TAG transport in the gut mucosa and lactose synthesis when fat stimulates an increase in milk yield (Garnsworthy, 1997). In support of this hypothesis, lactose supplements were found to partially overcome depressions in milk protein content when calcium salts of palm oil FA replaced cereals in the diet (Garnsworthy, 1997). Further studies indicated that increases in dietary rumen undegradable protein were capable of maintaining milk protein concentrations when milk yield was increased using rumen protected fat, while a combination of protected rapeseed and lactose proved to be even more effective (Garnsworthy, 1997).

Table 5 Milk production responses of lactating cows to dietary lipid supplements

Lipid	Forage	Inclusion (g/kg DM)	Milk (kg/day)	Milk protein		Milk fat		Reference
				content (g/kg)	output (g/day)	content (g/kg)	output (g/day)	
Rapeseed oil	GS	29	-2.1	-0.3	-70	-6.7	-250	Ryhänen et al., 2005
Rapeseed oil	MS	33	+0.8	-0.7	+3	-2.8	-80	Loor et al., 2002
Rapeseed oil	LS/BS	69	+2.7	+2.0	+109	-8.1	-22	Chelikani et al., 2004
Rapeseed oil[b]	MS/GS	49	+0.9	-4.8	-36	-1.6	-131	Givens et al., 2009
Rapeseed oil	RCS	91	+1.2	-1.0	+14	-1.0	+30	Halmemies-BF et al., 2011
Milled rapeseeds[b]	MS/GS	100	+1.9	-0.3	+41	+1.0	+99	Givens et al., 2009
Milled rapeseeds[b]	MS/GS	128	-0.3	+0.5	+14	-0.9	-50	Kliem et al., 2011
Milled rapeseeds[b]	MS/GS	168	-0.2	+1.6	+53	-2.3	-101	Kliem et al., 2011
Milled rapeseeds[b]	MS/GS	207	+0.5	-0.6	-3	-2.5	-89	Kliem et al., 2011
Whole rapeseeds[b]	MS/GS	100	-1.9	+0.3	-58	+3.5	+54	Givens et al., 2009
Soyabean oil	GS	27	1.8	-1.2	42	0.2	82	Shingfield et al., unpublished
Soyabean oil	MS	35	0.4	-0.1	10	-6.7	-189	Jenkins et al., 1996
Sunflower oil	MS	37	-0.8	-1.2	-59	-3.0	-104	Kalscheur et al., 1997
Sunflower oil	GS	50	2.0	-2.3	24	-3.1	38	Shingfield et al., 2008
Sunflower oil	RCS	92	+1.2	-0.4	+37	-3.2	-47	Halmemies-BF et al., 2011
Camelina oil	RCS	91	+0.1	-0.7	-21	-0.3	+9	Halmemies-BF et al., 2011
Camelina expeller	RCS	93	+1.1	-1.5	+1	-2.9	-33	Halmemies-BF et al., 2011

Mean response[a]

Table 5. Contd

Lipid	Forage	Inclusion (g/kg DM)	Milk (kg/day)	Milk protein		Milk fat		Reference
				content (g/kg)	output (g/day)	content (g/kg)	output (g/day)	
Linseed oil	GS	16	1.8	-1.1	41	-0.8	69	Offer et al., 1999
Linseed oil	GS	27	0.6	-0.7	2	0.7	34	Shingfield et al., unpublished
Linseed oil	MS	58	-4.1	+0.7	-126	-8.8	-335	Martin et al., 2008
Linseeds	MS	164	-1.5	+0.6	-32	+4.3	+81	Akraim et al., 2007
Linseeds	MS	124	-1.5	+0.6	-38	+4.3	+31	Martin et al., 2008
Extruded linseeds	MS	168	-2.6	-0.7	-110	-5.8	-293	Akraim et al., 2007
Extruded linseeds	MS	212	-2.2	-0.7	-89	-5.8	-211	Martin et al., 2008
Fish oil	GS	16	0.4	-3.0	-35	-10.9	-167	Offer et al., 1999
Fish oil	GS	31	3.2	-3.8	7	-15.0	-250	Keady et al., 2000
Fish oil	GS/MS	37	-4.5	-2.4	-198	-10.0	-358	Ahnadi et al., 2002
Fish oil	MS	17	1.5	-0.9	16	-13.3	-300	Chilliard and Doreau, 1997
Fish oil	MS/IH	30	-4.3	0.0	-136	-6.7	-311	Donovan et al., 2000
Palm oil fatty acids	LH/IS	18	+3.1	-0.1	+90	+4.9	+286	Mosley et al.,2007
Palm oil fatty acids	LH/IS	36	+3.3	-0.4	+69	+6.2	+302	Mosley et al.,2007
Palm oil fatty acids	LH/IS	52	+3.3	-0.8	+107	+4.4	+393	Mosley et al.,2007

Mean response[a]

[a]Responses calculated as the difference between treatment controls and lipid supplemented diets.
[b]Control diet contained calcium salts of palm oil fatty acids.
GS, grass silage; LH, lucerne hay; LS, lucerne silage; MS, maize silage; RCS, red clover silage.

MILK FAT CONTENT

Fat is the most variable constituent in milk, and is generally increased when supplemental fats are fed with high forage-high fibre diets, but decreased when lipids rich in PUFA are included in low fibre-high concentrate diets (Table 5). Irrespective of the composition of the basal ration, supplements of fish oil or marine algae lower milk fat content and yield in a dose dependent manner (Table 5). In the absence of changes in rumen fermentation or major pathways of fatty acid biohydrogenation, dietary fat supplements elevate milk fat concentrations as a result of an increase in the supply of long chain fatty acids available to the mammary gland for milk fat synthesis (Shingfield *et al.*, 2010a). In contrast, fat supplements that induce changes in rumen fermentation patterns and alter ruminal biohydrogenation pathways invariably result in diet-induced milk fat depression (MFD). Decreases in milk fat due to diets causing MFD often occur within a few days, and in extreme cases milk fat secretion can be lowered by more than half, with little or no change in the yields of milk, milk protein or lactose (Bauman and Griinari, 2003; Shingfield and Griinari, 2007). During diet-induced MFD the secretion of all fatty acids in milk is typically decreased, with the reductions being disproportionately higher for fatty acids synthesized de novo (Bauman and Griinari, 2003).

Diet-induced milk fat depression

Several theories have been proposed to explain diet-induced MFD. The major theories have suggested that decreases in milk fat arise from 1) lowered acetate and β-hydroxybutyrate production in the rumen limiting mammary *de-novo* fatty acid synthesis, 2) increased production of propionate and glucose stimulating insulin secretion causing fatty acids to be preferentially partitioned towards adipose tissue rather than the mammary gland, 3) inhibition of *de-novo* fatty acid synthesis by methylmalonate arising from decreases in vitamin B_{12} and increased propionate synthesis in the rumen or 4) direct inhibition by *trans* fatty acids (TFA) arising from incomplete biohydrogenation of dietary unsaturated fatty acids in the rumen (Bauman and Griinari, 2001, 2003). More recently, Gama *et al.* (2008) found that MFD induced by diets containing fish oil was associated with average melting point of milk fatty acids and proposed that MFD was related to the need to maintain milk fat fluidity.

Early studies reported that decreases in milk fat output for cows fed on diets causing MFD were associated with an increase in milk *trans* 18:1 concentrations (refer to Bauman and Griinari, 2001). Following reports that diet-induced MFD was associated with an increase in milk *trans*-10 18:1 content (Griinari *et al.*, 1998; Piperova *et al.*, 2000) and that *trans*-10, *cis*-12 CLA inhibits milk fat synthesis (Baumgard *et al.*, 2000), the biohydrogenation theory of MFD was proposed (Bauman and Griinari, 2001) which states that "under certain dietary conditions the pathways of biohydrogenation are altered to produce unique fatty acid intermediates which are potent inhibitors of milk fat synthesis" (Figure 3).

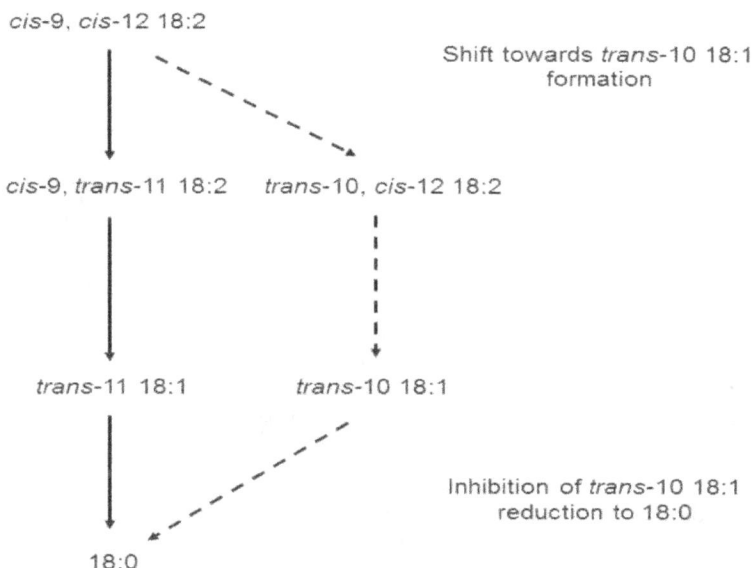

Figure 3. Selected pathways of linoleic acid metabolism in the rumen (adapted from Bauman and Griinari, 2001). Dashed arrows indicate the changes in ruminal biohydrogenation that occur on diets causing milk fat depression.

Of all the hypotheses developed to explain diet-induced MFD, the biohydrogenation theory appears to be the most robust and offers a more convincing explanation for MFD over a wider range of diets. *Trans*-10, *cis*-12 CLA formed during isomerisation of 18:2n-6 (Wallace *et al.*, 2007) is the only biohydrogenation intermediate to have been infused at the abomasum over a range of doses and shown unequivocally to inhibit milk fat synthesis in lactating cows (Figure 4).

However, increases in ruminal outflow of *trans*-10, *cis*-12 CLA, do not explain the decreases in milk fat synthesis in all cases of diet-induced MFD, with the implication that additional biohydrogenation intermediates and/or mechanisms must be involved (Shingfield and Griinari, 2007). Experiments involving infusion of a mixture of CLA isomers at the abomasum have provided evidence that *trans*-9, *cis*-11 CLA and *cis*-10, *trans*-12 CLA inhibit milk fat synthesis in the lactating cow, but further studies are required to confirm these intermediates contribute to

MFD in vivo (Shingfield and Griinari, 2007). Support for the role of *trans*-9, *cis*-11 CLA in MFD with fish-oil diets was provided by the study of Gama *et al.* (2008), in which increases in *trans*-9, *cis*-11 CLA explained more than 80% of MFD.

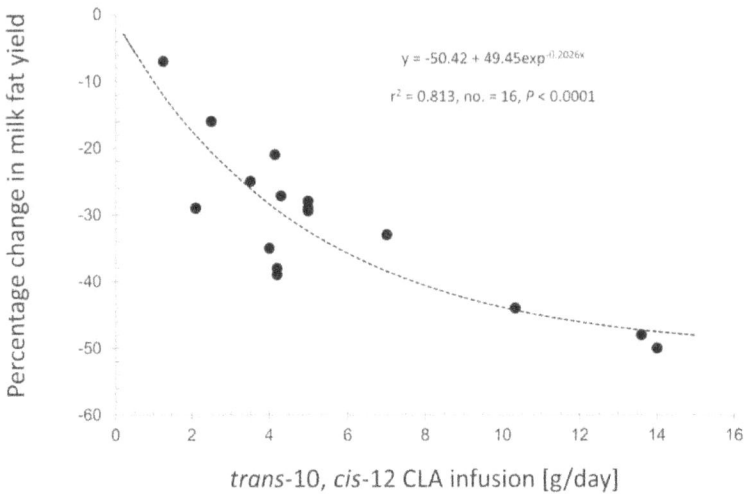

Figure 4. Relationship between abomasal infusions of *trans*-10, *cis*-12 conjugated linoleic acid (CLA) and relative changes in milk fat yield reported in 11 experiments with lactating cows (derived from Shingfield and Griinari, 2007).

Over a wide range of diets causing MFD, increases in milk fat *trans*-10 18:1 concentrations have been consistently reported (Figure 5). However, abomasal infusion of 42.6 g/d of relatively pure (95%) *trans*-10 18:1 in free fatty acid form in lactating cows over a 4-d period was shown to enrich *trans*-10 18:1 concentration in milk from 0.47 to 1.11 g/100 g fatty acids but have no effect on milk fat secretion, with the implication that *trans*-10 18:1 does not exert anti-lipogenic effects (Lock, Tyburczy, Dwyer, Harvatine, Destaillats, Mouloungui, Candy and Bauman, 2007). Owing to the relatively low recovery in milk fat it has been postulated that the associated increases in milk fat *trans*-10 18:1 content to post-ruminal infusions were too small to allow reliable detection of the effects on milk fat synthesis (Kadegowda *et al.*, 2008). Under certain conditions, *trans*-10 18:1 concentrations in bovine milk during MFD approach or exceed 10 g/100 g fatty acids (Figure 5). A recent experiment demonstrated that post-ruminal infusions of a mixture of 18:1 fatty acid methyl esters providing 92.1 g/d of *trans*-10 18:1 in lactating cows over a 5 d period resulted in reductions of 21.3% in milk fat content and 19.5% in milk fat yield (Shingfield, Sæbø, Sæbø, Toivonen and Griinari, 2009). Even though no direct cause and effect could be established, the lack of MFD associated with other constituent methyl esters implicated *trans*-10 18:1 as the most probable candidate responsible for the inhibitory effects on milk fat synthesis. Further studies are required to allow unambiguous conclusions on the role of *trans*-10 18:1 and other biohydrogenation intermediates on milk fat synthesis in lactating cows.

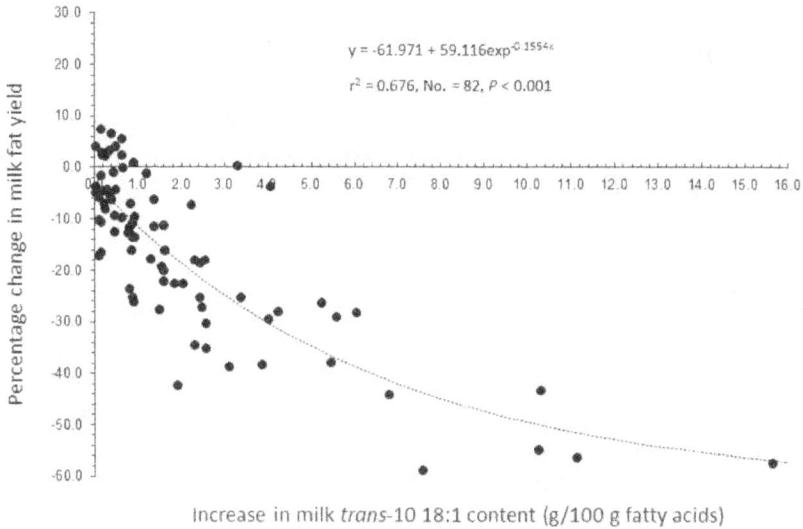

Figure 5. Association between increases in milk fat *trans*-10 18:1 content and corresponding changes in milk fat yield based on 82 comparisons between treatment groups and corresponding controls (adapted from Shingfield *et al.*, 2010a).

Altering milk fatty acid composition

There is increasing evidence from clinical and biomedical studies that diet plays an important role in the onset and development of chronic disease in the human population including cancer, cardiovascular disease (CVD), insulin resistance and obesity (WHO/FAO, 2003). Studies in human subjects have indicated that medium-chain SFA and TFA in the diet increase CVD risk, with the risk associated with TFA consumption being higher than SFA (WHO/FAO, 2003; Shingfield, Chilliard, Toivonen, Kairenius and Givens, 2008b) Excessive intakes of SFA may also be associated with lowered insulin sensitivity, which is a key factor in development of the metabolic syndrome and diabetes (Funaki, 2009). In an attempt to lower the economic and social burden of chronic disease, public health nutrition guidelines recommend a population-wide decrease in the intake of total fat, SFA and TFA, and an increase in consumption of the long-chain PUFA, 20:5n-3 and 22:6n-3. In industrialised countries, milk and dairy products are the main source of 12:0 and 14:0 in the human diet, and collectively ruminant-derived foods contribute significantly to total 16:0 and TFA consumption (Shingfield *et al.*, 2008b). However, developing public health policies promoting a decrease in the consumption of milk, cheese, butter and ruminant meat ignores the value of these foods as a versatile source of high quality protein, vitamins, minerals and bioactive lipids. Altering the fatty acid composition of milk fat, rather than simply promoting a population-wide decrease in the intake of milk and dairy products, represents one means to lower SFA intakes and increase *cis* mono- and PUFA in the human diet without requiring changes in consumer eating habits, while at the same time maintaining the potential benefits associated with the macro and micro nutrients in these foods.

Milk fat synthesis

It is well established that tissue lipids and milk fat in ruminants contain much higher proportions of saturates compared with dietary intake that is due, at least in part, to extensive lipolysis and subsequent hydrogenation of ingested unsaturated fatty acids in the rumen. Milk fat contains more than 400 different fatty acids, but SFA of chain lengths from 4 to 18 carbon atoms, *cis*-9 16:1, *cis*-9 18:1, isomers of *trans* 18:1 and 18:2n-6 are the most abundant (Jensen, 2002). Milk fat typically contains a high proportion of SFA (0.70-0.75) and monounsaturated fatty acids and small amounts of PUFA (0.05) (Lock and Shingfield, 2004). Fatty acids incorporated into milk TAG are derived from uptake of preformed fatty acids in arterial blood and synthesis of fatty acids in the mammary gland *de novo* (Chilliard *et al.*, 2007). Fatty acid synthesis *de novo* accounts for all 4:0 to 12:0, most of the 14:0 (ca. 95%) and about 50% of 16:0 secreted in milk, whereas all 18-carbon and longer chain fatty acids are made available following mammary extraction of plasma NEFA and TAG that originate from the absorption of fatty acids in the small intestine and body fat reserves (Chilliard *et al.*, 2007).

Mammary gland epithelial cells contain the stearoyl-CoA desaturase (SCD) complex, an enzyme that catalyses oxidation of fatty acyl CoA esters resulting in the introduction of a *cis* double bond between carbon atoms 9 and 10. Stearoyl and palmitoyl-CoA are the preferred substrates for SCD with 18:0 to *cis*-9 18:1 representing the major precursor:product of SCD in the bovine mammary epithelial cell (Palmquist *et al.*, 2005). Endogenous synthesis through activity of SCD in the mammary gland accounts for 0.90 of *cis*-9 14:1, 0.50 to 0.55 of *cis*-9 16:1, 0.60 of *cis*-9 18:1, and 0.70 to 0.95 of *cis*-9, *trans*-11 CLA secreted in milk fat (Palmquist *et al.*, 2005; Shingfield *et al.*, 2010a).

Using fat supplements to alter milk fat composition

Due to the high proportion of SFA in milk fat, some of which are known risk factors for cardiovascular diseases and insulin resistance, there has been increased interest in lowering the medium-chain saturates and increasing the concentration of specific unsaturated fatty acids in milk, either for production of added value products or in attempt to improve the public perception of the nutritional value of milk and dairy products.

Nutrition is the major environmental factor regulating milk fatty acid composition (Dewhurst, Shingfield, Lee and Scollan, 2006; Chilliard *et al.*, 2007; Shingfield *et al.*, 2008b). Animal genetics also influence milk fatty acid composition (Arnould and Soyeurt, 2009). Supplementing the diet with plant oils, oilseeds, fish oil, marine algae and rumen protected lipid supplements can be used to influence milk fat composition. However, the extent to which it is possible to enrich specific dietary unsaturated fatty acids in milk is largely dependent on the extent of biohydrogenation in the rumen. Often attempts to alter milk fatty acid composition, particularly using marine lipids and fat supplementation of low forage-high concentrate diets are accompanied by MFD (Table 5).

Dietary plant oil or oilseed supplements result in dose-dependent decreases in concentration and secretion of 10- to 16-carbon fatty acids in bovine milk with no major differences in milk 12:0, 14:0 and 16:0 concentration responses to oils enriched in *cis*-9 18:1, 18:2n-6 or 18:3n-3 (Table 6). These changes arise due to an increase in the supply of long chain fatty acids ($\geq$ 16-carbon atoms) that directly inhibit fatty acid synthesis de novo in the mammary gland (Shingfield *et al.*, 2010a). Decreases in medium-chain SFA do not occur in isolation, but are accompanied by increases in the relative abundance of 18:0, *cis*-9 18:1 and total *trans* 18:1 isomers (Table 6). Supplementing the diet with plant lipids enriched in 18:2n-6 or 18:3n-3 typically increases milk fat *cis*-9, *trans*-11 CLA concentrations, depending on inclusion rate and composition of the basal diet. Enrichment of *cis*-9 18:1 in milk of ruminants fed on diets containing oils and oilseeds arises from direct incorporation of *cis*-9 18:1 escaping biohydrogenation in the rumen and increases in the amount of 18:0 available for absorption and desaturation to *cis*-9 18:1 via the activity of SCD in the intestinal mucosa, mammary gland and adipose tissue. Increases in the amount of *trans*-11 18:1 leaving the rumen accounts for the majority of milk fat *cis*-9, *trans*-11 CLA enrichment in ruminants fed on diets containing plant oils and oilseeds (Palmquist *et al.*, 2005).

Since PUFA are not synthesized by ruminant tissues, the concentration of 18:2 n-6 and 18:3 n-3 in milk is dependent on the amounts of these fatty acids absorbed from the small intestine and partitioned towards the mammary gland. Milk 18:2n-6 concentration typically varies between 2.0 and 3.0 g/100 g fatty acids, but rarely

Table 6 Effect of dietary plant-based lipid supplements on bovine milk fatty acid composition

Lipid source	Oil (g/d)	Forage	F:C[a]	Milk fatty acid composition				
				4:0	6:0	8:0	10:0	12:0
Control	0	LH/LS	44:56	2.95	2.02	1.18	2.68	3.06
Palm oil by-product	476			3.09	1.88	0.99	2.12	2.42
Palm oil by-product	887			3.09	1.77	0.89	1.85	2.11
Palm oil by-product	1248			3.03	1.72	0.85	1.78	2.04
Control	0	MS/GH	48:52	3.35	2.67	1.51	3.46	3.94
Sunflower oil	957			2.31	1.21	0.54	1.20	1.65
Control	0	MS	27:73	3.28	2.70	1.62	4.26	5.14
Sunflower oil	755			1.84	1.03	0.48	1.16	1.81
Control	0	GH	65:35	3.40	2.65	1.73	3.95	4.47
Linseed oil	588			3.88	2.27	1.41	2.41	2.51
Control	0	GH	35:65	3.57	2.80	1.89	4.28	4.76
Linseed oil	612			2.96	1.62	0.97	2.38	2.80
Control	0	GH	64:36	2.96	2.31	1.43	3.54	4.22
Linseed oil	1050			2.82	1.76	0.84	1.77	1.96
Control	0	Pasture	(5)	1.87	1.40	0.97	2.33	2.83
Rapeseed oil	500			1.58	0.99	0.59	1.29	1.63
Sunflower oil	500			1.38	0.87	0.53	1.15	1.52
Linseed oil	500			1.67	1.06	0.65	1.41	1.75
Control	0	RCS	55:45	3.35	1.76	1.23	3.19	3.91
Rapeseed oil	310			3.54	1.72	1.14	2.75	3.24
Sunflower oil	280			3.58	1.71	1.14	2.76	3.24
Camelina oil	300			3.57	1.69	1.14	2.72	3.20
Camelina expeller	210			3.67	1.69	1.09	2.57	3.08
Ca salts of Palm oil	950	MS/GS	50:50	3.30	2.30	1.30	2.70	2.90
Whole rapeseed	1186	(75:25)		3.30	2.50	1.50	3.30	3.60
Milled rapeseed	1147			3.10	2.20	1.20	2.40	2.60
Rapeseed oil	1044			2.70	1.80	0.90	1.90	2.20
Control	0	MS/ LH	69:31	2.69	2.16	1.33	2.74	3.95
Whole linseed	1311	(88:12)		2.69	2.01	1.23	2.37	3.15
Extruded linseed	943			2.57	1.82	1.06	2.06	2.54

[a]Forage:concentrate ratio of the diet (on a dry matter basis). For studies in grazing cows the amount of concentrate supplements fed (kg/d) is reported in parentheses; [b]*cis*-9, *trans*-11 conjugated linoleic acid; GS, grass silage; GH, grass hay; LH, lucerne hay; LS, lucerne silage; MS, maize silage; RCS, red clover silage.

				(g/100g total fatty acids)				
14:0	*16:0*	*18:0*	*cis-9 18:1*	*trans 18:1*	*18:2n-6*	*CLA[b]*	*18:3n-3*	*Reference*
9.79	30.7	9.12	21.2	2.26	3.59	0.46	0.50	Mosley *et al.* 2007
8.63	39.1	6.83	19.3	1.79	3.17	0.40	0.41	
7.96	44.0	5.79	17.9	1.54	2.99	0.34	0.36	
7.89	45.6	4.95	17.4	1.44	3.11	0.30	0.36	
12.1	32.3	8.63	16.6	2.80	2.19	0.55	0.21	Roy *et al.*,2006
7.06	18.9	13.6	28.3	11.5	2.34	0.93	0.20	
12.8	28.7	5.77	14.9	5.19	2.96	0.60	0.09	
7.36	19.1	6.27	19.4	23.7	4.59	1.17	0.15	
13.1	29.4	7.05	15.3	2.69	1.75	0.62	0.78	Loor *et al.*, 2005
9.72	17.2	14.8	23.8	9.02	1.62	1.34	1.00	
12.7	25.7	6.17	14.9	5.00	2.69	0.81	0.76	
8.77	18.7	8.07	14.4	12.1	2.30	2.54	1.59	
13.1	34.9	6.99	14.2	2.11	1.58	0.54	0.74	Roy *et al.*, 2006
8.29	17.1	12.8	20.6	12.2	1.16	2.89	0.74	
10.2	24.1	14.3	22.1	4.95	1.12	1.19	0.60	Rego *et al.*, 2009
6.90	18.0	17.3	30.6	7.51	0.98	1.14	0.38	
6.61	18.2	16.8	29.6	8.78	1.25	1.61	0.42	
7.09	17.0	16.8	26.5	9.67	0.99	1.54	0.53	
13.0	32.4	7.63	13.2	4.02	2.08	0.44	1.1	Halmemies-BF
11.8	27.3	10.4	17.3	5.2	1.99	0.56	1.02	*et al.*, 2011
11.7	26.5	10.9	16.6	5.55	2.55	0.64	0.99	
11.6	27.1	9.86	16.5	4.91	2.10	0.57	1.17	
11.9	26.8	7.33	13.5	8.28	1.98	1.02	1.06	
10.0	34.5	9.80	18.6	4.10	2.25	0.57	0.25	Givens *et al.*,
11.7	31.1	10.8	17.0	3.20	1.76	0.44	0.23	2009
9.60	21.6	15.5	23.0	6.40	1.73	0.86	0.27	
8.70	19.8	14.6	24.3	10.0	1.78	1.31	0.22	
11.4	33.6	9.40	18.7	3.18	1.92	0.59	0.27	Akraim *et al.*,
9.15	24.4	14.2	21.8	6.61	1.70	0.84	0.95	2007
9.95	23.3	14.4	22.0	8.91	1.62	1.12	1.20	

Table 7 Effect of dietary fish oil and marine algae supplements on bovine milk fatty acid composition

Supplement	Oil (g/d)	Milk fatty acid composition (g/100g total fatty acids)						
		4:0	6:0	8:0	10:0	12:0	14:0	16:0
Control[a]	-	1.80	1.00	0.64	1.76	2.70	9.88	40.2
Fish oil[a]	250	1.81	0.93	0.59	1.58	2.36	10.3	39.6
Tuna oil[a]	95	1.80	1.00	0.63	1.68	2.48	9.93	39.5
Control	0	3.2	2.0	1.3	3.1	3.7	11.3	27.1
Menhaden fish oil	290	2.9	1.7	1.0	2.4	3.0	10.4	25.2
Menhaden fish oil	470	2.6	1.4	0.8	1.8	2.3	9.3	26.1
Menhaden fish oil	612	2.9	1.5	0.8	1.9	2.3	9.3	26.6
Control	0	3.9	2.5	1.5	3.5	4.0	12.1	29.4
Menhaden fish oil	432	3.9	2.3	1.3	2.8	3.2	11.4	27.6
Control	0	4.22	2.23	1.11	2.22	2.40	10.2	24.0
Mackerel oil	250	2.22	1.66	1.08	2.81	3.39	13.3	32.3
Control	0	1.91	1.92	1.28	3.43	4.27	13.9	34.2
Menhaden	270	1.83	1.75	1.23	3.54	4.49	14.8	31.8
Control	0	2.00	1.31	1.66	4.14	5.08	13.3	30.7
Menhaden fish oil	127	1.94	1.21	1.51	3.65	4.44	12.9	29.7
Control[a]	0	3.5	2.2	1.3	2.9	3.2	10.5	28.4
Marine algae[a]	910	3.6	2.0	1.1	2.5	3.0	11.8	33.0
Control[a]	0	3.9	2.3	1.6	3.0	3.7	11.3	28.9
Marine algae[a]	600	3.5	1.9	1.2	2.4	3.2	11.2	28.4
Control	0	4.65	2.80	1.35	2.71	2.49	9.35	28.8
Marine algae	201	4.69	1.94	1.09	1.98	2.07	8.01	27.7

[a]Milk fatty acid concentration g/100 g fat.
NR, not reported.

Milk fatty acid composition (g/100g total fatty acids)								
18:0	*cis-9 18:1*	*trans 18:1*	*18:2n-6*	*CLA[2]*	*18:3n-3*	*20:5n-3*	*22:6n-3*	*Reference*
12.3	18.8	2.23	2.03	0.16	0.72	0.09	0.04	Offer *et al.*,
6.74	5.67	19.6	2.52	1.55	0.74	0.11	0.08	1999
10.5	16.7	6.97	1.81	0.52	0.71	0.11	0.07	
9.4	16.5	2.4	3.1	0.18	0.60	0.05	0.02	Donovan *et*
7.0	14.5	6.1	2.4	0.36	1.58	0.22	0.06	*al.*, 2000
4.4	11.4	12.9	2.0	0.24	2.23	0.32	0.26	
4.0	10.9	12.1	2.4	0.22	1.90	0.40	0.20	
10.4	16.1	1.8	2.6	0.54	0.40	0.05	0.04	AbuGhazaleh
8.1	15.1	3.8	2.2	0.85	0.88	0.24	0.26	*et al.*, 2002
15.4	22.2	4.14	1.88	0.51	0.42	0.05	0.00	Shingfield *et*
3.50	5.93	13.2	2.01	2.41	0.45	0.11	0.10	*al.*, 2003
8.69	15.8	3.01	1.88	0.56	0.28	0.08	0.04	Loor *et al.*,
2.71	6.05	13.8	2.01	3.20	0.31	0.36	0.17	2005
7.04	17.8	1.68	2.83	0.52	0.54	0.12	0.03	Bharathan *et*
6.53	18.9	2.25	2.84	0.90	0.53	0.19	0.04	*al.*, 2008
12.2	23.2	2.4	2.8	0.54	0.37	NR	0.00	Franklin *et al.*,
4.3	13.0	12.8	2.7	0.47	2.62	NR	0.46	1999
10.2	21.4	2.9	2.2	0.32	0.51	0.05	0.04	Offer *et al.*,
7.7	18.1	8.8	2.4	0.36	0.92	0.09	0.30	2001
10.2	22.1	2.04	1.89	0.48	0.50	NR	0.09	Boeckaert *et*
3.59	17.6	11.6	1.37	1.00	0.42	NR	1.10	*al.*, 2008

exceeds 3.5 g/100 g fatty acids, even when oils rich in 18:2n-6 are fed (Table 6). Other than grass or legume forages, linseed (flaxseed) and more recently camlina, are the most common oilseeds used to increase milk 18:3 n-3 content. Irrespective of diet composition or form of lipid supplement, the potential to increase 18:3n-3 in milk varies between 0.1 and 0.9 g/100 g fatty acids (Table 6).

Ruminant milk typically contains < 0.1 g/100 g fatty acids of 20:5n-3 and trace amounts of 22:6n-3 (Table 7). Numerous experiments have examined the use of dietary fish oil, fish meal or marine algae supplements to increase 20:5n-3 and 22:6n-3 in ruminant milk. Irrespective of the source of marine lipid, composition of basal diet or ruminant species studied, enrichment of 20:5 n-3 and 22:6 n-3 in milk fat rarely exceeds a combined total of 1.2 g/100 g fatty acids and induce minor changes in 12:0, 14:0 and 16:0 concentration (Table 7). The inability to substantially increase long chain n-3 PUFA in milk is due to the extensive biohydrogenation of these fatty acids in the rumen (Shingfield *et al.*, 2010b) and the relatively low efficiency of transfer from the small intestine into milk of 20:5n-3 (14.3 to 33.0%) and 22:6n-3 (13.3 to 25.0%) (Palmquist, 2009).

Supplements of plant oils, oilseeds and marine lipids not only increase *trans* 18:1 content, but also alter the abundance of specific TFA in milk. Increases in dietary intakes of *cis*-9 18:1, 18:2 n-6 and 18:3 n-3 can be expected to specifically enrich *trans* 6-8 18:1, *trans* 10-12 18:1 and *trans*-11-16 18:1, respectively (Chilliard *et al.*, 2007; Shingfield *et al.*, 2008b). Increases in *trans* 18:1 due to fish oil and marine lipid supplements are associated with elevated *trans*-6 to -15 18:1 concentrations and lowered *trans*-16 18:1 concentration (Shingfield *et al.*, 2008b). Bovine milk contains several non-conjugated *trans* 18:2 fatty acids, but the concentration and isomer distribution differs compared with hydrogenated plant oils, margarines and edible oils (Shingfield *et al.*, 2008b). For typical diets containing no additional lipid supplements, total *trans* 18:2 in ruminant milk varies between 0.32 and 0.91 g/100 g fatty acids, but concentrations can approach or exceed 2.0 g/100 g fatty acids when plant oil or oilseeds are fed (Shingfield *et al.*, 2008b; Rego, Alves, Antunes, Rosa, Alfaia, Prates, Cabrita, Fonseca and Bessa, 2009; Halmemies-Beauchet-Filleau, Kokkonen, Lampi, Toivonen, Shingfield and Vanhatalo, 2011).

Implications and conclusions

Dietary fat supplements increase the energy concentration of the diet and, depending on the amount and composition, can be used not only to support higher milk yields, but also to improve dairy cow body condition, health and fertility. The extent to which dietary lipids influence physiological processes is to a large extent dependent on the transformations that occur in the rumen. Significant advances have been made during the last decade in characterizing intermediates formed during ruminal biohydrogenation of unsaturated fatty acids, the mechanisms involved, and some of the bacterial species responsible. One or more intermediates formed during ruminal biohydrogenation of 18-carbon unsaturated fatty acids are known to directly inhibit milk fat synthesis, but further investigations are required to fully explain the association between ruminal lipid metabolism and milk fat synthesis. Furthermore, the metabolic fate of 20:5n-3 and 22:6n-3 in the rumen and the biological activity of the intermediates formed remains uncertain. In moderate amounts, sources of PUFA do not adversely influence carbohydrate digestion in the rumen, but may lower rumen ammonia concentrations and enteric methane production. At inclusion rates above 50g/kg diet DM, fat supplements can be expected to induce adverse effects on rumen function and milk production. Dietary fat supplements can be used to alter milk fatty acid composition to be more in line with public health policies that recommend population-wide decreases in consumption of SFA and higher intakes of PUFA. However, unless fed in rumen protected form, fats rich in unsaturated fatty acids also increase milk TFA concentrations and alter the relative abundance of specific TFA isomers. Provided there are sufficient economic incentives, further progress towards altering milk fat composition to be more in line with public health recommendations may be achieved through genomic-based selection and formulation of diets to exploit this genetic potential.

References

AbuGhazaleh, A.A., Schingoethe, D.J., Hippen, A.R. and Whitlock, L.A. (2002) Feeding fish meal and extruded soybeans enhances the conjugated linoleic acid (CLA) content of milk. *Journal of Dairy Science*, **85**, 624-631.

Ahnadi, C.E., Beswick, N., Delbecchi, L., Kennelly, J.J. and Lacasse, P. (2002) Addition of fish oil to diets for dairy cows. II. Effects on milk fat and gene expression of mammary lipogenic enzymes. *Journal of Dairy Research*, **69**, 521-531.

Akraim, F., Nicot, M.C., Juaneda, P. and Enjalbert, F. (2007) Conjugated linolenic acid (CLnA), conjugated linoleic acid (CLA) and other biohydrogenation intermediates in plasma and milk fat of cows fed raw or extruded linseed. *Animal*, **1**, 835–843.

Arnould, V.M.-R. and Soyeurt, H. (2009) Genetic variability of milk fatty acids. *Journal of Applied Genetics*, **50**, 29-39.

Bauman, D.E. and Griinari, J.M. (2001) Regulation and nutritional manipulation of milk fat: low-fat milk syndrome. *Livestock Production Science*, **70**, 15-29.

Bauman, D.E. and Griinari, J.M. (2003) Nutritional regulation of milk fat synthesis. *Annual Reviews in Nutrition*, **23**, 203-227.

Baumgard, L.H., Corl, B.A., Dwyer, D.A., Sæbø, A. and Bauman, D.E. (2000) Identification of the conjugated linoleic acid isomer that inhibits milk fat synthesis. *American Journal of Physiology*, **278**, R179-R184.

Beauchemin, K.A., Kreuzer, M., O'Mara, F. and McAllister, T.A. (2008) Nutritional management for enteric methane abatement: a review. *Australian Journal of Experimental Agriculture*, **48**, 21–27.

Bharathan, M., Schingoethe, D.J., Hippen, A.R., Kalscheur, K.F., Gibson, M.L. and Karges, K. (2008) Conjugated linoleic acid increases in milk from cows fed condensed corn distillers solubles and fish oil. *Journal of Dairy Science*, **91**, 2796-2807.

Boeckaert, C., Vlaeminck, B., Dijkstra, J., Issa-Zacharia, A., Van Nespen, T., Van Straalen, W. and Fievez, V. (2008) Effect of dietary starch or micro algae supplementation on rumen fermentation and milk fatty acid composition of dairy cows. *Journal of Dairy Science*, **91**, 4714-4727.

Chelikani, P.K., Bell, J.A. and Kennelly, J.J. (2004) Effects of feeding or abomasal infusion of canola oil in Holstein cows 1. Nutrient digestion and milk composition. *Journal of Dairy Research*, **71**, 279-287.

Chilliard, Y. and Doreau, M. (1997) Influence of supplementary fish oil and rumen-protected methionine on milk yield and composition in dairy cows. *Journal of Dairy Research*, **64**, 173-179.

Chilliard, Y., Glasser, F., Ferlay, A., Bernard, L., Rouel, J. and Doreau, M. (2007) Diet, rumen biohydrogenation and nutritional quality of cow and goat milk fat. *European Journal of Lipid Science and Technology*, **109**, 828-855.

Dewhurst, R.J., Scollan, N.D., Youell, S.J., Tweed, J.K.S. and Humphreys, M.O. (2001) Influence of species, cutting date and cutting interval on the fatty acid composition of grasses. *Grass and Forage Science*, **56**, 68-74.

Dewhurst, R.J., Shingfield, K.J., Lee, M.R.F. and Scollan, N.D. (2006) Increasing the concentrations of beneficial polyunsaturated fatty acids in milk produced by dairy cows in high-forage systems. *Animal Feed Science and Technology*, **131**, 168-206.

Donovan, D.C., Schingoethe, D.J., Baer, R.J., Ryali, J., Hippen, A.R. and Franklin, S.T. (2000) Influence of dietary fish oil on conjugated linoleic acid and other fatty acids in milk fat from lactating dairy cows. *Journal of Dairy Science,* **83**, 2620-2628.

Doreau, M., Aurousseau, E., and Martin, C. (2009a) Effect of linseed lipids fed as rolled seeds, extruded seeds or oil on organic matter and crude protein digestion in cows. *Animal Feed Science and Technology*, **150**, 187-196.

Doreau, M. and A. Ferlay (1994) Digestion and utilisation of fatty acids by ruminants. *Animal Feed Science and Technology*, **45**, 379-396.

Doreau, M. and A. Ferlay (1995) Effect of dietary lipids on nitrogen metabolism in the rumen: a review. *Livestock Production Science*, **43**, 97-110.

Doreau, M., Laverroux, S., Normand, J., Chesneau, G. and Glasser, F. (2009b) Effect of linseed fed as rolled seeds, extruded seeds or oil on fatty acid rumen metabolism and intestinal digestibility in cows. *Lipids*, **44**, 53-62.

Franklin, S.T., Martin, K.R., Baer, R.J., Schingoethe, D.J. and Hippen, A.R. (1999) Dietary marine algae (Schizochytrium sp.) increases concentrations of conjugated linoleic, docosahexaenoic and trans vaccenic acids in milk of dairy cows. *Journal of Nutrition*, **129**, 2048–2054.

Funaki, M. (2009) Saturated fatty acids and insulin resistance. *Journal of Medical Investigation*, **56**, 88-92.

Gama, M.A.S., Garnsworthy, P.C., Griinari, J.M., Leme, P.R., Rodrigues, P.H.M., Souza, L.W.O. and Lanna, D.P.D. (2008) Diet-induced milk fat depression: Association with changes in milk fatty acid composition and fluidity of milk fat. *Livestock Science*, **115**, 319–331.

Garnsworthy, P. C. (1997). Fats in dairy cow diets. In *Recent Advances in Animal Nutrition – 1997*, pp. 87-104. Edited by P.C. Garnsworthy and J. Wiseman. Nottingham University Press, Nottingham.

Glasser, F., Schmidely, P., Sauvant, D. and Doreau, M. (2008) Digestion of fatty acids in ruminants: a meta-analysis of flows and variation factors: 2. C18 fatty acids. *Animal*, **2**, 691-704.

Giger-Reverdin, S., Morand-Fehr, P. and Tran, G. (2003). Literature survey of the influence of dietary fat composition on methane production in dairy cattle. *Livestock Production Science*, **82**, 73–79.

Givens, D.I., Kliem, K.E., Humphries, D.J., Shingfield, K.J. and Morgan, R. (2009) Effect of replacing calcium salts of palm oil distillate with rapeseed oil, milled or whole rapeseeds on milk fatty acid composition in cows fed maize silage-based diets. *Animal*, **3**, 1067-1074

Grainger, C. and Beauchemin, K.A. (2011) Can enteric methane emissions from ruminants be lowered without lowering their production? *Animal Feed Science and Technology*, **166**, 308–320.

Griinari, J.M., Dwyer, D.A., McGuire, M.A., Bauman, D.E., Palmquist, D.L. and Nurmela, K.V.V. (1998) Trans-octadecenoic acids and milk fat depression in lactating dairy cows. *Journal of Dairy Science*, **81**, 1251-1261.

Halmemies-Beauchet-Filleau, A., Kokkonen, T., Lampi, A.M., Toivonen, V., Shingfield, K.J. and Vanhatalo, A. (2011) Effect of plant oils and camelina expeller on milk fatty acid composition in lactating cows fed red clover silage based diets. *Journal of Dairy Science*, **94**, 4413-4430.

Harfoot, C.G. and Hazlewood, G.P. (1988) Lipid metabolism in the rumen. In *The Rumen Microbial Ecosystem*, pp. 285–322. Edited by P.N. Hobson. Elsevier Applied Science Publishers, London, UK.

Hristov, A.N., Domitrovich, C., Wachter, A., Cassidy, T., Lee, C., Shingfield, K.J., Kairenius, P., Davis, J. and Brown, J. (2011) Effect of replacing solvent-extracted canola meal with high-oil traditional canola, high-oleic acid canola, or high-erucic acid rapeseed meals on rumen fermentation, digestibility, milk production, and milk fatty acid composition in lactating dairy cows. *Journal of Dairy Science*, **94,** 4057-4074.

Hristov, A. N. and Jouany J.-P. (2005) Factors affecting the efficiency of nitrogen utilization in the rumen. In *Nitrogen and Phosphorus Nutrition of Cattle and Environment*, pp. 117–166. Edited by A. N. Hristov and E. Pfeffer. CAB International, Wallingford.

Hristov, A.N., Vander Pol, M., Agle, M., Zaman, S., Schneider, C., Ndegwa, P., Vaddella, V.K., Johnson, K., Shingfield, K.J. and Karnati, S.K.R. (2009) Effect of lauric acid and coconut oil on ruminal fermentation, digestion, ammonia losses from manure, and milk fatty acid composition in lactating cows. *Journal of Dairy Science*, **92,** 5561-5582.

Jenkins, T.C. and Bridges, W.C. (2007) Protection of fatty acids against ruminal biohydrogenation in cattle. *European Journal of Lipid Science and Technology*, **109,** 778-789.

Jenkins, T.C., Wallace, R.J., Moate, P.J. and Mosley, E.E. (2008) BOARD-INVITED REVIEW: Recent advances in biohydrogenation of unsaturated fatty acids within the rumen microbial ecosystem. *Journal of Animal Science*, **86,** 397-412.

Jenkins, T.C., Bateman, H.G. and Block, S.M. (1996) Butylsoyamide increases unsaturation of fatty acids in plasma and milk of lactating dairy cows. *Journal of Dairy Science,* **79,** 585-590.

Jensen RG 2002. The composition of bovine milk lipids: January 1995 to December 2000. *Journal of Dairy Science*, **85,** 295-350.

Kadegowda, A.K., Piperova, L.S. and Erdman, R.A. (2008) Principal component and multivariate analysis of milk long-chain fatty acid composition during diet-induced milk fat depression. *Journal of Dairy Science*, **91,** 749-759.

Kairenius, P., Toivonen, V. and Shingfield, K.J. (2011) Identification and ruminal outflow of long-chain Fatty Acid biohydrogenation intermediates in cows fed diets containing fish oil. *Lipids*, **46,** 587-606.

Kalscheur, K.F., Teter, B.B., Piperova, L.S. and Erdman, R.A. (1997) Effect of fat source on duodenal flow of trans-C18:1 fatty acids and milk fat production in dairy cows. *Journal of Dairy Science,* **80,** 2115-2126.

Keady, T.W.J., Mayne, C.S. and Fitzpatrick, D.A. (2000) Effects of supplementation of dairy cattle with fish oil on silage intake, milk yield and milk composition. *Journal of Dairy Research*, **67**, 137-153.

Kliem, K.E., Shingfield, K.J., Humphries, D.J. and Givens, D.I. (2011) Effect of replacing calcium salts of palm oil distillate with incremental amounts of conventional or high oleic acid milled rapeseed on milk fatty acid composition in cows fed maize silage based diets. *Animal*, **5**, 1311-1321.

Lee, Y.J. and Jenkins, T.C. (2011) Biohydrogenation of linolenic acid to stearic acid by the rumen microbial population yields multiple intermediate conjugated diene isomers. *Journal of Nutrition*, **141**, 1445-1450.

Lock, A.L. and Shingfield, K.J. (2004) Optimising milk composition. In *Dairying- Using Science to Meet Consumers' Needs*, Occasional Publication No. 29 of the British Society of Animal Science, pp. 107-188. Edited by E. Kebreab, J. Mills and D.E. Beever. Nottingham University Press, Nottingham.

Lock, A.L., Tyburczy, C., Dwyer, D.A., Harvatine, K.J., Destaillats, F., Mouloungui, Z., Candy, L. and Bauman, D.E. (2007) Trans-10 octadecenoic acid does not reduce milk fat synthesis in dairy cows. *Journal of Nutrition*, **137**, 71-76.

Loor, J.J., Ferlay, A., Ollier, A., Doreau, M. and Chilliard, Y. (2005) Relationship among *trans* and conjugated fatty acids and bovine milk fat yield due to dietary concentrate and linseed oil. *Journal of Dairy Science*, **88**, 726-740.

Loor, J.J., Herbein, J.H. and Jenkins, T.C. (2002) Nutrient digestion, biohydrogenation, and fatty acid profiles in blood plasma and milk fat from lactating Holstein cows fed canola oil or canolamide. *Animal Feed Science and Technology*, **97**, 65-82.

Loor, J.J., Ueda, K., Ferlay, A., Chilliard, Y. and Doreau, M. (2004) Biohydrogenation, duodenal flow, and intestinal digestibility of trans fatty acids and conjugated linoleic acids in response to dietary forage concentrate ratio and linseed oil in dairy cows. *Journal of Dairy Science*, **87**, 2472–2485.

Lourenço, M., Ramos-Morales, E. and Wallace, R.J. (2010) The role of microbes in rumen lipolysis and biohydrogenation and their manipulation. *Animal*, **4**, 1008-1023.

Machmüller, A. (2006) Medium-chain fatty acids and their potential to reduce methanogenesis in domestic ruminants. *Agriculture, Ecosystems and Environment*, **112**, 107–114.

Maia, M.R.G., Chaudhary, L.C., Figueres, L. and Wallace, R.J. (2007) Metabolism of polyunsaturated fatty acids and their toxicity to the microflora of the rumen. *Antonie van Leeuwenhoek*, **91**, 303-314.

Martin, C., Morgavi, D.P. and Doreau, M. (2010) Methane mitigation in ruminants: from microbe to the farm scale. *Animal*, **4**, 351–365.

Martin, C., Rouel, J., Jouany, J.P., Doreau, M. and Chilliard, Y. (2008). Methane output and diet digestibility in response to feeding dairy cows crude linseed, extruded linseed, or linseed oil. *Journal of Animal Science*, **86,** 2642–2650.

McKain, N., Shingfield, K.J. and Wallace, R.J. (2010) Metabolism of conjugated linoleic acids and 18:1 fatty acids by ruminal bacteria: products and mechanisms. *Microbiology*, **156,** 579-588.

Mosley, S.A., Mosley, E.E., Hatch, B., Szasz, J.I., Corato, A., Zacharias, N., Howes, D. and McGuire, M.A. (2007) Effect of varying levels of fatty acids from palm oil on feed intake and milk production in Holstein cows. *Journal of Dairy Science*, **90,** 987-993.

Nam, I.S. and Garnsworthy, P.C. (2007) Biohydrogenation of linoleic acid by rumen fungi compared with rumen bacteria. *Journal of Applied Microbiology*, **103,** 551-556.

Noci, F., O'Kiely, P., Monahan, F.J., Stanton, C. and Moloney, A.P. (2005b) Conjugated linoleic acid concentration in M. longissimus-dorsi from heifers offered sunflower oil-based concentrates and conserved forages. *Meat Science*, **69,** 509–518.

Offer, N.W., Marsden, M., Dixon, J., Speake, B.K. and Thacker, F.E. (1999) Effect of dietary fat supplements on levels of n-3 polyunsaturated fatty acids, trans acids and conjugated linoleic acid in bovine milk. *Animal Science*, **69,** 613-625.

Offer, N.W., Marsden, M. and Phipps, R.H.E. (2001) Effect of oil supplementation of a diet containing a high concentration of starch on levels of trans fatty acids and conjugated linoleic acids in bovine milk. *Anim Science*, **73,** 533-540.

Or-Rashid, M.M., Wright, T.C. and McBride, B.W. (2009) Microbial fatty acid conversion within the rumen and the subsequent utilization of these fatty acids to improve the healthfulness of ruminant food products. *Applied Microbiology and Biotechnology*, **84,** 1033–1043.

Palmquist, D.L. (2009) Omega-3 fatty acids in metabolism, health, and nutrition and for modified animal product foods. *The Professional Animal Science*, **25,** 207–249.

Palmquist DL, Lock AL, Shingfield KJ and Bauman DE 2005. Biosynthesis of conjugated linoleic acid in ruminants and humans. In *Advances in Food and Nutrition Research, Volume 50*, pp 179-217. Edited by S. Taylor. Elsevier Academic Press, US.

Piperova, L.S., Teter, B.B., Bruckental, I., Sampugna, J., Mills, S.E., Yurawecz, M.P., Fritsche, J., Ku, K and Erdman, R.A. (2000) Mammary lipogenic enzyme activity, trans fatty acids and conjugated linoleic acids are altered in lactating dairy cows fed a milk fat- depressing diet. *Journal of Nutrition*, **130,** 2568-2574.

Rego, O.A., Alves, S.P., Antunes, L.M.S., Rosa, H.J.D., Alfaia, C.F.M., Prates,

J.A.M., Cabrita, A.R.J., Fonseca, A.J.M. and Bessa, R.J.B. (2009) Rumen biohydrogenation-derived fatty acids in milk fat from grazing dairy cows supplemented with rapeseed, sunflower, or linseed oils. *Journal of Dairy Science*, **92**, 4530-4540.

Roy, A., Ferlay, A., Shingfield, K.J. and Chilliard, Y. (2006) Examination of the persistency of milk fatty acid composition responses to plant oils in cows given different basal diets, with particular emphasis on trans-C18:1 fatty acids and isomers of conjugated linoleic acid. *Animal Science*, **82**, 479–492.

Ryhänen, E.L., Tallavaara, K., Griinari, J.M., Jaakkola, S., Mantere-Alhonen, S. and Shingfield, K.J. (2005) Production of conjugated linoleic acid enriched milk and dairy products from cows receiving grass silage supplemented with a cereal-based concentrate containing rapeseed oil. *International Dairy Journal*, **15**, 207-217.

Schmidely, P., Glasser, F., Doreau, M. and Sauvant, D. (2008) Digestion of fatty acids in ruminants: a meta-analysis of flows and variation factors. 1. Total fatty acids. *Animal*, **2**, 677-690.

Shingfield, K.J., Ahvenjärvi, S., Toivonen, V., Vanhatalo, A., Huhtanen, P. and Griinari, J.M. (2008a) Effect of incremental levels of sunflower-seed oil in the diet on ruminal lipid metabolism in lactating cows. *British Journal of Nutrition*, **99**, 971-983.

Shingfield, K.J., Bernard, L., Leroux, C. and Chilliard, Y. (2010a) Role of trans fatty acids in the nutritional regulation of mammary lipogenesis in ruminants. *Animal*, **4**, 1140-1166.

Shingfield, K.J., Chilliard, Y., Toivonen, V., Kairenius, P. and Givens, D.I. (2008b) Trans fatty acids and bioactive lipids in ruminant milk. In *Bioactive Components of Milk, Advances In Experimental Medicine and Biology, Volume 606*, pp 3-65. Edited by Z. Bösze. Springer, New York.

Shingfield, K.J. and Griinari, J.M. (2007) Role of biohydrogenation intermediates in milk fat depression. *European Journal of Lipid Science and Technology*, **109**, 799-816.

Shingfield, K.J., Lee, M.R.F., Humphries, D.J., Scollan, N.D., Toivonen, V., Beever, D.E. and Reynolds, C.K. (2011) Effect of linseed oil and fish oil alone or as an equal mixture on ruminal fatty acid metabolism in growing steers fed maize silage based diets. *Journal of Animal Science*, **89**, 3728-3741.

Shingfield, K.J., Kairenius, P. Ärölä, A., Paillard, D., Muetzel, S., Ahvenjärvi, S., Vanhatalo, A., Huhtanen, P., Toivonen, V., Griinari, J.M. and Wallace, R.J. (2012). Dietary fish oil supplements modify ruminal biohydrogenation, alter the flow of fatty acids at the omasum, and induce changes in the ruminal *Butyrivibrio* population in lactating cows. *Journal of Nutrition*, **142**, 1437-1448.

Shingfield, K.J., Lee, M.R.F., Humphries, D.J., Scollan, N.D., Toivonen, V., Reynolds, C. and Beever, D.E. (2010b). Effect of incremental amounts of fish oil in the diet on ruminal lipid metabolism in growing steers. *British Journal of Nutrition*, **104**, 56-66.

Shingfield, K.J., Reynolds, C.K., Lupoli, B., Toivonen, V., Yurawecz, M.P., Delmonte, P., Griinari, J.M., Grandison, A.S. and Beever, D.E. (2005a) Effect of forage type and proportion of concentrate in the diet on milk fatty acid composition in cows given sunflower oil and fish oil. *Animal Science*, **80**, 225-238.

Shingfield, K.J., Sæbø, A., Sæbø, P.-C., Toivonen, V. and Griinari, J.M. (2009) Effect of abomasal infusions of a mixture of octadecenoic acids on milk fat synthesis in lactating cows. *Journal of Dairy Science*, **92**, 4317-4329.

Shingfield, K.J., Salo-Väänänen, P., Pahkala, E., Toivonen, V., Jaakkola, S., Piironen, V. and Huhtanen, P (2005b) Effect of forage conservation method, concentrate level and propylene glycol on the fatty acid composition and vitamin content of cows' milk. *Journal of Dairy Research*, **72**, 349-361.

Sinclair, K.D. and Garnsworthy, P.C. (2010). Fatty acids and fertility in dairy cows. In *Recent Advances in Animal Nutrition – 2009*, pp. 1-19. Edited by P.C. Garnsworthy and J. Wiseman. Nottingham University Press, Nottingham.

Steward, C.S., Flint, H.J. and Bryant, M.P. (1997) The rumen bacteria. In *The Rumen Microbial Ecosystem*, pp. 10-72. Edited by P.N. Hobson and C.S. Steward. Blackie Academic and Professional, London.

Toral, P.G., Shingfield, K.J., Hervás, G., Toivonen, V. and Frutos, P. (2010) Effect of fish oil and sunflower oil on rumen fermentation characteristics and fatty acid composition of digesta in ewes fed a high concentrate diet. *Journal of Dairy Science*, **93**, 4804-4817.

Ueda, K., Ferlay, A., Chabrot, J., Loor, J.J., Chilliard, Y. and Doreau, M. (2003) Effect of linseed oil supplementation on ruminal digestion in dairy cows fed diets with different forage: concentrate ratios. *Journal of Dairy Science*, **86**, 3999–4007.

Vanhatalo, A., Kuoppala, K., Toivonen, V. and Shingfield, K.J. (2007) Effects of forage species and stage of maturity on bovine milk fatty acid composition. *European Journal of Lipid Science and Technology*, **109**, 856-867.

Vlaeminck, B., Fievez, V., Cabrita, A.R.J., Fonseca, A.J.M. and Dewhurst, R.J. (2006) Factors affecting odd- and branched-chain fatty acids in milk: A review. *Animal Feed Science and Technology*, **131**, 389-417.

Wallace, R.J., McKain, N., Shingfield, K.J. and Devillard, E. (2007) Isomers of conjugated linoleic acids are synthesized via different mechanisms in ruminal digesta and bacteria. *Journal of Lipid Research*, **48**, 2247-2254.

WHO/FAO (World Health Organization/Food Agricultural Organization) 2003.

Diet, nutrition and the prevention of chronic diseases. Report of a joint WHO/FAO Expert Consultation. WHO Technical Report series 916, Geneva, Switzerland, WHO, 148 pp.

Woods, V.B. and Fearon, A.M. (2009) Dietary sources of unsaturated fatty acids for animals and their transfer into meat, milk and eggs: A review. *Livestock Science* **126,** 1–20.

Wu, Z. and Huber, J.T. (1994) Relationship between dietary-fat supplementation and milk protein-concentration in lactating cows - a review. *Livestock Production Science*, **39,** 141-155.

5

RATION FORMULATION FOR DAIRY COWS: LEAST COST VERSUS LEAST ENVIRONMENTAL IMPACT

P C GARNSWORTHY AND J M WILKINSON
School of Biosciences, University of Nottingham, Sutton Bonington Campus, Loughborough, Leicestershire LE12 5RD, UK

Introduction

Governments have made international commitments to reduce greenhouse gas emissions (GHGE) and the United Kingdom government has set a target of an 80% reduction in emissions of GHGE by the year 2050 compared to the baseline of 1990 (Office of Public Sector Information, 2011). In the context of food production at the farm level, this largely involves reducing emissions of nitrous oxide from agricultural soils and manures, and methane from enteric fermentation and manures (IPCC, 2006; MacCarthy et al., 2011).

Ruminant livestock are less efficient at converting dietary N into N in animal product than pigs and poultry (Wilkinson and Audsley, 2012) and in the context of milk production, grazed pasture alone does not provide a diet balanced for milk production because its ratio of effective rumen degradable protein (ERDP) to ME is too high. Thus at pasture the grazing animal is offered high-protein herbage which is associated with low nitrogen use efficiency (NUE), defined as N in milk as a percentage of total dietary N input (Dewhurst, 2006). Furthermore, daily dry matter intake (DMI) from grazed pasture is restricted to around 16 kg DM/cow (Leaver, 1983). Consequently, in pasture-based systems not only are annual milk yields restricted to 4 to 5 thousand litres per cow, but NUE is also unacceptably low (Dewhurst, 2006). In contrast, by supplementing grazed and conserved forages with nutritionally balanced concentrates, milk yields in mixed housing/grazing systems can average 6 to 8 thousand litres, rising to 10 to 12 thousand litres per cow in some continuously housed systems (Wilkinson et al., 2011).

Diets for highly productive dairy cows can include raw materials such as cereal grains, which potentially could be eaten directly by humans. This leads to debate about the competition between livestock and humans for land and other resources needed to grow crops. In the drive to increase efficiency of feed use, concentrate feeds of high nutrient concentration have been developed, which can comprise predominantly cereal grains mixed with the meal residues from the removal of oil from oilseed crops, particularly soyabean meal. A high proportion of these crops is potentially consumable as human food or used to produce soaps, cosmetics and paints (e.g. palm oil and linseed oil).

There are environmental issues associated with the production of oilseed crops such as soyabeans and palm seeds, which are causing international concern. Increased pressure on human-edible feeds, such as cereal grain and soyabean meal, for humans and non-ruminants places greater emphasis on efficiency of feed use by dairy cows (Wilkinson, 2011).

The ability of dairy cows to convert grassland herbage and forage crops into milk is likely to become of greater significance in terms of global human food production as the population of the planet increases in future decades (Godfray et al., 2010). The conservation of forages as silage is an important source of nutrients for dairy cows in many countries of the world (Wilkinson and Toivonen, 2003) because it enables crops to be available for use either throughout the year or in periods of restricted seasonal availability of pastures for grazing due to drought or cool weather. However, the consumption of concentrate (compound and blended) feed per cow and annual milk yield per cow both increased substantially in the United Kingdom from 1990 to 2010 and there was no change in the amount of milk produced per unit of concentrate (DEFRA, 2011). Estimated UK production of conserved forage also increased between 1990 and 2010 despite a substantial reduction in the population of dairy cows during the period (Wilkinson and Wray, 2012), implying less reliance on grazed pasture in 2010 than in 1990.

Changes in ration formulation affect cost per kg total diet DM, NUE, GHGE per kg of feed DM, total daily feed DMI, methane production per cow, methane per kg of DM consumed and hence GHGE per kg milk. Least cost ration formulation is the most common approach to dairy cow nutrition adopted by the animal feed industry. An understanding of relationships between the economic cost of rations and their environmental cost is essential in order to develop new approaches to dairy cow feeding which are both economically and environmentally robust.

In this paper the effects on NUE and GHGE per kg milk of implementing theoretically a range of nutritional strategies relevant to conventional systems of milk production operated on farms in northern Europe and America are explored using the Ultramix ration formulation programme (AGM Systems Ltd, Romsey, UK). Organic options are not considered here because they have been explored elsewhere (e.g. Olesen et al., 2006; Williams et al., 2006; Weiske and Michel, 2007). Ration formulations for cows giving a range of daily milk output are considered in terms of N losses as nitrous oxide, nitrate, and ammonia with emphasis on differences between urine and faecal excretion routes. Factors affecting methane emissions are also discussed together with interactions between methane and N emissions. Feed conversion efficiency (kg milk per kg feed DM, ME and MP) is explored in terms of both gross efficiency and human-edible efficiency.

Material and methods

NITROGEN SUPPLY AND EXCESS

Equations of the Feed into Milk applied feeding system for dairy cows (FiM; Thomas, 2004) were used as a starting point for diet formulation. These equations allow prediction of DMI and calculations of requirements and supply of metabolisable energy (ME) and metabolisable protein (MP) at the animal level. A rumen model enables calculation of nitrogen supply to rumen microorganisms in relation to predicted fermentation of feed materials to yield ATP, and hence calculation of microbial crude protein (MCP) supply. Diets were formulated to meet ME and MP requirements for various classes of cow and for various feeding systems, as detailed later.

In the FiM system, MP supply is calculated from flows of digestible microbial true protein and digestible undegradable protein at the small intestine. Requirements for MP are calculated from milk protein yield, pregnancy, live-weight change and endogenous nitrogen losses in urine, faeces, hair and scurf. By definition, protein that is not digested or metabolised is excreted in faeces or urine. Nitrogen excretion was, therefore, calculated from the FiM MP equations by summing the indigestible and non-metabolisable fractions at each step (Figure 1). Urinary nitrogen losses included endogenous urinary protein, excess effective rumen degradable protein (ERDP), microbial non-protein nitrogen, and the difference between net protein and MP required for milk protein synthesis. An adjustment was made for the non-protein nitrogen (urea) content of milk to allow for this alternative route of nitrogen excretion. Faecal nitrogen losses included endogenous faecal protein, acid-detergent insoluble nitrogen, indigestible undegradable protein, and indigestible microbial true protein. An adjustment was made for endogenous protein absorbed from the hind-gut, as indicated in FiM. Equations for these calculations are in Appendix 1.

Nitrogen use efficiency was calculated as total nitrogen output in milk divided by total nitrogen intake.

CARBON FOOTPRINT OF FEEDS

A value for the carbon footprint (CFP) of each raw material was obtained from the Dutch FeedPrint database (Vellinga et al., 2012). Each CFP includes carbon dioxide equivalents (CO_2-eq) released during growing the crop (e.g. seed, pesticides, green manure, crop residues, organic manure, fertilizer, fuel for cultivation), storing the crop (including crop losses during storage), transporting the crop (to processing, feed mill and farm), and processing the crop (e.g. drying, grinding).

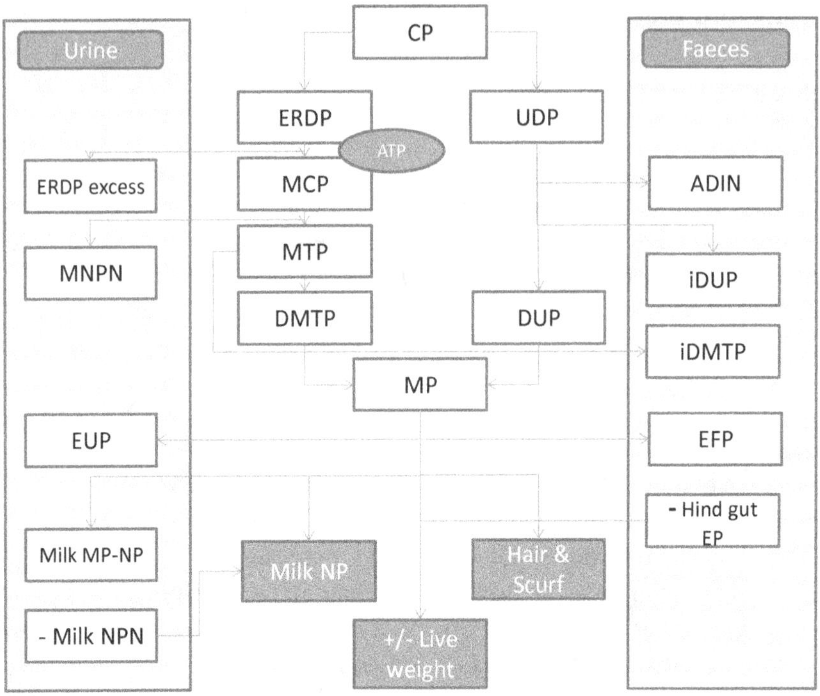

Figure 1. Flow of nitrogen from dietary crude protein intake to fractions in urine, faeces, milk and body tissue. (For abbreviations, see Appendix 1)

It also includes allowances for land use (changes in management) allocated on the basis of long-term equilibrium (e.g. 200 years for permanent grassland) and land-use change (e.g. deforestation) allocated on a global basis, so as not to penalise unduly individual crops or land that has been in cultivation for many years. Values for each raw material are Dutch averages that allow for potentially different CFP of imported and home-grown commodities according to the balance of trade and countries of origin. For co-products, such as soyabean meal and sugar beet pulp, CFP components are allocated to primary and secondary products on the basis of economic value. For compound feeds, CFP is calculated from CFP and typical proportions of individual ingredients, plus the additional CFP from processing (e.g. mixing and pelleting) into compound feeds.

For grass and grass silages, CFP values in the FeedPrint database were 50 to 60% higher than UK values due to differences in N application and DM content of silages. For these forages, therefore, CFP values from the Cranfield life-cycle analysis model were used (E. Audsley: personal communication). For feed production emissions, UK grazed grass receiving 108 kg fertiliser N/ha was given a value of 329 g CO_2e/kg DM; UK grass silage receiving 301 kg N/ha was given a value of 304 g CO_2e/kg DM . For compatibility with CFP values of other feeds, emissions due to land use and land-use change in the FeedPrint database were added as 69 g CO_2e/kg DM for grazed grass and 78 g CO_2e/kg DM for grass silage.

HUMAN-EDIBLE PROPORTIONS OF FEEDS

To provide a metric that can be used to evaluate competition for land use between human food and animal feed, Wilkinson (2011) allocated values to different categories of raw materials according to their potential use for human food. Grass and forages were allocated a value of zero; cereals, pulses and soyabean products were allocated 0.8; other oilseeds, cereal co-products and food by-products, such as sugar beet pulp, were allocated 0.2.

METHANE EMISSIONS

Two approaches were adopted to predict methane emissions by cows that would be fed on the formulated diets. The first approach was to assign methane factors to each raw material for calculating the proportion of gross energy that is lost as methane. Methane factors were obtained from the UK Tables of Nutritive Values and Chemical Composition of Feedingstuffs (Rowett, 1990).

The second approach was to use a prediction equation based on composition and predicted intake of the formulated diet. The equation chosen was that of Yates et al. (2000), which has shown reasonable agreement with our on-farm measurements of methane emissions by high-yielding dairy cows. The equation is:

Methane output (MJ/d) = 1.36 + 1.21 DMI − 0.825 CDMI + 12.8 NDF

where CDMI is concentrate intake (kg DM per day) and NDF is neutral-detergent fibre concentration (kg/kg total diet DM).

RAW MATERIALS

A database of feeds was constructed which contained a range of ingredients often used in diets for dairy cows (Appendix 2). Compositional data were obtained from the FiM database and augmented with data from the Trident Feeds website (www.tridentfeeds/products) and Rowett (1990). Prices of straights (raw material feeds) for June 2012 were obtained from the websites of Farmers Weekly (www. fwi.co.uk/prices-trends) and DairyCo (www.dairyco.org.uk/datum/farm-inputs/feed-prices/uk-feed-prices.aspx); forage prices used were: grazed grass £10/t fresh weight; grass silage £25/t fresh weight; maize silage £22/t fresh weight.

DIET SPECIFICATIONS

Across all diets, the following cow specifications were kept constant: live weight = 650 kg; lactation number = 2; stage of lactation = 9 weeks post-calving; milk fat concentration = 39 g/kg; milk protein concentration = 31 g/kg.

Diets were formulated at three levels of milk yield: 40, 30 and 20 l/d, for which maximum live-weight changes were -0.6, -0.5 and 0 kg/d respectively.

A maximum constraint was imposed on diet formulations for DMI, calculated using FiM equations. Minimum constraints were imposed for ME and MP requirements, also calculated using FiM equations. To ensure that nitrogen supply did not limit microbial protein synthesis, the ratio of ERDP to MCP was constrained to a minimum of 1.0. To minimise the risk of acidosis, and to encourage rumination and butterfat synthesis, rumen stability value (RSV) balance was constrained to a minimum of +20 and the proportion of total DMI derived from forage DM was constrained to a minimum of 0.4.

Intakes of forages were not constrained. Maximum intakes of individual non-forage raw materials were constrained to 4 kg/d, except sugar beet pulp, which was constrained to a maximum of 5 kg/d, and protected fat, which was constrained to a maximum of 0.5 kg/d. Diets were not formulated for mineral and vitamin requirements, so a fixed quantity of mineral and vitamin supplement was included at 0.2 kg/d.

DIET FORMULATION

For each milk yield level, diets were formulated on a least-cost basis to represent different feeding systems. These feeding systems were grass silage plus compound feeds, grass silage plus straights, maize silage plus grass silage and straights, and grazed grass plus straights. For systems involving grass silage, silage of higher quality was offered to cows with milk yields of 40 l/d than to cows with milk yields of 30 or 20 l/d.

Results and discussion

COMPOUNDS AND STRAIGHTS

Formulations for diets based on grass silage plus either compound feed or straights are in Table 1. As expected, forage to concentrate ratio was inversely proportional to milk yield and daily cost increased with milk yield. Quantities of raw materials in each diet depended on the raw materials offered, raw material composition, and constraints imposed. For example, at the milk yield level of 40 l/d, the diet based on silage plus straights contained more silage and less concentrates than the diet based on silage plus compound because straights were available with higher ME concentration (e.g. bypass fat, soyabean meal) and higher CP concentration (e.g. soyabean and rapeseed meals) than the single compound offered. This enabled a combination of straights to meet constraints at a lower concentrate inclusion level than a single compound. In the 40-litre straights diet, soyabean meal was included at its maximum level because not only did soya have a higher CP concentration than the compound, it also had a higher ME concentration. In any formulation, raw materials that address two constraints simultaneously (e.g. ME and MP concentrations) will always be selected preferentially.

Table 1. Cost and formulation of diets based on grass silage plus either compound feed or straights at three levels of milk yield

Feeding System	*Compound*			*Straights*		
Milk yield level (l/d)	*40*	*30*	*20*	*40*	*30*	*20*
Cost (£/d)	3.48	2.91	2.07	2.96	2.91	2.04
Raw materials (kg/d)						
Grass silage average		55	56		31	44
Grass silage good	32			41		
Compound feed	12.9	6.4	2.8			
Wheat				4	1.3	
Barley				0.7	4	4
Sugarbeet pulp					5	1.7
Rapeseed meal				0.3		
Soyabean meal				4	0.8	
Bypass fat				0.3	0.3	
Minerals				0.2	0.2	0.2

For all diets, total nitrogen excretion (g/day) increased with increasing milk yield, as expected from increasing MP requirements (Figure 2). At yield levels of 20 and 30 l/d, total nitrogen excretion was greater for compound diets than for straights diets; at 40 l/d, however, total nitrogen excretion was less for compound diets than for straights diets. This is because least cost formulation will oversupply some nutrients (e.g. protein) if this satisfies requirements for a more expensive nutrient (e.g. energy) at lower overall cost. When the FiM system was introduced, the more precise specification of protein requirements as MP rather than RDP and UDP in the AFRC (1984) system led to a general reduction in total protein concentrations of diets for dairy cows (Diana Allen: personal communication).

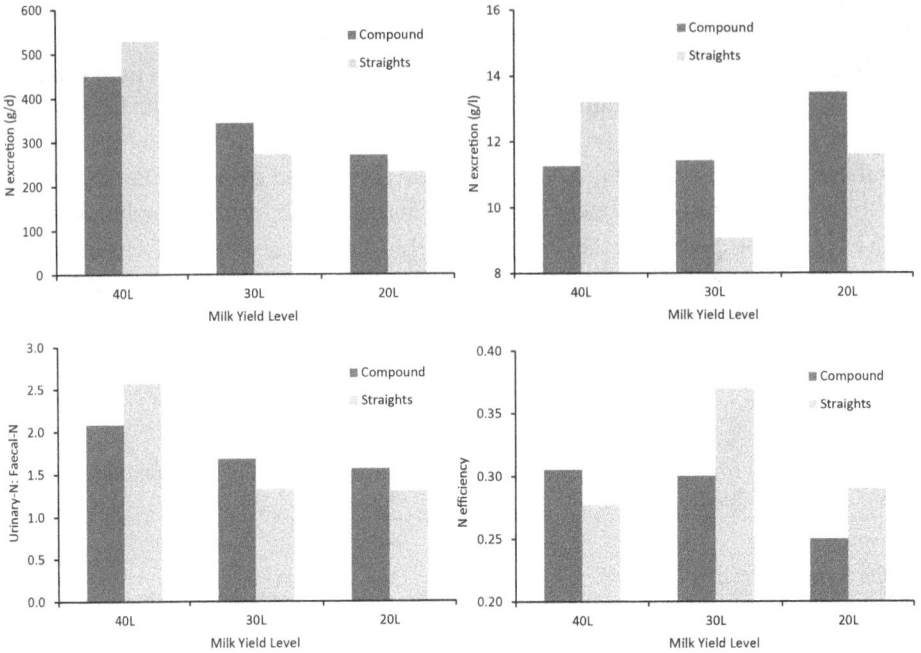

Figure 2. Nitrogen excretion and efficiency for diets formulated at least cost from grass silage plus either compound feed or straights to supply nutrient requirements for dairy cows with milk yields of 40, 30 or 20 l/d.

When considered per unit of product, nitrogen excretion decreased with increasing milk yield, apart from the diet based on straights at 40 l/d (Figure 2). The ratio of urinary nitrogen to faecal nitrogen increased with increasing yield level. This is due mainly to increased MP requirements at higher yield levels because metabolic urinary protein (non-metabolised absorbed protein) increases in direct proportion to MP supply (Thomas, 2004). The ratio of urinary to faecal nitrogen is likely to affect GHGE because volatile nitrogen (urine N) is more likely to generate ammonia, whereas faecal nitrogen is more likely to contribute to nitrous oxide emissions. Ammonia does not contribute directly to GHGE, although some may contribute indirectly to nitrous oxide emission following subsequent deposition on soil. Quantities of nitrogen lost after excretion depend on manure handling and storage methods, but the less excreted, the less available to cause pollution.

Overall NUE was similar for compound diets at 30 and 40 l/d, and for the straights diet at 20 l/d. The compound diet at 20 l/d had the lowest NUE and the straights diet at 30 l/d had by far the highest NUE. It must be emphasised that these findings apply only to the circumstances of this exercise. In practice, compound feeds might be formulated differently for different yield levels and milk protein concentration (hence protein output) normally varies with yield level. Nevertheless, the exercise does demonstrate that considerable variation in NUE can be predicted for different scenarios.

The carbon footprint (CFP), expressed per litre of milk produced, did not vary much across the different milk yield levels. The CFP of diets based on compound feed was greater than those based on straights due to the extra carbon released during processing of compound feeds (Figure 3).

Percentage of human-edible raw materials decreased with increasing milk yield level and was greater for diets based on straights than for diets based on compound feed. This reflects the inclusion of wheat, barley and soya in the list of straights offered, all of which could be replaced by human-inedible co-products if desired, but at greater cost for the overall diet due to the lower concentrations of nutrients in these co-products.

Predicted methane emissions per litre of milk decreased with increasing yield level, as expected. The decrease predicted when compound feed is replaced by straights at the lower milk yield levels reflected the increase in proportion of concentrates in these diets.

FORAGE SOURCES

For comparison with the diets based on grass silage plus straights, further sets of diets were formulated based on either grazed grass or a mixture of maize and grass silages (Table 2).

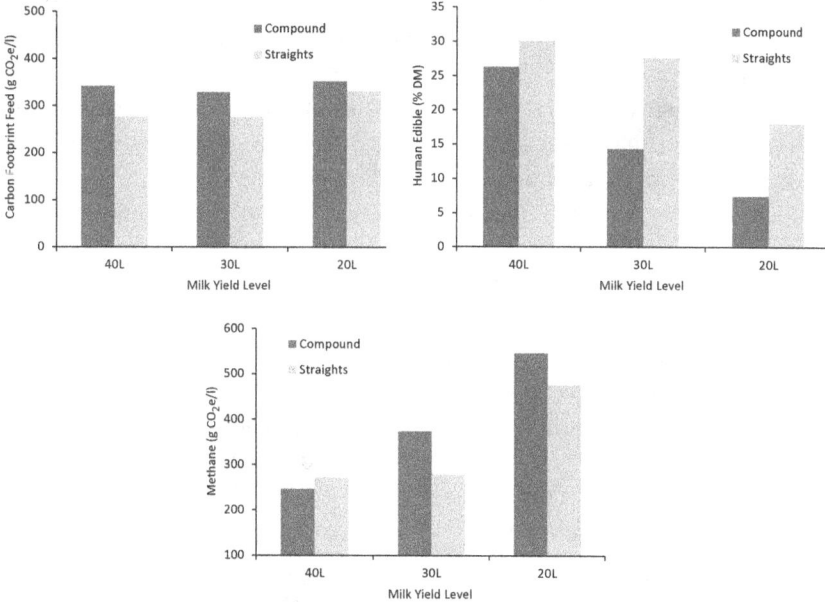

Figure 3. Carbon footprint, human-edible percentage and predicted methane emissions for diets formulated at least cost from grass silage plus either compound feed or straights to supply nutrient requirements for dairy cows with milk yields of 40, 30 or 20 l/d.

Table 2. Cost and formulation of diets based on either grazed grass or a mixture of maize and grass silages plus straights at three levels of milk yield

Feeding System	Grazing			Maize/Grass silage		
Milk yield level (l/d)	40	30	20	40	30	20
Cost (£/d)	3.19	2.03	1.37	3.08	2.44	1.93
Raw materials (kg/d)						
Grazed grass	51	60	52			
Maize silage				45	40	32
Grass silage average					14	11
Grass silage good				12		
Wheat	4.0	3.1				
Barley	4.0	1.0	4.0	3.8	0.8	4.0
Sugarbeet pulp	0.8		0.9		1.6	
Wheatfeed					4.0	1.2
Soyabean meal	2.4	1.1		3.3		
Urea					0.2	0.1
Bypass fat	0.6	0.5	0.1	0.3		
Minerals	0.2	0.2	0.2	0.2	0.2	0.2

At the lowest yield level (20 l/d), the grazed grass and the maize silage diets used similar ingredients (mainly barley plus either sugarbeet pulp or wheatfeed) to the grass silage diet. As yield level increased, increasing proportions of concentrates containing increasing proportions of cereals and soya were required. This emphasises the fact that, although cereals and soya are relatively high in price per tonne, they are more economic than co-products for supplying high quality nutrients when constraints are tight because they are cheaper per unit of ME and MP.

As in the previous exercise, nitrogen excretion (g/d) and the ratio of urinary to faecal nitrogen increased with increasing milk yield level (Figure 4). Grazed grass and maize silage diets were similar for all nitrogen parameters within yield levels. Diets based on grass silage, however, showed considerable variation in all parameters compared with the other forage sources; at 40 l/d, the grass silage diet had much greater excretion (g/d and g/l) and lower NUE; at 30 l/d, the grass silage diet had slightly lower excretion (g/l) and greater NUE. This illustrates the effects of step changes in dietary ingredients that can occur when conducting least cost formulations at different levels of milk yield.

Carbon footprint of feed ingredients, expressed per litre of milk produced, decreased consistently when moving from grazed grass to grass silage to maize silage (Figure 5). This is consistent with the differences in CFP of the three forages (Appendix 2).

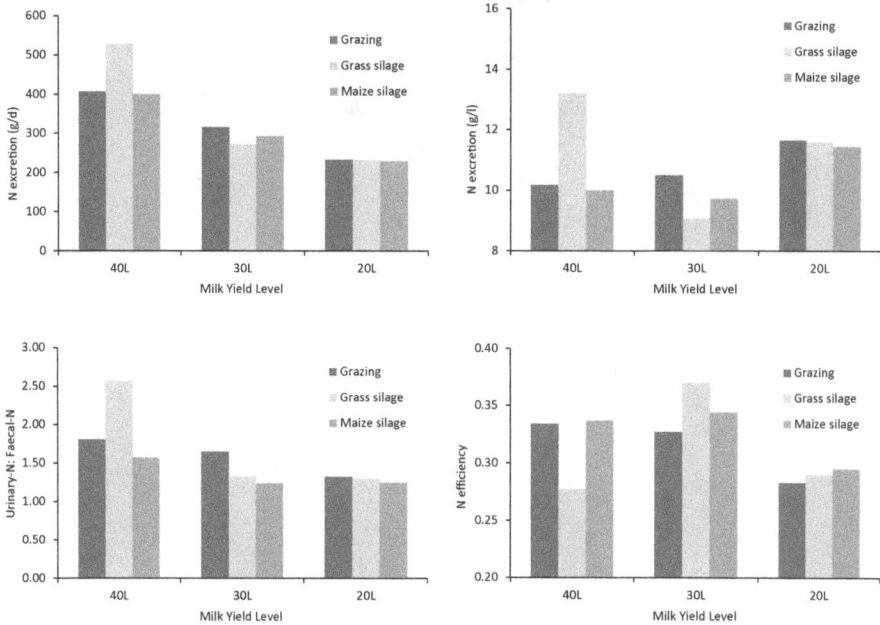

Figure 4. Nitrogen excretion and efficiency for diets formulated at least cost from grazed grass, grass silage, or maize silage, plus straights to supply nutrient requirements for dairy cows with milk yields of 40, 30 or 20 l/d.

Percentage of human-edible raw materials decreased with increasing milk yield level and decreased consistently when moving from grazed grass to grass silage to maize silage. The human-edible percentage was particularly low for the maize silage diet at a yield level of 30 l/d, in which the straights were mostly co-products.

Predicted methane emissions per litre of milk (Figure 5) decreased with increasing yield level, in agreement with other studies; for example, the recent DairyCo report on the carbon footprint of 415 British dairy herds (DairyCo, 2012). Comparison of forages, however, produced some unexpected results; methane emissions were predicted to be greater for diets based on maize silage, particularly at the highest level of milk yield. Many studies have shown that maize silage reduces methane emissions compared with grass silage (e.g. Tamminga et al., 2007: Garnsworthy et al., 2012). The explanation for the apparent conundrum lies in the prediction equation used in the current study, in which one of the main drivers for methane is concentrate intake. Concentrate intake is inversely related to methane emissions, so predicted methane per litre of milk increased as the proportion of concentrates decreased from 40% of DMI for grazed grass to 30% for maize silage.

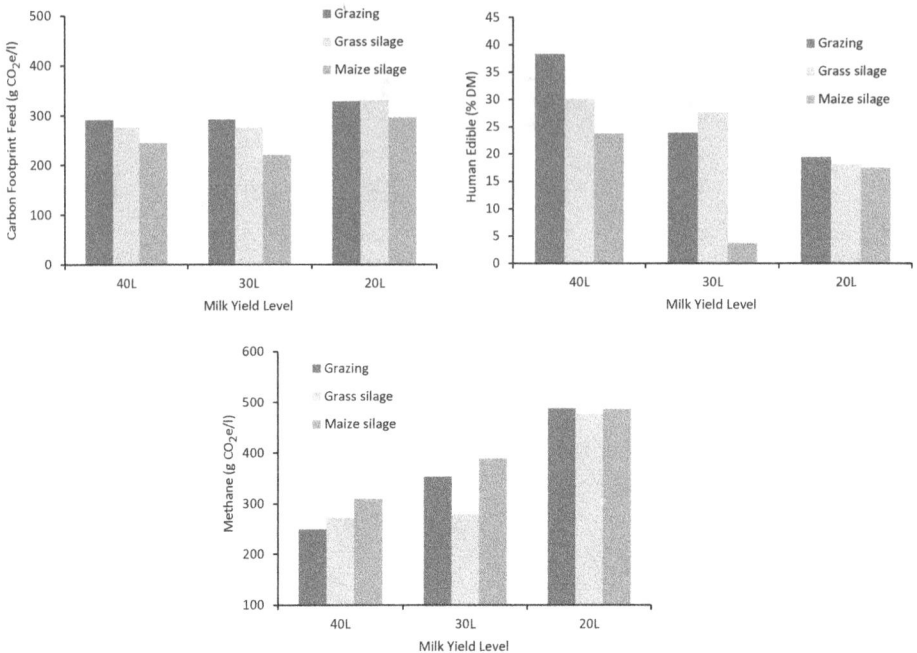

Figure 5. Carbon footprint, human-edible percentage and predicted methane emissions for diets formulated at least cost from grazed grass, grass silage, or maize silage, plus straights to supply nutrient requirements for dairy cows with milk yields of 40, 30 or 20 l/d.

FORMULATING FOR LEAST ENVIRONMENTAL COST

To test the scope for lowering CFP of diets, the diet based on maize silage at a yield level of 40 l/d was taken as a baseline diet (Base) and CFP was imposed as a constraint with progressively lower values until no feasible solution could be found to the formulation. The resulting diet (Low-C; Table 3) had a CFP that was 25% lower than that of the baseline diet. The Low-C diet, however, had a much reduced forage content (although still >0.4 of total DM) to make room for high proportions of straights with low CFP. Another diet was formulated (Low-C2) in which the proportion of forage was constrained to the same as the baseline diet, but sources of forage and straights could vary, thereby testing the scope for lowering CFP of concentrates. Diet Low-C2 had a CFP 18% lower than that of the baseline diet and relied on raw materials with high nutrient density (soyabean meal and bypass fat) for reductions in CFP. Both diets with reduced CFP were slightly more expensive than the baseline diet (+8% for Low-C; +2% for Low-C2). This illustrates the basic principle that any effective constraint (i.e. it affects the formulation) increases costs; it also indicates that reducing CFP can cost money.

Table 3. Cost and formulation of diets based on maize and grass silages plus straights at a milk yield level of 40 l/d and designed for lowest carbon footprint of the whole diet (Low-C) or the concentrate portion of the diet (Low-C2)

	Carbon footprint target		
	Base	*Low-C*	*Low-C2*
Cost (£/d)	3.08	3.37	3.13
Raw materials (kg/d)			
Maize silage	45	26	47
Grass silage good	12	7	10
Brewers grains fresh		7	7
Barley	3.8		
Sugarbeet pulp		5.3	0.2
Molasses		2.0	2.0
Wheatfeed		2.7	
Wheat DDGS		0.5	
Soyabean meal	3.3		2.8
Rapeseed meal		1.9	
Bypass fat	0.3	0.3	0.5
Minerals	0.2	0.2	0.2
Carbon footprint (g/l)	244	183	200
Human-edible DM (g/kg)	237	118	179
Nitrogen use efficiency (g/kg)	337	374	348
Methane (g CO_2-eq/l)	309	252	313

The value for CFP of soyabean meal used in the current study is 1,056 g/kg DM (Appendix 2), which is comprised of 625 g/kg DM derived from growing, processing and transporting the crop, and 431 g/kg DM derived from land use and land-use change. This CFP is considerably lower than the value used in some studies (e.g. 7,690 g/kg for Brazilian soyabean meal in FAO, 2010) due to a difference in allocation of land-use change. Whereas analyses such as FAO (2010) relate land use back to the original natural vegetation, e.g. tropical rainforest or natural grassland, FeedPrint acknowledges that soya, like other crops, is mostly grown on land which had been in production for more than 20 years (Vellinga et al., 2012). Carbon released by deforestation or cultivation of natural grassland, therefore, should be shared amongst all subsequent land uses up to the present day. Furthermore, land use change should be considered on a global scale because changes in the growing area of one crop affects the areas of other crops, both locally and globally – "land-use change assessment of a single crop is useless" (Vellinga et al., 2012). If it is assumed that all soyabean meal is sourced from land recently converted to arable cropping, its CFP is 7,690 g/kg, and the CFP of the 40 litre diet based on grass silage plus straights increases from 276 to 951 g per litre of milk. If soyabean meal is excluded from that diet, it is replaced by rapeseed meal, wheat-DDGS and wheatfeed, at an increase in cost of 4 % and a decrease in NUE of 3 %. The CFP of the diet also decreases from 276 to 268 g per litre of milk.

As well as reducing CFP, diets Low-C and Low-C2 also improved proportion of human-edible feed, NUE, and predicted methane emissions compared with the least cost base diet (Figure 6). Therefore, if lowering any one of these environmental parameters were to be supported by price incentives, the additional costs of formulating to that constraint could provide added benefits in other areas. At present, however, reductions in greenhouse gas emissions and in nitrogen excretion remain government targets rather than those of individual milk producers.

A common aspiration of milk producers is to increase milk yield per cow. Indeed, average milk yield per cow has increased progressively in the UK over the period 1990 to 2010 (DEFRA, 2011). Comparison of the four contrasting diets formulated for 40 litres with the comparable diets formulated for 20 litres/cow revealed an increase in average cost per litre of 71.5 % (Tables 1 and 2). Despite the higher cost, the higher milk output gave environmental gains in terms of reductions in methane/litre and in CFP/litre for the straights diets (Figures 3 and 5) in agreement with practice on UK farms (DairyCo, 2012), However, because of the higher N input from the diets formulated for 40 litres, there was generally no benefit to NUE

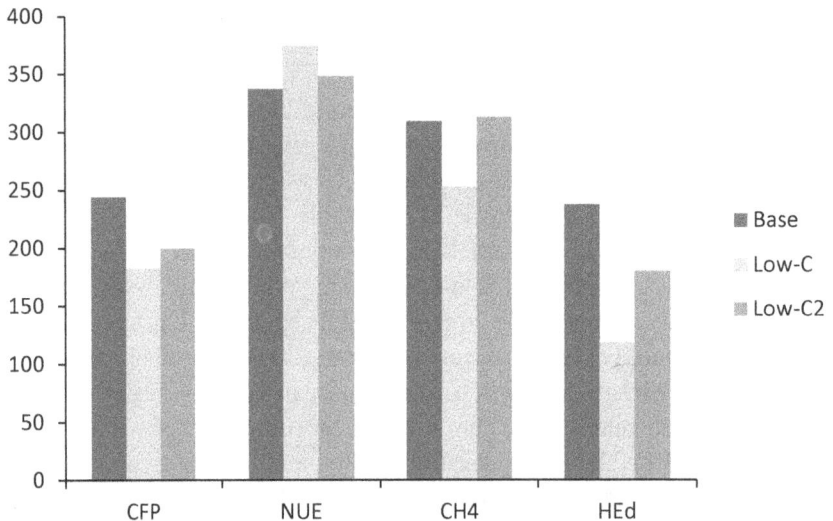

Figure 6. Carbon footprint (CFP; g/l milk), nitrogen use efficiency (NUE; g/kg), predicted methane emissions (CH4; g CO_2-eq/l milk) and human-edible percentage (HEd; g DM/kg total DM) for diets formulated at least cost from maize and grass silages plus straights to supply nutrient requirements for dairy cows with a milk yield of 40 l/d. Base = baseline diet; Low-C = diet with lowest carbon footprint of all ingredients; Low-C2 = diet with lowest carbon footprint of concentrate ingredients.

of increasing milk yield per cow (Figure 4) apart from the compound diets based on grass silage (Figure 2).

Conclusions

The results of this exercise demonstrate that formulating diets for dairy cows on the basis of least cost can lead to step changes in inclusion levels of ingredients when compared across forage systems and yield levels. Consequently, a range of values was predicted for each measure of environmental impact. It must be stressed that the diets are shown to illustrate principles and should not be used in practice without consulting a nutritionist. Formulations depend upon the compositional matrix of raw materials, constraints imposed and prices of raw materials, which can all vary in different scenarios.

The main finding of the study is that equations to predict nitrogen excretion, carbon footprint of raw materials, methane emissions and proportions of human-edible feed ingredients can all be incorporated into models for least cost diet formulation. Equations can be challenged, as can the underlying equations that predict nutrient requirements, and further equations could be incorporated to predict other parameters. Nevertheless, current predictions are within the normal ranges observed in research trials and commercial practice.

Changes in impact measures are linked across scenarios (through changes in efficiency), so an improvement in one measure is often accompanied by improvements in other measures. Each of the impact measures can be used as a constraint to iteratively reduce the environmental impact of milk production. Any constraint will, however, increase the cost of the resulting diet. Some impact reductions, such as lower methane emissions and improved NUE, can have indirect financial benefits which will partially offset increased diet costs. In general, however, reductions in environmental impacts are likely to require price incentives to achieve widespread uptake.

Acknowledgements

This work was supported by DairyCo under the Health, Welfare and Nutrition Research Partnership. We would like to thank: Alan Munford (AGM Systems Ltd) for providing FiM equations for use in Ultramix models; Theun Vellinga (Wageningen UR Livestock Research) for providing a link to the FeedPrint database and for valuable explanations of CFP calculations; Eric Audsley (Cranfield University) for providing UK values for CFP of grass and silage; and

Tim Davies (Kite Consulting Services) for providing comparative data from his carbon footprint models.

References

AFRC (1984) *The Nutrient Requirements of Ruminant Livestock - Protein.* CAB, Farnham Royal.

DairyCo (2012) *Greenhouse Gas Emissions on British Dairy Farms: DairyCo Carbon Footprinting Study: Year One.* DairyCo, Kenilworth, UK.

DEFRA (2011) *Agricultural Statistics and Climate Change.* http://www.defra. gov.uk/statistics/foodfarm/enviro/climate/ Accessed 17 November 2011.

Dewhurst, R. (2006) Manipulating cow diets to reduce nutrient waste to the environment. *Proceedings of the 2006 South Island Dairy Event.* http:// www.side.org.nz Accessed 12 January 2012.

FAO (2010) *Greenhouse Gas Emissions from the Dairy Sector: A Life Cycle Assessment.* Food and Agriculture Organization of the United Nations, Rome, Italy.

Godfray, H.C.J., Beddington, J.R., Crute, I.R., Haddad, L., Lawrence, D., Muir, J.F., Pretty, J., Robinson, S., Thomas, S and Toulmin, C. (2010) Food security: The challenge of feeding 9 billion people. *Science,* **327,** 812-818.

Intergovernmental Panel on Climate Change (IPCC) (2006) *2006 IPCC Guidelines for National Greenhouse Gas Inventories,* Prepared by the National Greenhouse Gas Inventories Programme. Edited by H. S.Eggleston, L. Buendia, K. Miwa, T. Ngara and K. Tanabe. IGES, Japan.

Leaver, J.D. (1983) *Milk Production: Science and Practice.* Longman, Harlow, UK.

MacCarthy, J., Thomas, J., Choudrie, S., Thistlethwaite, G., Passant, N, Murells, T.P., Watterson, J.D., Cardenas, L and Thomson, A. (2011) *UK Greenhouse Gas Inventory, 1990-2009.* AEA Technology plc, Harwell, UK.

Office of Public Sector Information (2011) *Climate Change Act 2008.* http:// www.legislation.gov.uk/ukpga/2008/27/contents Accessed 4 January 2012.

Olesen, J.E., Schelde, K., Weiske, A., Weisberg, M.R., Asman, W.A.H., and Drurhuus, J. (2006) Modelling greenhouse gas emissions from European conventional and organic dairy farms. *Agriculture Ecosystems and Environment,* **112,** 207-220.

Rowett (1990) *UK Tables of Nutritive Values and Chemical Composition of Feedingstuffs.* Rowett Research Services Ltd, Aberdeen, UK.

Tamminga, S., Bannink, A., Dijkstra, J. and Zom, R. (2007) *Feeding Strategies to Reduce Methane Losses from Cattle.* Report 34, Animal Sciences group,

Wageningen UR, Lelystad, The Netherlands. 44pp.

Thomas, C. (2004) *Feed Into Milk: A New Applied Feeding System for Dairy Cows*. Nottingham University Press, Nottingham.

Vellinga, Th.V., Blonk, H., Marinussen, M., van Zeist, W.J. and de Boer, I.J.M. (2012) *Methodology used in feedprint: a tool quantifying greenhouse gas emissions of feed production and utilization*. Wageningen UR Livestock Research, Lelystad, The Netherlands.

Weiske, A. and Michel, J. (2007) *Greenhouse gas emissions and mitigation costs of selected mitigation measures in agricultural production*. MEACAP WP3 D15a. http://www.ieep.eu/assets/589/wp3__d15a__ghg_and_mitigation.pdf Accessed 04 January 2012.

Wilkinson, J.M. (2011) Redefining efficiency of feed use by livestock. *Animal,* **5**, 1014-1022.

Wilkinson, J.M. and Audsley, E. (2012) Options from life-cycle analysis for reducing greenhouse gas emissions from crop and livestock production systems. *International Journal of Agricultural Management* (Submitted)

Wilkinson, J.M., Garnsworthy, P.C. and Huxley, J.N. (2011) Continuous housing of cows: challenges and opportunities. *Advances in Animal Biosciences,* **2**, 230.

Wilkinson, J.M. and Toivonen, M.I. (2003) *World Silage: A Survey of Forage Conservation Around the World*. Chalcombe Publications, Lincoln, UK.

Wilkinson, J.M. and Wray, A.E. (2012) Ruminant feed production in the United Kingdom in 1990 and 2010. *Advances in Animal Biosciences,* **3**, 14.

Williams, A.G., Audsley, E. and Sandars, D.L. (2006) Determining the environmental burdens and resource use in the production of agricultural and horticultural commodities. *Main Report. Defra Research Project IS0205*. Cranfield University, Bedford, UK.

Yates, C.M., Cammell, S.B., France, J. and Beever, D.E. (2000) Prediction of methane emissions from dairy cows using multiple regression analysis. *Proceedings British Society of Animal Science 2000*, 94.

Appendix 1 – Equations used to calculate N excretion

The following equations were derived from equations used to calculated MP requirements and supply in the Feed into Milk system (Thomas, 2004).

Values taken directly from FiM are:

Dry matter intake (DMI)
Effective rumen degradable protein (ERDP)
Microbial crude protein (MCP)
Metabolisable protein requirement for milk (MPmilk) and pregnancy (MPpreg)
Net protein requirement for milk (NPmilk) and pregnancy (NPpreg)
Digestible undegraded protein (DUP)
Digestible microbial true protein (DMTP)
Acid-detergent insoluble nitrogen (ADIN)

URINARY EXCRETION

Endogenous urinary protein (EUP) = $4.1 \times W^{0.75}$
Surplus effective rumen degradable protein (ERDPsurplus) = ERDP – MCP
Metabolic urinary protein (MUP) = (MPmilk – NPmilk) + (MPpreg – NPpreg)
Microbial non-protein nitrogen (MNPN) = $0.25 \times$ MCP
Endogenous protein balance (EPbal) = $2.34 \times$ DMI
Milk non-protein nitrogen (NPNmilk) = $0.05 \times$ milk protein yield
Total urinary nitrogen excretion = (EUP + ERDPsurplus + MUP + EPbal)/6.25 + MNPN - NPNmilk

FAECAL EXCRETION

Metabolic faecal protein (MFP) = $30 \times$ DMI
Indigestible microbial true protein (iDMTP) = $0.75 \times$ MCP
Indigestible undegraded protein (iDUP) = DUP/9
Endogenous protein absorbed from hind gut (EPHG) = $0.125 \times$ DMTP
Total faecal nitrogen excretion = (MFP + iDMTP + iDUP - EPHG)/6.25 + ADIN

Appendix 2 – Feed prices and composition

	UK Price[1] (£/t)	DM (g/kg)	ME (MJ/kg DM)	CP (g/kg DM)	CFP (g/kg DM)
Grazed grass	20	200	11.2	155	398
Grass silage average	25	250	10.1	135	341
Grass silage good	25	310	11.8	151	334
Maize silage	22	260	11.0	90	253
Dairy compound feed	240	870	13.5	207	926
Wheat	175	876	13.6	130	589
Barley	150	860	13.2	141	594
Sugarbeet pulp	160	890	12.5	107	330
Wheatfeed	162	860	12.0	180	359
Wheat DDGS	270	920	13.7	348	797
Brewers grains	37	284	11.3	208	45
Molasses	175	750	12.7	140	157
Rapeseed meal	230	885	11.9	406	714
Soyabean meal	342	885	14.0	542	1056
Urea	600	950	0.0	2300	3490
Bypass fat	620	1000	38.0	0	1763
Minerals	470	990	0.0	0	0

[1] At June 2012.

6

SUCCESSFUL FEED COMPOUNDING IN A COMPETITIVE MARKET

BERND SPRINGER
Senior editor, Feed Magazine/Kraftfutter, Mainzer Landstraße 251, 60326 Frankfurt, Germany

Introduction

How can the compound feed industry work successfully? German feed compounders do not earn a lot, but it is enough to keep the industry growing and becoming the biggest compound feed industry in Europe. In this chapter I want to share with you some ideas about the factors that led the industry into the successful present and hopefully further successful future.

Animal husbandry in Germany

Germany has good conditions for animal husbandry. There is no other explication available why in this country overall milk and meat production is increasing. Since the year 2000, growth was about 30 per cent for pig meat production and 70 per cent for poultry production. For beef, however, there was a slight decrease in production. This is in contrast to overall trends in meat production for Europe as a whole. Looking at the period from 1976 up to today, in Europe we had only a 6 per cent growth in meat production. So a constantly increasing share of the 50 million tonnes of meat which are produced in Europe annually comes from Germany; in other countries meat production is shrinking. Until the year 2000, Germany was a net importer of meat. Since then, in the case of pork it has developed into a net exporter; about 1 million tonnes of pig meat and co-products are exported each year.

Milk production shows a positive trend across Europe. German milk producers benefit from an increasing global trade in dairy products. In spite of milk quotas,

German milk production increased from 27 million tonnes in 2005 to 29.8 million tonnes in 2011. In the competition with other milk producing regions, however, Germany is confronted with impacts of the global dairy market. The regional centres of dairy cattle farming in Germany lie in the south and the north-west of the country. Of the total 4.2 million cows, nearly 30 percent (1.25 million cows) are kept in Bavaria in the south and almost 20 percent (0.8 million cows) in Lower Saxony in the north. The movements on the milk quota exchange show that production is migrating from some locations in South Germany and increasing in the federal states of Lower Saxony and North Rhine-Westphalia.

Most German pig farms are located in Lower Saxony and North Rhine-Westphalia, where nearly 60 percent of the 11.2 million fattening pigs in the country are to be found. The numbers of both layer hens and egg-producing poultry farms have shrunk considerably in Germany in the last three years (to 35.3 million layer hens in 2010). By contrast, the number of broilers has risen to 67.5 million. Altogether poultry farming for meat production has increased by over 90 percent since 1990, driven by turkey production, which has grown by 125 percent.

Structure of the compound feed industry in Germany

The compound feed industry is tied to the location of its customers and experiences any changes in the structure of livestock and poultry farming at first hand. This pressure to adapt generates a sustained process of concentration in the compound feed industry. In 2002 there were 420 business establishments in Germany, but by 2010 the number had dropped to 332. Reasons for the decline in the number of business establishments are to be found above all in the growing pressure of competition due to surplus capacities – despite the growing number of animals and Germany's rising level of self-sufficiency in processed animal products. In recent years this structural change has been aggravated chiefly by tight competition on the commodities market. Extreme price fluctuations – both upward and downward – represent an enormous increase in the risk potential for feed producers. Accordingly, the process of concentration is likely to continue in the next few years and lead to a further decline in the number of plants producing compound feed.

Over the past 20 years there have been distinct shifts between the size categories of businesses and a growing concentration of compound feed production among the major producers is becoming apparent. The growth threshold for business establishments currently lies at an annual production level of 100,000 t and more. In the business year 2009/2010 the 34 establishments in the size category above 200,000 t produced 45.1 percent of the total volume of compound feed, while in the business year 1991/1992 this figure was below 30 percent. One side effect of the structural adjustments in the compound feed industry is that the small plants remaining have become more strongly oriented to producing special varieties of compound feed, while the larger producers primarily supply the market with compound feed ranges for the key productive livestock and poultry species.

Inhomogeneous customer needs

Apart from the different forms of animal husbandry, compound feed suppliers also have to cater to a broad spectrum of customer characters. These range from "production technicians" possessing a high level of nutritional knowledge, who expect high-level expert consultancy on feeding issues, to pure "users and economists", who want to be presented with the right solution so that everything "simply works" without going into any great detail themselves. Of course there is the whole spectrum in between these extremes. Accordingly, competition on the compound feed market is to a great extent a competition between sales forces, whose recipe for success lies in addressing customers in the right way.

Where are the returns?

Even in times of relatively high food prices, margins at the individual stages of the food chain are low. The income of farmers through selling their livestock in 2009 was 2.8 billion Euro for cattle, 6.2 billion for pigs, 1.6 billion for poultry, 7.1 billion for milk, and 0.7 billion for eggs. Margins are particularly low for the actual production stage. Of the total revenues of 18.4 billion Euros in 2009, farmers spent 5.4 billion Euros on compound feed, which was only 45 per cent of total feed costs; and the low margin problem continues in the directly upstream feed industry.

In mid-June 2012, German feed compounders sold dairy cow feed for 275 Euro per tonne, pig fattening feed for 277 Euro per tonne, piglet feed for 362 Euro per tonne and layer feed for 350 Euro per tonne. At the same time, feed compounders had to buy feed wheat for 219 Euro per tonne, maize for 213 Euro per tonne and soyabean meal for 410 Euro per tonne. Consequently, there is only a small difference of about 50 Euro per tonne between raw material price and selling price. With this 50 Euro, compounders have to pay buildings, electricity, waste management, additives, storing, mixing and transport.

Despite the low margin, feed compounders are partners of agriculture on two fronts: they absorb raw materials from the field and supply farms with efficient feedstuffs. Germany's feed industry has consolidated and perfected its role as partner in recent years. There are admittedly repeated and even cut-throat price wars at sales-team level that slash the margins for the compound feed producers and are used to switch some customers to a new supplier. However, stable, problem-oriented customer relations predominate, in which the feed adviser who knows his customers well can help to stabilise their incomes. The playing field covers the right balance between selling crops and taking farm-produced feedstuffs into storage, solving sub-acute health problems in the animal populations, developing special feeding concepts geared to specific farms, supporting the choice of the right genetics and exploiting them optimally by diets designed to suit, and much more besides.

Although 10 to 20 years ago compound feed plants located close to ports (sites such as Hamburg, along the Rhine and the main rivers) enjoyed an advantage in procuring raw materials, this plays a lesser role today because compound feed now contains up to 50 percent grain. This raw material is largely produced and provided on the domestic market. In the face of foreseeable rising competition with the food market, however, raw materials not suitable for use as foods will become more important for compound feed production again, and port locations will regain some of their former advantage.

Challenges encountered in feeding animals

World population is predicted to grow to 9 billion people in 2050, which will consume 465 million tonnes of meat and more than 1 billion tonnes of milk. Obviously feed production has to increase as well. Directly and indirectly, the success of the compound feed industry depends on the European agricultural policy. At the moment, alongside its main task of achieving a successful agricultural reform, Europe's agricultural policy is faced with implementing the ban on cage keeping of layer hens in all countries. There is still need for action in several countries. Until all the Member States follow the regulations regarding keeping, substantial market distortions will remain, especially in the market for processing eggs. One further challenge for the entire agricultural sector is the call for sustainable production methods. The feed industry must keep an eye on the requirements of food processors and the supply of certified products – and the differences between certificates – especially when procuring raw materials. The feed industry is faced with all these tasks, alongside its daily challenge of providing its customers with low-cost, high-performance feed and surviving in the highly competitive market.

Some further challenges in feeding animals occur, which feed producers and animal farmers will need to solve in a spirit of partnership. The first is to reduce the use of medicines and at the same time improve the health status of high-performing animal populations through multi-phase feeding, buffers, feed acids, additives, enzymes, amino acids and so on. The feed producers are important partners of livestock farmers and veterinarians when it comes to keeping herds and flocks healthy. It has been demonstrated that by providing a nutrient specification in line with needs, rations adapted to the performance phase of the animals, and suitable additives (on a probiotic basis or made from plant raw materials) the use of medicaments can be reduced. However, it is important to publicise these findings among veterinarians.

The next challenge is to harness more fibre as digestible energy through feed processing or use of additives. To react to the growing competition with food raw materials it becomes important to use more co-products in rations, for instance using distillers dark grains with solubles (DDGS) and perhaps algae. In livestock production, feed costs contribute 50 to 70 per cent of total production costs and the major cost components are energy and protein sources. Nowadays nutritionists are facing challenges in feed formulation since ingredient prices are increasing due to a tight supply-demand situation. Bio-fuel production competes increasingly with the use of cereals and oilseeds for food and feed production. On the other hand, increased biofuel production results in increased supply of co-products, such as DDGS and rapeseed meal that find their way into animal feed. Limitations apply, however, particularly for usage of DDGS products in animal feed, mainly due to low and variable available lysine content and significant variation in product quality. The quality of DDGS is related to fermentation conditions, drying temperature and the amount of solubles added back to the product. Available or standardized ileal digestible lysine (SID) content is a key parameter and needs to be known for each batch of DDGS in order to avoid impediments in animal performance when using this co-product in feed formulation.

Further challenges include: hygiene requirements, for instance to control salmonella or mycotoxins; increasing energy efficiency, both in the production of compound feed and through optimisation of feed energy digestibility. Feed energy digestibility can be improved by optimal ration formulation, multi-phase feeding, and additives that moderate digestion by conveying nutrients to the crucial sections of the digestive tract (for instance by coating of ingredients with special lipids). Ongoing research is looking at effective use of the mode of action of phytogenic additives, such as palatants, flavour and digestion enhancers.

In addition, compound feed producers must continue to invest in technologies that increase working precision and reduce labour needs (for instance by automation). Here the German feed millers are at the forefront, with a state of the art university research and common industry research (for instance the International Research Institute of Feed Technology (IFF) in Braunschweig-Thune, Germany, where new technologies can be tested at laboratory and plant scale). Sustainability will be an important topic too. An EU directive already specifies the use of sustainable biomass for biofuels and certification makes it possible to distinguish on global markets between sustainable biomass and biomass without any evidence of sustainability. There is still a lack of any such statutory specification for foods and feeds. However, in its coalition agreement, the German Federal Government proposed to extend sustainability standards to all markets.

7

EU FEED ADDITIVE REGISTRATION AND REVIEW PROCESSES: IMPACT ON NEW PRODUCT DEVELOPMENT

ELINOR MCCARTNEY
Pen and Tec Consulting S.L, Barcelona, Spain

Introduction

Meeting current and future regulatory requirements in the European Union (EU) for feed and feed additives is a major challenge for businesses operating in this sector. As a result of the EU White Paper on Food Safety, published in 2000, there have been sweeping changes to legislation concerning the food chain, especially feed and feed additives. The 2003 EU feed additive regulation (Regulation EC [N°] 1831/2003) replaced the former 1970 feed additive Directive 70/524/EEC and introduced a new system for assessing feed additive dossiers.

The current evaluation procedure involves the European Commission (EC) the European Union Reference Laboratory (EURL), the European Food Safety Authority (EFSA) and the Standing Committee on the Food Chain and Animal Health – Nutrition Section (SCFCAH), which includes delegations from all 27 EU Member States ('Comitology').

The new feed additive regulation, Regulation (EC) N° 1831/2003, re-categorised feed additives and created new functional groups such as amino acids, silage agents and urea. Technological feed additives have been expanded to include mycotoxin inactivators, and work is underway to create a new feed hygiene additive category.

The ban on antibiotic growth promoters in the EU was completed in January 2006, although coccidiostats and histomonostats remain as feed additives. Maintaining approvals under current legislation presents considerable challenges for all operators in this business sector.

Around 12,000 active substances or products were notified in 2004 under the new feed additive regulation. November 2010 was the re-evaluation deadline for most of these notifications, resulting in the submission of around 450 re-evaluation dossiers, many still under EFSA scrutiny. The majority of these active substances and products had never been subjected to an EU assessment according to current standards of safety, quality and efficacy. The new feed additive register was first published in November 2005 and is regularly updated. The EC has started to delete a large number of active substances from this register since no re-evaluation dossiers were submitted and, for example, has recently published regulations withdrawing many silage additives.

The more recent pioneering feed regulation, Regulation (EC) N° 767/2009, allows certain nutritional and physiological claims on feeds and provides for an informal, web-based register, as well as a formal community catalogue of feed materials, which is updated by EU regulation from time to time.

This chapter reviews EU food chain legislation, examines both procedures and data requirements relating to animal nutrition, and discusses the main issues that confront companies in this important industry sector. The key elements of a successful feed additive dossier are illustrated. Creative marketing examples are given, showing how an understanding of the legal environment affects new product development.

EU feed legislation: how and when it all began

Most of the first half of the 20th Century in Europe was marked by wars and hunger, but by the end of the century, consumer preferences and food safety emerged as key drivers of EU legislation and have remained a strong focus for European regulatory authorities in the early years of the 21st Century (Figure 1).

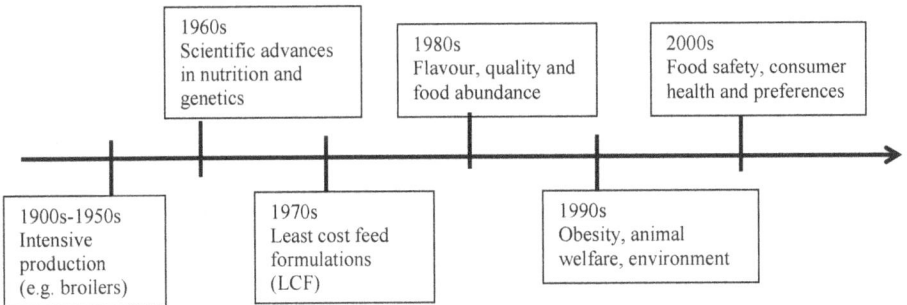

Figure 1. Changing European focus with respect to the food chain, 1900s to 2000s

In the era after the Second World War the EU regulatory environment concerning the food chain was dominated by pharmaceutical thinking, which still persists to a large extent. Since 2000, and as a result of the EU White Paper on Food Safety (EC, 2000), Europe has harmonised food and feed legislation, by using more nutritional ('non-drug') approaches and applying HACCP (Hazard Analysis and Critical Control Points) principles and traceability to food safety. Table 1 highlights some of the main 'STEEPLE' factors that influence European regulatory approaches and how scientific cultures have shifted over time.

Table 1. STEEPLE factors and transition from pharmaceutical to food cultures

STEEPLE factors	Cultures
Social	Human pharmaceuticals
Technological	Antibiotics for veterinary use
Economic	Coccidiostats
Ethical	Antibiotic growth promoters (AGPs)
Political	Alternative feed additives for animals
Legal	Food nutrition and health claims
Ecological	Environmental focus

The key drivers for current legal trends with respect to feed materials and feed additives include various food chain scares such as:

- 'mad cow disease' (BSE – bovine spongiform encephalopathy),

- dioxins and PCBs (polychlorinated biphenyls),

- increasing concerns with respect to antimicrobial resistance (AMR) in the food chain,

- food poisoning outbreaks associated with *Campylobacter*, *Salmonella* and other enteropathogens.

The occurrence of these food scandals and crises, both perceived or real, led to the establishment of EFSA in January 2002. However, some of the most important drivers of new laws relating to animal nutrition were the perceptions of the EC, Member States and consumers that unscrupulous operators were placing toxic feed materials on the European market. Examples of such intentional or unintentional criminal acts include:

- dioxins/PCBs from industrial oils,

- hormone-containing waste fermentation products from pharmaceutical manufacturing,

- heavy metals in trace mineral compounds not suitable for food chain use, e.g. zinc oxide imported for use in ceramics,

- dried slaughterhouse waste, e.g. faeces sold as 'urea'.

In fact, EU consumers have been shown to be poor at determining real risks to health, as shown in a French food safety survey carried out in 2000 (Table 2). The top three consumer concerns in relation to food safety were BSE (mentioned by 52% consumers), genetically modified organisms (GMOs, mentioned by 32% of consumers) and water pollution (mentioned by 27% consumers). In fact, poor hygiene in feed mills, on the farm, at slaughterhouses, and during food transport, processing and storage are arguably of much greater importance to consumer health, bearing in mind that *Campylobacters* and *Salmonella* are the most important food poisoning organisms in the EU (EFSA 2012a). Table 2 illustrates that consumers tend to worry about what is in the news, and in 2000 'mad cows' and GMOs were hitting the headlines.

Table 2. 2000 French survey on food safety (Brufau, personal communication)

Consumer concerns	% in top 3
BSE	52%
GMOs	32%
Water pollution	27%
Listeria	26%
Break in cold chain	24%
Hormones in beef cattle	22%
Dioxins	21%
Antibiotics in animal production	17%
Contamination of farmland	16%
Chemical treatment of cereals	14%
Salmonella	13%
Poor kitchen hygiene	10%
Food past sell by date	9%
Colours, preservatives	6%

Table 3 illustrates that in 2012 Europeans are not dying from GMOs and 'mad cows'. Neither are today's Europeans dying from hunger, unlike over 2 million children around the world. Europeans today are dying from excess, diseases associated with overconsumption of fatty, salty and sweet foods, obesity and associated bad habits such as smoking, drinking, and insufficient, regular exercise.

Antimicrobial resistance

European scientists and legislators are worried about antimicrobial resistance, but what is meant by antimicrobial resistance? Figure 2 represents one scheme produced by the EURL (EURL, 2007). Regulators and their advisors (e.g. EFSA, 2012b) often used the lowest *in vitro* breakpoints (MICs, minimal inhibitory

Table 3. Main causes of death, global and EU

Causes of death	N° of deaths/year
Global hunger	8M[1]
Global HIV/AIDS	2M[2]
Global Malaria	0.9M[2]
Cancer (EU-27[6])	369,500[3]
Circulatory and heart disease (EU-27)	336,000[3]
Suicide (EU-27)	46,000[3]
Road traffic accidents (EU-27)	40,000[3]
Infections/parasites (EU-27)	34,000[4]
HIV (EU-27)	<350[4]
BSE (UK only)	<5[5]
GMOs	0

[1]FAO 2008; [2]WHO 2008; [3]EC 2011 [4]Eurostat 2009; [5]SCENIHR 2006; [6]EU-27 population to age 65 years

concentrations) to categorise bacteria as resistant. However, most veterinarians and doctors are aware that *in vitro* MICs do not always correlate with clinical effectiveness.

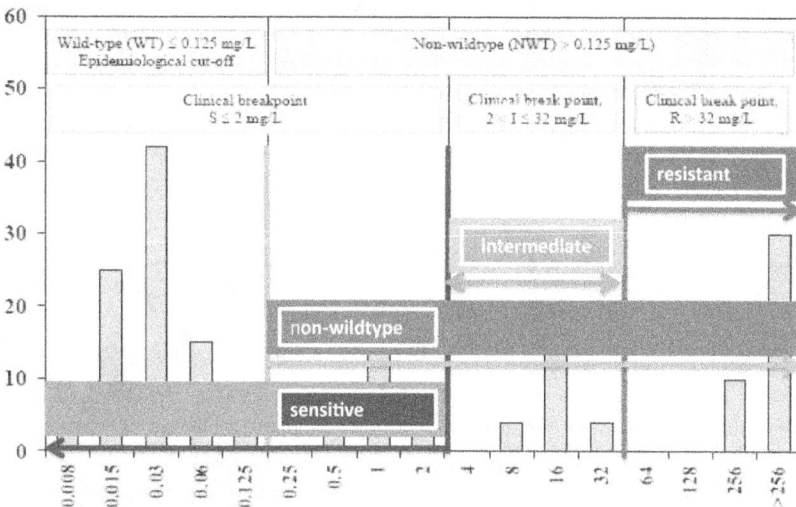

WT = Wild type organisms, i.e micro-organisms without phenotypically detectable antimicrobial resistance to the drug in question

Figure 2. Illustration of antimicrobial resistance via *in vitro* MICs (EURL, 2007)

Scandinavia and the EU ban on antibiotic growth promoters (AGPs)

Denmark and other Scandinavian countries were successful in driving the EU to ban AGPs in animal feed using data such as shown in Figure 3. Until the mid-1990s substantial amounts of avilamycin were used in Denmark as an AGP in broilers. From 1997 the Danes implemented a voluntary ban on AGPs, after which resistance to avilamycin in marker strains of *Enterococcus faecium* fell dramatically. Hence it seems clear that antimicrobial use promotes AMR and a reduction in antimicrobial use results in a reduction in AMR. It is important to note that pigs never harboured *E. faecium* strains resistant to avilamycin as the use of avilamycin in pigs in Denmark was essentially zero. Notably, DANMAP began recording human AMR data in 2002, much later than the database on animal AMR, and perhaps indicative of the received wisdom that use of antimicrobials in animals is the main cause of AMR in humans.

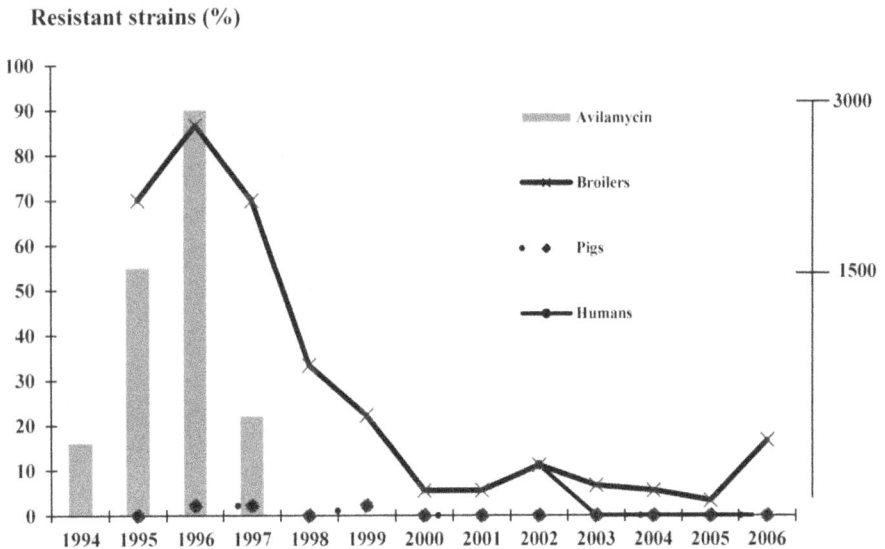

Figure 3. Danish avilamycin consumption and resistance in *E. faecium* marker strains (DANMAP, 2006)

Figure 4 shows a dramatic drop in AGP consumption in Denmark between 1994 and 2000 (DANMAP, 2006). The total Danish consumption of antibiotics in food animals fell by 15% from around 130 tonnes in 1990 to around 110 tonnes in 2006, a substantial overall reduction, especially taking into account that Danish food animal production rose in the same time period by around 8% (Figure 5). However, Figure 4 also shows a worrying trend in increased use of veterinary antibiotics from 2000 onwards. The Danish experience has been replicated in all

EU Member States since the completion of the EU-wide AGP ban in 2006. Thus the first effect of EU legislation to ban AGPs has been increased consumption of veterinary antibiotics. The second effect has been innovations in veterinary antibiotics, notably the development of long-acting injectable formulations for both farm and companion animals.

Consumption (tonne actives)

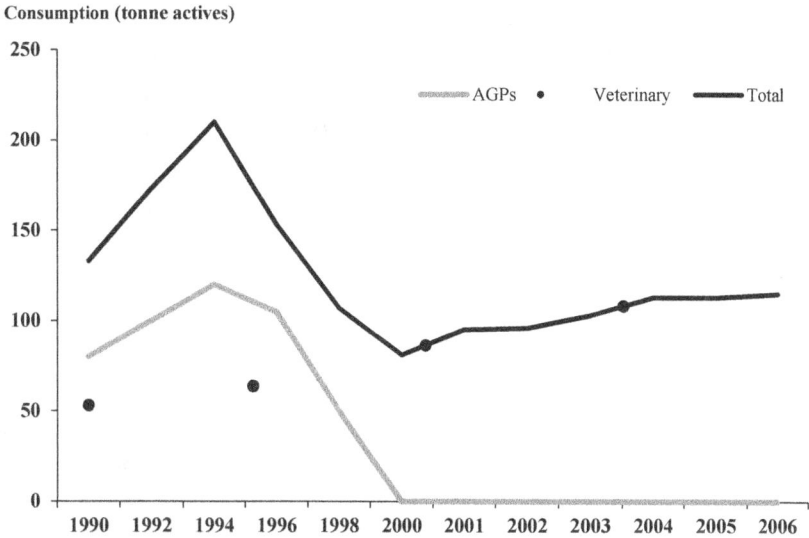

Figure 4. Antimicrobial consumption in Denmark, 1990-2006 (DANMAP, 2006)

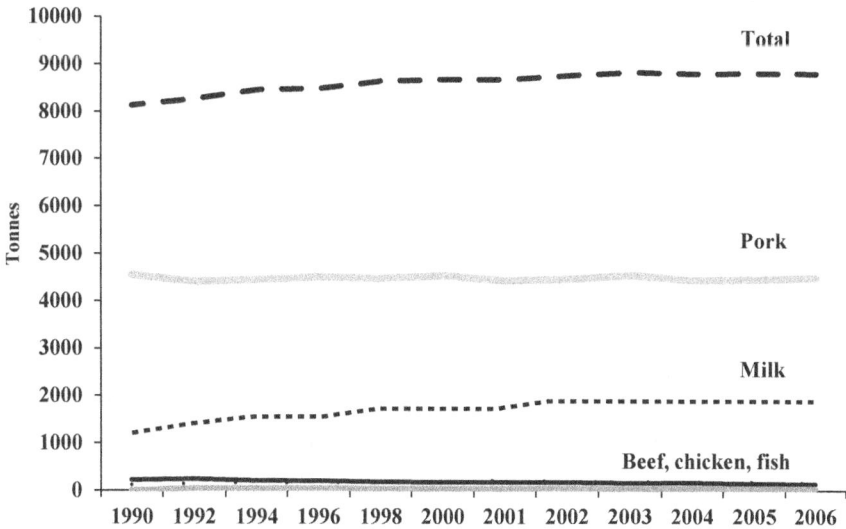

Figure 5. Danish food production from 1990-2006 (DANMAP, 2006)

Since the completion of the EU AGP ban in 2006, the emphasis of regulators and scientists has shifted to the role of veterinary antibiotic use in food animals as a risk factor contributing to AMR in humans (Figure 6). The European Medicines Agency (EMEA) estimates that AMR is responsible for around 25,000 deaths per year in the EU; a serious health problem, especially in the light of the scarcity of new, effective antibiotics (Figure 7). Data from McKenna (2011) show that the number of new systemic antibiotic agents has declined since 1980, particularly for beta-lactams and quinolones. This is a real cause for concern, as it would appear that AMR is increasing in a world with fewer new antibiotics. As Figure 8 suggests, however, much of human AMR arises with the use of antibiotics in the community and hospitals (EMEA, 2009).

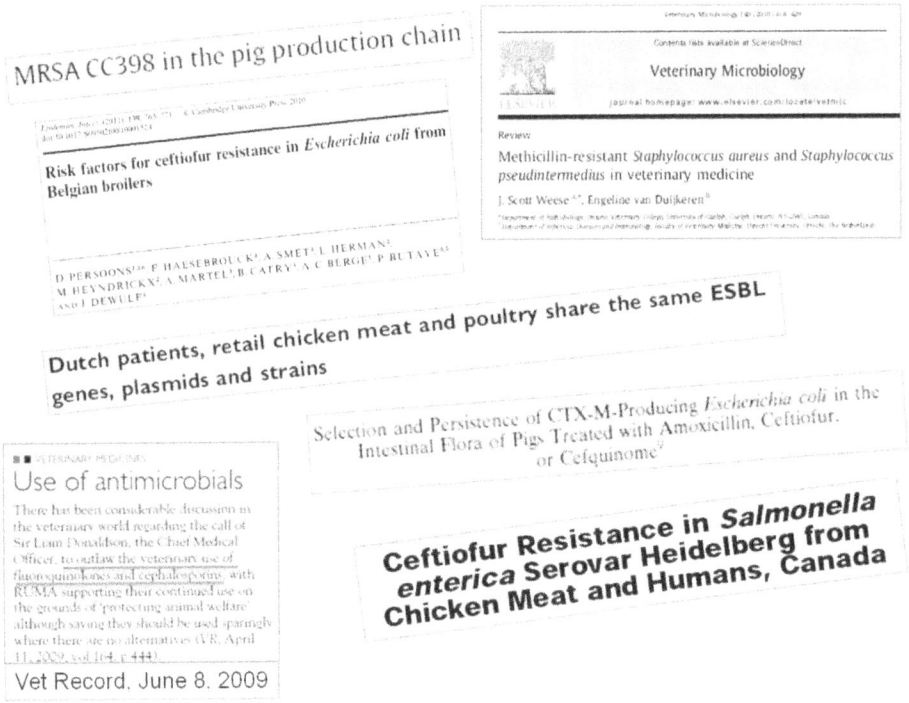

Figure 6. Emphasis on AMR in food animals in the scientific press

Mark Twain attributed to Benjamin Disraeli, a British Prime Minister in Victorian times, the expression *'There are lies, damned lies and statistics'*, and a review of Figures 2 to 8 illustrates the multiple and differing conclusions that can be drawn from the same data sets. The link between AMR and feed legislation can most likely be traced to politics, since consumer preferences now drive food chain policies and politics in the EU. The EU AGP ban may be the thin end of a very long political wedge that is currently putting pressure on the use of veterinary antibiotics in

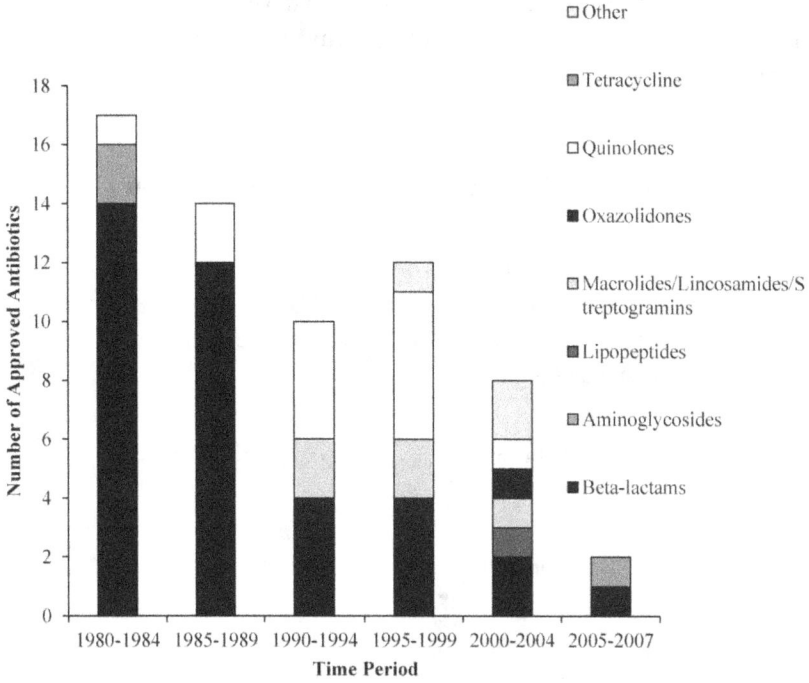

Figure 7. New antibiotics since 1980 (McKenna, 2011)

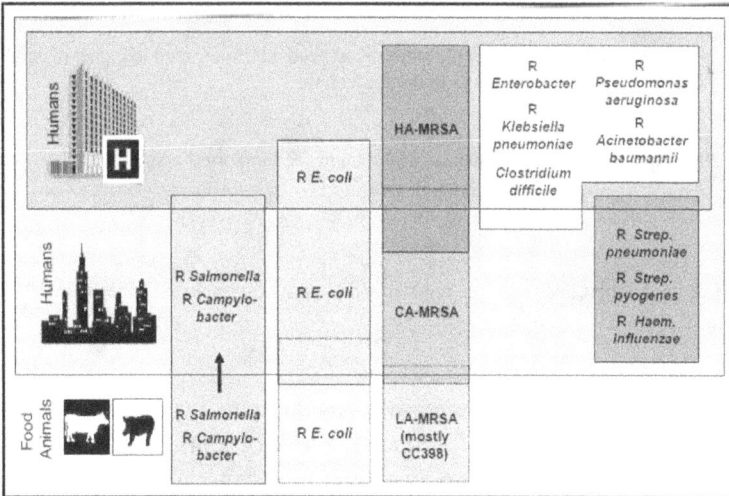

Figure 8. Compartments of antimicrobial resistance (ECDC/EMEA, 2009)

both food and non-food animals. This pressure will have repercussions far beyond animal nutrition and the use of antimicrobial drugs to treat infections in animals and humans.

The EU response: the rebirth of food and feed legislation

The EU responded to consumer concerns on food chain safety with a key document, the EU White Paper on Food Safety, published in 2000. The White Paper on Food Safety instigated a complete review of all food and feed legislation in the EU, lasting more than a decade (Figure 9).

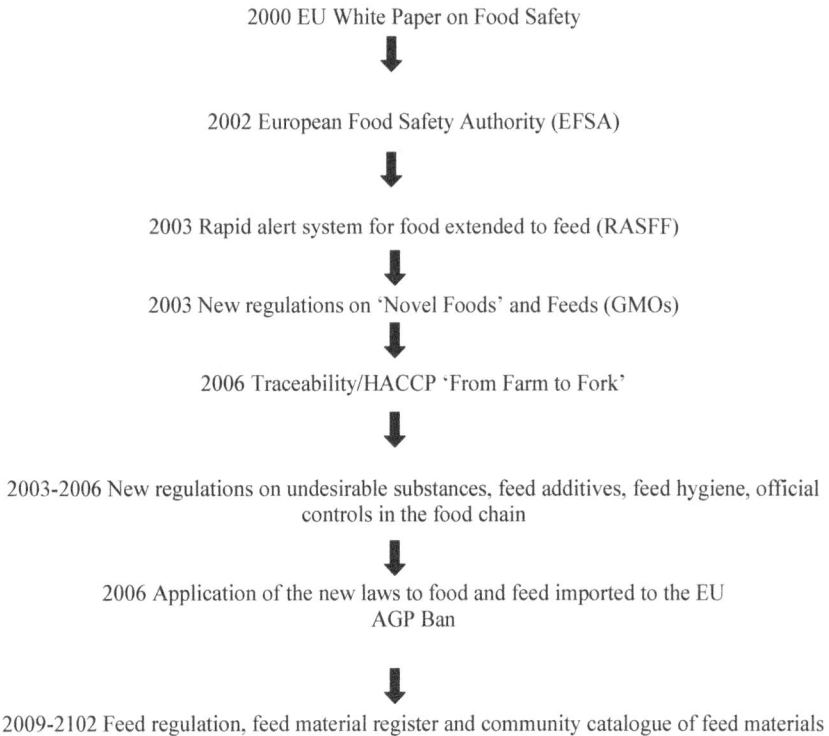

2000 EU White Paper on Food Safety

↓

2002 European Food Safety Authority (EFSA)

↓

2003 Rapid alert system for food extended to feed (RASFF)

↓

2003 New regulations on 'Novel Foods' and Feeds (GMOs)

↓

2006 Traceability/HACCP 'From Farm to Fork'

↓

2003-2006 New regulations on undesirable substances, feed additives, feed hygiene, official controls in the food chain

↓

2006 Application of the new laws to food and feed imported to the EU
AGP Ban

↓

2009-2102 Feed regulation, feed material register and community catalogue of feed materials

Figure 9. EU legislative response, 2000-2012

Despite inadvertently stimulating increased consumption of veterinary antibiotics, the abolition of AGPs in the EU has produced several benefits. It has promoted the incorporation of better quality, more digestible feed materials into animal diets, and driven innovation in feed additives, allowing the development of improved feed enzymes, new prebiotics and probiotics, as well as products based on herbs, spices, essential oils and other AGPAs (antibiotic growth promoter alternatives). Increasingly, fat and other coating systems are used to improve delivery to target gut sites and/or to improve the stability and shelf-life of active substances. Additionally, the EU AGP ban, supported with legislation on animal welfare and control of *Salmonella* spp. has stimulated interest and efforts in improved farm hygiene and husbandry; drivers which extend beyond EU borders to third country suppliers, notably Brazil.

Feed additive regulation: out with the old and in with the new

A well as completing the AGP ban, the new feed additive regulation, Regulation (EC) N° 1831/2003, reclassified amino acids, urea and silage additives as feed additives. The new regulation also required re-evaluation of all existing feed additives and introduced 10-year renewals to feed additive authorisations. All applications now require deposition of a sample of the feed additive in question, and/or access to strain deposits in the case of live micro-organisms. Validation and verification of analytical methods for active substance/s in feed additives must be carried out, and documentation is reviewed by the EURL. The new regulation defines a feed additive as a substance or preparation that may be given in feed, water or by other means (e.g. oral bolus) with the purpose of improving feed, animal products or animal colour. A feed additive may also satisfy nutritional needs, improve the environment, or improve animal production, performance or welfare. Feed additives other than coccidiostats and histomonostats may not claim to treat, prevent or cure disease, since those claims are veterinary claims (Table 4).

Table 4. Feed additive categories defined according to Regulation (EC) N° 1831/2003

Category	Function
Technological	Acts on feed, feedingstuffs, feed materials, e.g. preservatives, anti-oxidants, emulsifiers, stabilisers, thickeners, gelling agents, binders, anti-radionucleotides, anti-cakers, acidifiers, silage agents, denaturants, anti-mycotoxin substances.
Sensory	Adds colour to feed/animals or flavour to feeds.
Nutritional	Vitamins, pro-vitamins, trace elements, amino acids, urea.
Zootechnical	Improves feed digestibility, gut flora equilibrium or the environment. Includes non-antibiotic performance enhancers.
Coccidiostats and histomonostats	The only antimicrobials currently permitted as feed additives.

Obtaining EU authorisation for a feed additive

The main reference material for compiling a feed additive application ('dossier') includes Commission Regulations (EC) Nºs 1831/2003 and 429/2008 and various guidance documents from EFSA scientific panels. The Panel on Additives and Products or Substances used in Animal Feed (FEEDAP), the Panel on Genetically Modified Organisms (GMO) and the Panel on Biological Hazards (BIOHAZ) all have guidance documents publically available to applicants. Table 5 summarises the final dossier structure.

Table 5. Summary of the evaluation process and structure of the final dossier

EURL	EU	EFSA: (1 paper copy, 2 CDs)		
Cover letter Declaration form EU Annex I ←	Cover letter Application form (EU Annex I)	Part 1 Administrative	Part 2 Technical	Part 3 Confidential
3 reference samples (same lots) 3 reference standards	Administrative data	Cover letter	Section I Public Summary Scientific Summary List of Documents Confidential Information	Confidential parts
Certificate of ID/ analysis	Section I Public Summary	Application form (EU Annex I)	Section II Quality Annexes	From Section II
Pay EURL fees	Section I Scientific Summary	Contact details (Annex E)	Section III Safety Annexes	From Section III
Public Summary Scientific Summary	Section I Dossier index	Description and proposed use of additive Annex A (Register entry)	Section IV Efficacy Annexes	From Section IV
Obtain proof of payment or fee waiver	Section I Confidential parts	Completeness Checklist (Annex B)	Section V Post-market monitoring	All documents in English
Multi-tasking of dossiers is acceptable	EURL proof of payment or fee waiver	Declaration e-copy = paper copy	Sections II, III and IV must include bibliography	PDFs (<20 Mb)

The EU feed additive evaluation and authorisation process

This is a complex process summarised in Figure 10. The official application for EU authorisation of a feed additive is made to the EC, but the complete dossier is sent to EFSA, who acknowledge physical reception. Once EFSA has received formal instruction from the EC to evaluate the dossier, EFSA reviews the dossier for completeness, an administrative task that takes 30 working days. If the dossier is incomplete, EFSA responds with a 'MiP' (missing information parts) requesting the missing data. Once the dossier is considered complete and correctly formatted, EFSA sends a validation letter to indicate 'clock zero' which marks the start of the '6-month' evaluation period. From this point, EFSA then circulates the dossier to the EURL, the EC and the Member States. EFSA also requires confirmation from applicants that the public summary does not contain any confidential information and upon receipt of this confirmation publishes the public summary on the EFSA website. An EFSA working group (WG) is established of independent experts who evaluate the dossier from a scientific point of view. During the evaluation EFSA may issue a 'clock stop' in request for supplementary data or information ('SiN'). The applicant must respond to EFSA before the evaluation process can proceed. All WG

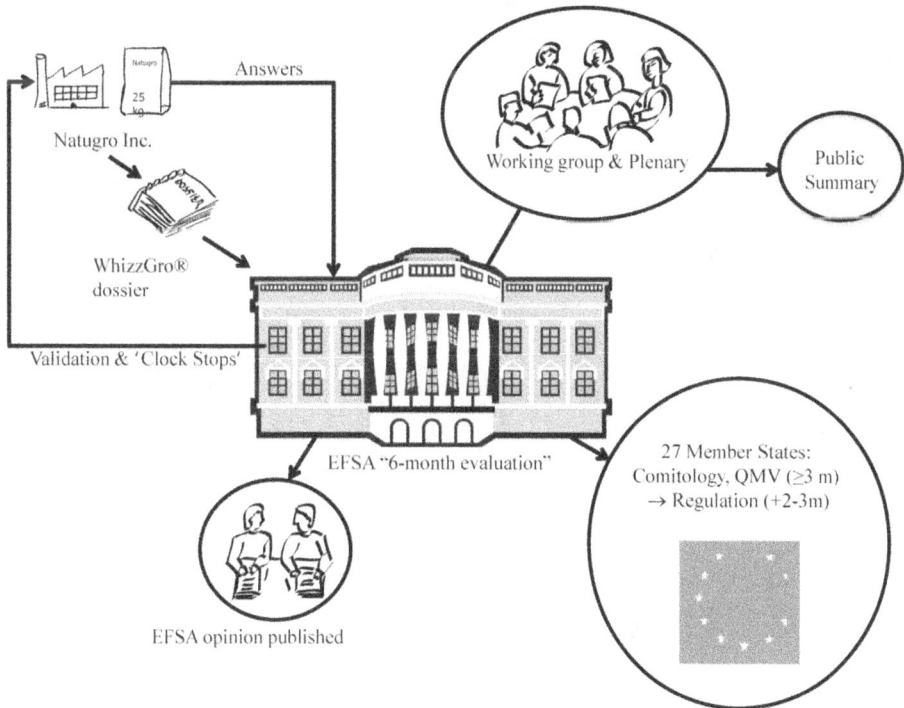

Figure 10. EU feed additive evaluation and authorisation process

experts are listed on the EFSA website as are FEEDAP and other EFSA scientific panel members. The independent scientists are supported by EFSA scientific and administrative staff.

The WG drafts a scientific opinion, which is reviewed, corrected and adopted at EFSA plenary meetings. Plenary meetings consist of 21 FEEDAP members, with staff from the EC, the EURL and EFSA attending as necessary. The EFSA opinion is published on the EFSA web page and circulated to the EC and Member States. Within 3 months of receipt of the EFSA opinion, a draft regulation to authorise or prohibit the feed additive is drawn up by the EC for debate by Member State delegates to SCFCAH. A Qualified Majority Vote (QMV) makes the final decision on authorisation or prohibition (Table 6). A successful QMV requires approval of at least 50% of Member States, and must also represent more than 60% of the EU population. The number of votes allocated to each Member State is determined by the country's population.

Table 6. The EU 27 Member States and QMV

SCFCAH votes	*Population (M)*	*N° votes*
Germany	82	29
UK	63	29
France	65	29
Italy	61	29
Spain	47	27
Poland	38	27
Romania	21	14
Netherlands	17	13
Greece	11	12
Czech Republic	11	12
Belgium	11	12
Hungary	10	12
Portugal	11	12
Sweden	9	9
Bulgaria	7	8
Austria	8	8
Slovakia	5	5
Denmark	6	5
Finland	5	5
Ireland	4	4
Lithuania	3	4
Latvia	2	2
Slovenia	2	2
Estonia	1	1
Cyprus	1	4
Luxembourg	0.5	4
Malta	0.5	3
EU 27	502	345

Best practices for a successful EU feed additive dossier

Planning ahead and developing an adequate strategic dossier plan to avoid problems arising later with EFSA, the EU and their Member States is essential (Table 7). At project start, it is essential to take time to consider commercial objectives envisaged for after EU authorisation, and to determine a correct and coherent legal definition of the candidate feed additive. The EU does not permit veterinary claims on feed additives. A veterinary claim is a claim to prevent, treat or cure disease. Should the product fall outside current feed additive definitions, the dossier evaluation will be delayed in 'Comitology' while Member States debate the 'new' classification. On the other hand, a 'pioneer' dossier can set new standards and break down regulatory obstacles. This is an opportunity to achieve an EU 'first' with concomitant marketing advantages. GMOs, zootechnical feed additives, coccidiostats and histomonostats are linked authorisations, where authorisations are exclusive to the applicant, thus protecting investments. Micro-organisms used as producer strains for enzymes, amino acids and vitamins, silage inoculants and probiotics are evaluated and authorised as strain-specific additives, which effectively protects these products from 'copycat' competitors. The most successful EU dossier projects are those where the applicant has invested resources in forward planning and a good data audit, beginning with safety issues. During the planning and data audit phases difficult questions may arise, for example the time and cost of data generation, the probability of technical and regulatory success, and how best to protect project investment. Nevertheless, it is better to deal with problems at this stage and make critical decisions, rather than later in the application process when considerable resources have been expended.

All relevant and current EFSA, EURL and EC documents should be collected prior to starting work on building the dossier. It is advisable to refer to recent published ESFA opinions for similar products as well as previous reports and opinions from both the Scientific Committee on Animal Nutrition (SCAN) and the Scientific Committee on Food (SCF), both EC predecessors of EFSA scientific panels. Other possible relevant references include publications from the Joint FAO/WHO Expert Committee on Food Additives (JECFA), the U.S. Food and Drug Administration (FDA) and the Environmental Protection Agency (EPA). It is recommended to carry out formal literature searches and frequently check for EFSA/EC web page updates to make sure you are using the latest guidelines and guidance.

A dossier with a negative opinion from EFSA on safety will not be presented for a positive QMV (authorisation) until the safety issue is resolved, or it may be presented for a negative QMV (prohibition). Increasingly, a dossier with a negative EFSA opinion on efficacy will not be subject to QMV until additional EFSA-compliant efficacy data are generated.

Table 7. EU dossier planning, iteration and key issues

Planning	Data audit	Expert advice	Iterate	Key issues
1. Safety	AMR issues?	Safety margins?	History of use and human/animal exposure?	Environmental studies required?
2. Efficacy	Target species, dose and 'claims'	Suitability of non-EU studies?	Difficulty of proof	Minimum effective dose?
3. Quality	i.e. validation/verification of analytical methods	e.g. product specification	CEN/ISO/AOAC methods	Stability, compatibility
4. Generate data	Key safety quality, efficacy data	Study design and statistics?	Frequent checks for EFSA/EU/EURL guidance updates	Check raw data and statistics
5. Reports	GLP, GCP, EFSA-compliant	Review in detail	In-house reports signed and study director	Negative or weak points
6. Annexes	Safety Annexes	Efficacy Annexes	Quality Annexes	Bibliography
7. Text	Safety text	Efficacy text	Quality text	Summary text (clarity and coherence)
8. Administration	EURL	EU	EFSA	Submit dossier

Notes - GLP: good laboratory practice; GCP: good clinical practice; CEN/ISO/AOAC: official and published analytical methods

The quality of dossier documentation is paramount to dossier success. Increasingly, regulators are demanding GLP-accredited studies (mandatory for laboratory animal safety studies) and GCP-type efficacy studies. Quality studies are preferably carried out in ISO 17025-accredited laboratories, using official EU methods, or CEN (European Committee for Standardization), ISO (International Organization for Standardization), or AOAC (Association of Official Agricultural Chemists) methods. EFSA requires, as a minimum, compliance with all relevant EFSA guidance documents. Table 8 gives an example of current minimum EFSA requirements for target animal safety and efficacy studies, and Figure 11 shows and extract from a mandatory EFSA dossier completeness check list, to be used prior to dossier submission.

Table 8. EFSA- compliance - elements required for tolerance/efficacy study protocols/ reports

Item	*Page*
1. Title page	
2. Table of Contents	
3. Summary (inserted in final report)	
4. Quality statement	
5. Target study dates and reporting requirements	
6. Materials and methods (including statistical models and techniques)	
7. Results (tables)	
8. Discussion and conclusions (text/bullet points)	
9. References	
10. Appendices: Curriculum vitae of study director and study monitor, Certificate/s of analysis of test feed additive/s, study feeds (proximate and additive active substance/s, Relevant external laboratory reports (e.g. blood and tissue analyses), Raw data, Statistical outputs, EFSA Annex C for efficacy and tolerance studies.	

In fact, the EFSA completeness checklist (Figure 10) is a useful tool, not only to help identify missing data or information, but also in detecting where justifications are required for missing data. For example, a long history of use in foods commonly consumed in the EU may help obviate the need for tissue residue studies. Opportunities to reduce data requirements and hence cost and time to EU approval can be found in the legal text of EU guidelines (Regulation EC [N°]

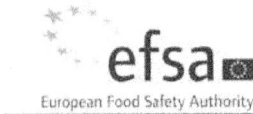

efsa ▪

European Food Safety Authority

FEEDAP UNIT

ANNEX B

COMPLETENESS CHECK LIST [1]

FAD-▮▮▮▮▮

ADMINISTRATIVE DATA OF APPLICANT(S)	
Name of the applicant or representative	

DESCRIPTION AND PROPOSED CLASSIFICATION OF THE ADDITIVE	
Additive name	
Trade name	
Category(-ies)	
Functional group(s)	
Animal species/category(ies)	

TYPE OF APPLICATION	
New additive/ New use (Article 4(1) of Regulation (EC) No 1831/2003)	☐
Authorisation of existing product (Article 10(2) or 10(7) of Regulation (EC) No 1831/2003)	☐
Modification of an authorisation (Article 13 (3) of Regulation (EC) No 1831/2003)	☐
Renewal of an authorisation (Article 14 of Regulation (EC) No 1831/2003)	☐

[1] **Disclaimer:** This check list is provided by the European Food Safety Authority as help in the authorisation process. However, users are reminded that the texts of Regulation (EC) No 429/2008 and 1831/2003 are the only authentic legal references and that the information in this check list does not constitute legal advice. The European Food Safety Authority does not accept any liability with regard to the content of this check list

© European Food Safety Authority, 2008

Figure 11. EFSA completeness check list

429/2008). For example, in the case of complex mixtures derived from plants EU guidelines permit key quality studies (e.g. stability and homogeneity in premixes and feeds) to be carried out with a major constituent, rather than every active substance in the mixture. Figures 12 and 13 show the a positive EFSA opinion and a successful EU authorisation for a zootechnical feed additive that improves weaned piglet performance and is based on nature-identical active substances embedded in a patented, oil-based protective matrix.

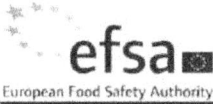

efsa■

European Food Safety Authority　　　　　　　　　　　　　　EFSA Journal 2010; 8(6):1633

SCIENTIFIC OPINION

Scientific Opinion on Safety and efficacy of AviPlus[s] as feed additive for weaned piglets[1]

EFSA Panel on Additives and Products or Substances used in Animal Feed (FEEDAP)[2,3]

European Food Safety Authority (EFSA), Parma, Italy

ABSTRACT

AviPlus[s] is based on a mixture of citric (25%) and sorbic (16.7%) acids, thymol (1.7%) and vanillin (1.0%). It is intended for use with weaned piglets at 1–3 g/kg complete feed. The applicant initially did not consider vanillin to be an integral component of AviPlus[s] and so did not monitor its concentration. Thus, it is assumed that vanillin was present at the specified concentration in the test substance used in the studies described. In the absence of any adverse effects at ten times the maximum recommended dose, the FEEDAP Panel considers that AviPlus[s] is safe for weaned piglets when used at the dose range proposed. As all the active components in AviPlus[s] occur naturally and are authorised for use in human food, the FEEDAP Panel considers that the use of the additive in animal feed is safe for consumers. The potential for irritation/sensitisation by dermal/ocular exposure cannot be fully excluded. No environmental assessment is considered necessary as the active components occur widely in nature and the use of the additive would not detectably add to the existing environmental load. Seven studies were provided to establish efficacy, three with the maximum and four the minimum recommended dose. Significant improvements in daily weight gain and feed to gain ratio were seen in all three studies with the maximum recommended dose. Benefits were seen at the minimum dose in only two of the four studies but a meta-analysis of the four studies showed an overall significant improvement in feed to gain ratio and a higher final bodyweight. Consequently, the FEEDAP Panel concludes that AviPlus[s] has the potential to increase the growth rate of piglets and improve feed to gain ratio with the minimum recommended dose.

Figure 12. Example of a positive EFSA opinion (EFSA, 2010)

The feed regulation, feed material register and catalogue of feed materials

The new feed regulation, Regulation (EC) Nº 767/2009, concerns feed labelling and marketing. It introduces a non-exclusive 'informal' list of feed ingredients, the web-based feed materials register, managed by feed industry organisations such as FEFAC (European Feed Manufacturers' Federation), and a formal, but

3.12.2010 ⟦ EN ⟧ Official Journal of the European Union L 317/3

COMMISSION REGULATION (EU) No 1117/2010

of 2 December 2010

concerning the authorisation of a preparation of citric acid, sorbic acid, thymol and vanillin as a feed additive for weaned piglets (holder of the authorisation Vetagro SpA)

(Text with EEA relevance)

THE EUROPEAN COMMISSION,

Having regard to the Treaty on the Functioning of the European Union,

Having regard to Regulation (EC) No 1831/2003 of the European Parliament and of the Council of 22 September 2003 on additives for use in animal nutrition (¹), and in particular Article 9(2) thereof,

Whereas:

(1) Regulation (EC) No 1831/2003 provides for the authorisation of additives for use in animal nutrition and for the grounds and procedures for granting such authorisation.

animal health, human health or the environment, and that this additive has the potential to increase the growth rate and improve the feed to gain ratio of the target species. The Authority does not consider that there is a need for specific requirements of post-market monitoring. It also verified the report on the method of analysis of the feed additive in feed submitted by the Community Reference Laboratory set up by Regulation (EC) No 1831/2003.

(5) The assessment of the preparation shows that the conditions for authorisation, as provided for in Article 5 of Regulation (EC) No 1831/2003, are satisfied. Accordingly, the use of this preparation should be authorised as specified in the Annex to this Regulation.

Figure 13. Example of a successful EU feed additive authorisation (EC, 2010)

still non-exclusive, catalogue of feed materials, updated annually by the EC. The feed regulation aims to improve feed labelling by increasing transparency while still protecting intellectual property. Feed ingredients are listed in descending order by weight, but full composition (% w/w) must be supplied to regulatory authorities on demand. Certain claims are permitted on feed and feed materials such as optimisation of nutrition and support of physiological functions. As for feed additives, veterinary claims to prevent, treat or cure disease are not permitted. Unlike feed additives, claims on feeds and feed materials are not subject to a pre-marketing authorisation, but feed claims must not be false or misleading. The data supporting feed claims must be available prior to marketing, must be made available to the EC and Member States on demand, and may be submitted to EFSA for review if the EC suspects that claims are false. In many cases the legal definitions classifying products as feeds or feed additives are ambiguous, complex and confusing, so comprehensive knowledge of the legislation avoids challenges by regulatory authorities. Often, a creative approach is necessary to meet commercial objectives, but still comply with the law.

Creative product development in animal nutrition

The quest to replace AGPs with cost-effective alternatives has stimulated creativity. Innovators have taken a new look at old and nature-identical substances with antiseptic, disinfectant, digestion- or appetite-stimulating effects. The nutritional quality of feed materials has been enhanced. Examples are Hamlet Protein® (Denmark), a soyabean derivative with anti-nutritional factors eliminated, and NuPro (Alltech®, USA), a high quality yeast protein. Both products are manufactured with proprietary processes to enhance appetence, digestibility and contribute to gut health. Patented coating systems have been developed to 'package' botanical active substances, both natural and nature-identical, and deliver them to targeted intestinal sites for maximum efficacy. Examples of such botanically-inspired zootechnical feed additives that enhance animal performance are FRESTA® *F* (Delacon Biotechnik GmbH, Austria) and AviPlus® (VetAgro SpA, Italy). FRESTA® *F* and AviPlus® are examples of pioneering products deliberately positioned and approved as zootechnical feed additives in order to differentiate the products from generic 'botanical' competitors, often sold as flavouring premixtures or complementary feeds. Thus, obtention of EU authorisation as a feed additive may now form part of the marketing mix. Figure 14 illustrates the mechanism of delivery of active substances from fat-coated micropearls that degrade as they pass through the gut and Figure 15 illustrates the data supporting the efficacy of the coating system.

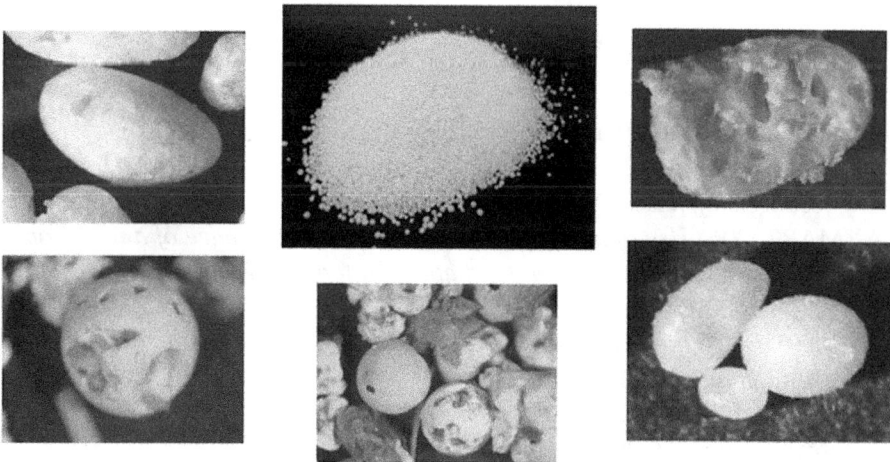

Figure 14. Slow delivery of active substances to the lower gut of weaned piglets (Piva et al., 2007)

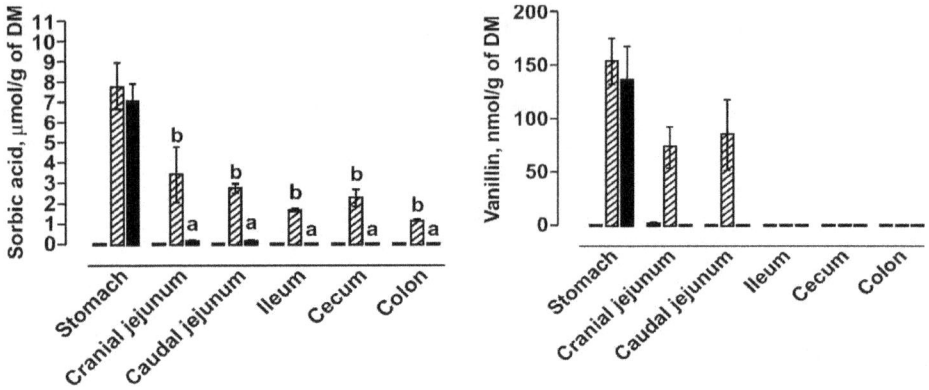

Sorbic acid concentrations in gastrointestinal tracts of pigs fed the control diet, pigs fed the control diet supplemented with a microencapsulated blend of organic acids and natural identical flavours (PB, striped bars), and pigs fed the control diet supplemented with the same blend of organic acids and natural identical flavours with the protective matrix powder but not coating the active ingredients (NPB, black bars). In control-fed pigs, sorbic acid was not detected in any section of the gastrointestinal tract. Data are shown as means ⊠ SEM (n = 5). [a,b]In the same segment of the gastrointestinal tract, different letters indicate $P <$ 0.05.

Vanillin concentrations in gastrointestinal tracts of pigs fed the control diet, pigs fed the control diet supplemented with a microencapsulated blend of organic acids and natural identical flavours (PB, striped bars), and pigs fed the control diet supplemented with the same blend of organic acids and natural identical flavours with the protective matrix powder but not coating the active ingredients (NPB, black bars). In control-fed pigs, vanillin was not detected in any section of the gastrointestinal tract. Data are shown as means ± SEM (n = 5).

Figure 15. Data illustrating slow-delivery of active substances (Piva et al., 2007)

References

Brufau, J, Personal communication to Elinor McCartney

Council Directive 70/524/EEC *of 23 November 1970 concerning additives in feeding-stuffs*, L 270, 14.12.1970, http://eur-lex.europa.eu/en/index.htm

DANMAP (2006) *Use of antimicrobial agents and occurrence of antimicrobial resistance in bacteria from food animals, foods and humans in Denmark*, ISSN 1600-2032.

EC (2000) *EU White Paper on Food Safety*, Commission of the European Communities, Brussels

EC (2003) *Regulation N° 1831/2003 of the European Parliament and of the Council of 22 September 2003 on additives for use in animal nutrition*, 2003R1831 01.09.2010 004.001 http://eur-lex.europa.eu/en/index.htm

EC (2008) *Commission Regulation N° 429/2008 of 25 April 2008 on detailed rules for the implementation of Regulation (EC) No 1831/2003 of the European Parliament and of the Council as regards the preparation and the presentation of applications and the assessment and the authorisation of feed additives*, 22.5.2008 L 133/1 http://eur-lex.europa.eu/en/index.htm

EC (2009) *Regulation N° 767/2009 of the European Parliament and of the Council of 13 July 2009 on the placing on the market and use of feed, amending European Parliament and Council Regulation (EC) No 1831/2003 and repealing Council Directive 79/373/EEC, Commission Directive 80/511/ EEC, Council Directives 82/471/EEC, 83/228/EEC, 93/74/EEC, 93/113/EC and 96/25/EC and Commission Decision*, 2004/217/EC, 1.9.2009 L229/1, http://eur-lex.europa.eu/en/index.htm

EC (2010) *Commission Regulation N° 1117/2010 of 2 December 2010 concerning the authorisation of a preparation of citric acid, sorbic acid, thymol and vanillin as a feed additive for weaned piglets (holder of the authorisation Vetagro SpA)*, 3.12.2010 L317/3 http://eur-lex.europa.eu/en/index.htm

EC (2011) *Europe in figures: Eurostat yearbook 2011*, Publications Office for the European Union, Luxembourg. ISSN 1681 4789

ECDC/EMEA (2009) *ECDC/EMEA Joint Technical Report: The Bacterial Challenge: time to react*, ECDC/EMEA Joint Working Group, Stockholm.

EFSA (2010) Panel on Additives and Products or Substances used in Animal Feed (FEEDAP); *Scientific Opinion on Safety and efficacy of AviPlus®* as feed additive for weaned piglets, EFSA Journal 2010; 8(6):1633. [15 pp.]. doi:10.2903/j.efsa.2010.1633. Available online: http://www.efsa.europa.eu

EFSA (2012a) Panel on Biological Hazards (BIOHAZ); *Scientific Opinion on a review on the European Union Summary reports on trends and sources zoonoses, zoonotic agents and food-borne outbreaks in 2009 and 2010 – specifically for the data on Salmonella, Campylobacter, verotoxigenic Escherichia coli, Listeria monocytogenes and foodborne outbreaks*, EFSA Journal 2012;10(6):2726 [25 pp.] doi:10.2903/j.efsa.2012.2726. Available online: http://www.efsa.europa.eu/efsajournalEFSA (2012b) Panel on Additives and Products or Substances used in Animal Feed (FEEDAP); *Guidance on the assessment of bacterial susceptibility to antimicrobials of human and veterinary importance*, EFSA Journal 2012;10(6):2740. [10 pp.] doi:10.2903/j.efsa.2012.2740. Available online: www.efsa.europa.eu/ efsajournal

EURL (2007) *Newsletter N°2 June 2007*, CRA-W Gembloux

Eurostat (2009) *Annual data on causes of death: standardized death rate per 100,000 inhabitants* http://appsso.eurostat.ec.europa.eu/nui/ [Last updated on 27/07/2012]

FAO (2008) *The State of Food Insecurity in the World*, Food and Agriculture Organisation of the United Nations, Rome. ISBN 978-92-5-106049-0

Grove-White, D. and Murray, R. (2009) Veterinary Medicines: Use of antimicrobials, *Veterinary Record*, **164**, 727 doi:10.1136/vr.164.23.727

McKenna, M. (2011) *New antibiotics: Not many and fewer all the time* [Internet] http://www.wired.com/wiredscience/2011/02/not-many-antibiotics/

Persoons, D., Haesebrouck, F., Smet, A., Herman, L., Heyndrickx, M., Martel, A., Catry, B., Berge, A.C., Butaye, P. and Dewulf, J. (2011) Risk factors for ceftiofur resistance in Escherichia coli from Belgian broilers. *Epidemiology and Infection,* **139**, 765-771 doi:10.1017/S0950268810001524

Piva, A., Pizzamiglio, V., Morlacchini, M., Tedeschi, M. and Piva, G. (2007) Lipid microencapsulation allows slow release of organic acids and natural identical flavors along the swine intestine, *Journal of Animal Science.* **85**, 486–493.

Scientific Committee on Emerging and Newly Identified health risks (SCENIHR) (2006) Opinion on *The Safety of Human-derived Products with regard to Variant Creutzfeldt-Jakob Disease* SCENIHR/005/06

Weese, J. S. and van Duijkeren, E. (2010) Methicillin-resistant Staphylococcus aureus and Staphylococcus pseudintermedius in veterinary medicine. *Journal of Veterinary Microbiology,* **140**, 418-429 doi:10.1016/j.vetmic.2009.01.039

WHO (2008) *Global burden of disease: 2004 update,* WHO Press, Geneva.

8

THE IMPACT OF BIOFUELS ON THE SUPPLY OF ANIMAL FEED RAW MATERIALS

N. WOOLF

AB Agri, 64 Innovation Way, Lynchwood, Peterborough, PE2 6FL, UK

Introduction

Much has been written and discussed concerning the various effects of Biofuels production. The intention of this paper is to provide an overview of the development of global Biofuels and an assessment of the effect of Biofuel production on the animal feed raw material market. Raw materials that are used either as Biofuel Feedstock as well as those becoming available as Biofuel Co-products are covered.

The global Biofuel industry has developed over the past couple of decades at differing speeds and on different scales in each continent for a number of reasons including Economic, Environmental and Political.

The definition of biofuel is:

A Gaseous, liquid, or solid substance of biological origin that is used as a fuel

(Collins English Dictionary)

On a more practical level this means a fuel from renewable resources; either ethanol fermentable biomass, from biodiesel from vegetable oil or biogas from the organic decomposition of organic materials. Co-fired biomass can also be included.

Many of these activities have an impact on the availability of animal feed raw materials and, while legislation has been drafted to promote the production of sustainable energy through subsidy support and mandatory schemes, the effect on supply to the animal feed sector in the form of tighter raw material supply lines, lower sitting stocks, broader demand for the portfolio of animal feed products and increased price volatility is perhaps unfairly connected to the growth of biofuels.

The biofuel sector requires input feedstock and mostly produces an output co-product.

EXAMPLE INPUT FEEDSTOCKS

1. Bio-ethanol - Grain, Sugar Beet
2. Bio-diesel – Oil from Rapeseed, Sunflower seed, Soybean and Palm fruit
3. Biogas – Any anaerobic digestible raw material, including Maize Silage and Food and Drink production 'co-products'
4. Biomass combustion – Any product with economically viable calorific value for use in either co-firing or dedicated biomass facilities. Current inputs include amongst others, Palm Kernel expellers, Olive Pulp pellets and Myscanthas.

EXAMPLE OUTPUT CO-PRODUCTS

- Bioethanol – (Distillers Dried Grains and Solubles ,Vinasses, Gluten Feed where the plant has been adapted for a wet milling process for vital gluten removal)
- Biodiesel – Rapeseed, Sunflower and Soybean meals. Palm Kernel Expeller
- Biogas – Digestate (Fertiliser)
- Biomass – N/A

In order to assess the effect of Biofuels on the supply of animal feed raw materials it is helpful to begin by looking at how Biofuels have evolved over recent years.

History of Biofuel

Biofuels have been in use since wood was first used as a fuel source. Liquid biofuel has been used from the earliest days of automotive industry development with ethanol and peanut oil being used to run petrol and diesel engines. In the main, biofuel development has taken place in a reactionary way. The Brazilian Ethanol industry developed during the 1970s as a result of the oil crisis. More recently, energy security drove growth in the US ethanol industry and greenhouse gas reduction targets became a significant driver for EU biofuel growth.

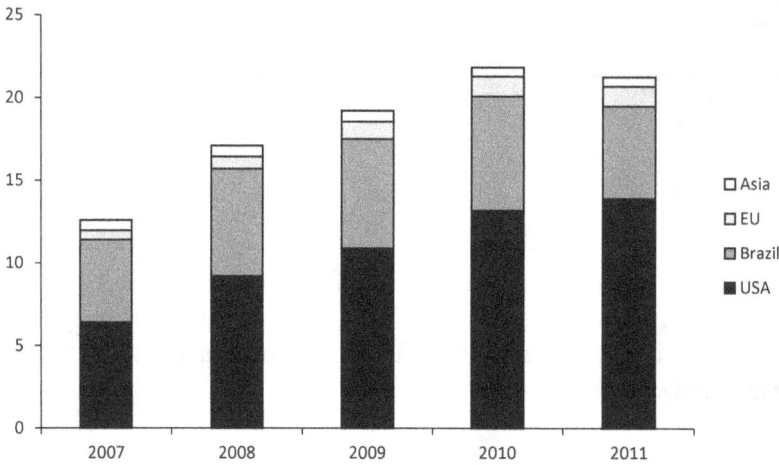

Figure 1 The balance of production by continent, emphasising the dominance of Brazil and USA as the major ethanol producers.(Units: Millions US Gallons per year)

Grain for Bio ethanol

In order to meet 2020 sustainability targets, ethanol production will require around 360 million tonnes of grain or grain equivalent. As an indication, total grain production in 2012/13 according to International Grain Council estimates as at April 2012 is due at 1.9 billion tonnes. If one assumes that global grain production improves only slightly, nearly 20% of all production will be required for ethanol production.

Table 1: World Grain production (million/t)

	08/09	*09/10*	*10/11*	*11/12*	*12/13**
Wheat	685	679	653	696	681
Maize	800	820	828	864	900
Other	317	300	272	281	295
Total	1802	1799	1753	1841	1876

*Projection

According to Global Market Analysis (Nov 2011), of the total 2011/2012 wheat production of 691 million tonnes, 131 million tonnes (11%) was forecast to go into 'other uses' including predominantly ethanol production.

Table 2: Global Market Analysis (Nov 2011) Wheat usage- million/t

Wheat	09/10	10/11	11/12
Total Utilisation	657	667	687
Food	464	469	474
Feed	120	124	131
Other	73	75	77

Of total 2011/2012 coarse grain production of 1151 million tonnes, 317 million tonnes (28%) was forecast to go into 'other uses', including a significant proportion into ethanol production. Around 40% of all maize grown in the USA is now used in the production of ethanol (around 130 million/t).

Table 3: Global Market Analysis (Nov 2011) Coarse grains usage- million/t

Coarse Grains	09/10	10/11	11/12
Total Utilisation	1127	1145	1155
Food	192	199	201
Feed	635	632	637
Other	300	314	317

Bioethanol (Brazil)

As indicated previously, commercial use of ethanol is not new. Mass production of ethanol began in earnest in the 1970s in Brazil using sugar cane. Brazilians had been blending small quantities of ethanol with imported gasoline until the 1973 oil crisis focused efforts toward increasing the production of ethanol. Today, Brazil remains the second largest producer of ethanol and for the time being the largest exporter. Figure 2 shows how the ethanol market has evolved in Brazil with the number of vehicles running on pure Ethanol and more recently as flex fuel vehicles (with both ethanol and gasoline reservoirs) increasing dramatically to become a large majority of all light vehicles on Brazilian roads today.

In Brazil, ethanol is produced for energy security and economic reasons rather than environmental sustainability. With Brazil having large scale availability of sugar cane, production costs are usually amongst the lowest in the world. Since 2008, high demand for sugar has dented the competitiveness of Brazilian ethanol, causing production to drop 20% in 2011. For the first time since the 1990s ethanol was imported from the USA and many flex fuel car drivers switched to using gasoline. As of early 2012, year on year production of ethanol in Brazil is 40% down.

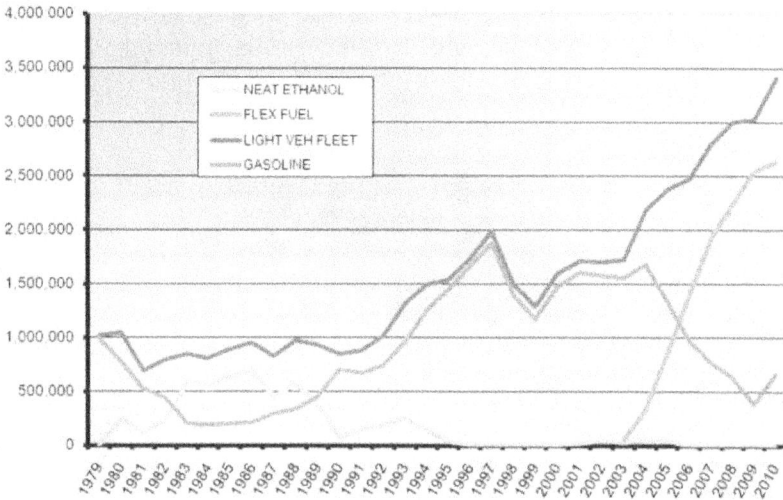

Figure 2 (Courtesy of ANFAVEA Brazil, 2010) – Ethanol/Gasoline/Flex-fuel balance in Brazilian Light Vehicle Fleet by year

The evolution of the Brazilian ethanol industry had limited impact on the supply of animal feed as the processing of sugar cane does not result in any significant animal feed co-product. The main co-products are cane debris, stalk and pulp which are possible feed stock for combustion purposes.

Bioethanol USA

Since 2005, the USA has become the world's largest producer of ethanol fuel. By 2010 the USA was producing nearly 50 billion litres of fuel and together with Brazil accounted for around 88% of global production. In the USA, the product is used predominantly in low level blends into conventional engine type vehicles and production is mainly from maize, with some wheat used in more northerly states. The supply of ethanol into the US gasoline market is currently around 10% having increased 1500% between 1990 and 2010.

The industry has grown massively since 2000, driven by federal legislation aimed at reducing oil consumption and enhancing energy security. As maize is the main feedstock, some of the challenges relate to the balance between production energy and its social and economic impacts. The increase in production of distillers dried grains and solubles (DDGS) from maize ethanol has had a huge impact on feeding livestock in the USA with demand for over 40% of the corn crop to be processed for Ethanol. As shown in Figure 3, US ethanol production is not purely about meeting requirements for energy security; it is a product openly traded in the global market, mainly to Brazil, with some being bought into the EU. However, the exported volume is still less than 10% of the overall volume produced.

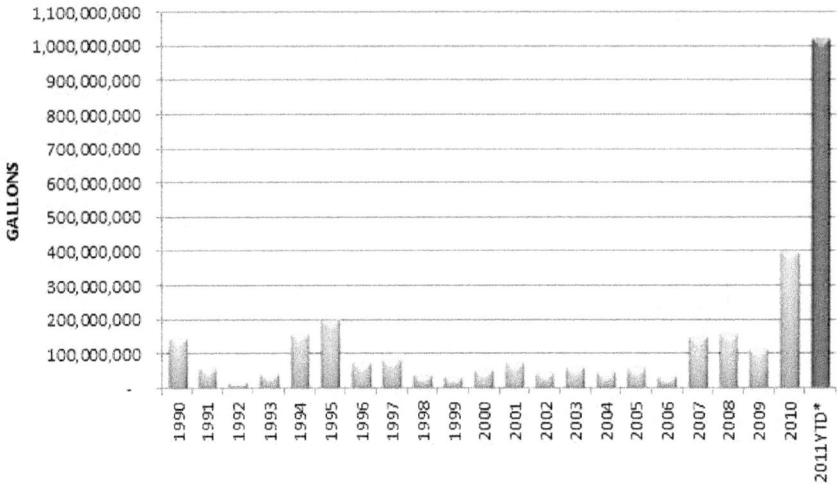

Figure 3 The growth in export of U.S. Ethanol (Courtesy of US Grains Council)

The huge increase in the availability of DDGS has seen a large scale switch from feeding maize to feeding DDGS, mainly to Cattle. The US Grains council has worked successfully to raise the profile of maize DDGS over recent years and to open up new markets for the product (see Table 4: US DDGS exports). Due to lower transport costs, Canada and Mexico utilise large volumes but large quantities are also exported to Asia. However, political interference in natural market flow has occurred in the Chinese market where imports have fallen due to internal lobbying from domestic DDGS producers suggesting such imports are undermining their own markets. A further challenge to the emerging DDGS export market has been seen in Europe where GM approval delays cause US produced DDGS to be a risky import option for a European shipper.

Against this backdrop, the US DDGS export market has developed sufficiently well and internal understanding and demand for the products has improved greatly. The economics of selling maize for ethanol and buying back higher protein DDGS nutrition has proven to be a convincing proposition to such an extent that whereas prior to 2009 US DDGS would usually trade at a significant discount into EU markets, there now exists in the main, virtual price parity between EU and US origin DDGS.

Table 4: Top 15 importers of US DDGS 2011 (Courtesy of US Grains Council)

Country	2010 YR	2011 YR	Jan/Feb 2011	Jan/Feb 2012	% Change	Net change
World total	9,027,043	7,649,202	1,333,778	1,219,281	-9	-114,497
Mexico	1,650,308	1,780,736	325,556	313,699	-4	-11,857
China	2,531,452	1,389,068	240,454	254,195	6	13,741
Canada	1,042,215	737,689	162,156	109,780	-32	-52,376
Vietnam	430,236	499,523	76,249	89,477	17	13,228
Japan	217,780	301,234	34,918	74,091	112	39,173
Korea, South	506,474	295,134	10,572	55,941	429	45,369
Indonesia	251,073	248,381	31,761	29,929	-6	-1,832
Taiwan	144,485	235,226	22,076	34,447	56	12,371
Israel	162,695	214,074	37,315	6,033	-84	-31,282
Thailand	291,070	203,152	54,628	25,031	-54	-29,597
Ireland	275,068	177,048	48,748	-	-100	-48,748
Morocco	133,135	168,284	25,858	12,939	-50	-12,919
Philippines	112,052	145,915	21,513	40,369	88	18,856
UK	115,860	122,501	22,364	-	-100	-22,364
Spain	39,893	120,221	36,379	-	-100	-36,379

Figure 4 clearly indicates DDGS and maize prices have moved upward since 2009 and this has driven a longer term development for US DDGS co-products as an economic alternative to feeding maize. In Europe, where feed compound manufacturers promote use of a broader range of raw materials, the correlation between grain and DDGS prices is less strong. Here, DDGS prices are predominantly valued for their protein content and as such are linked with other protein alternatives including rape meal, sunflower meal and soya bean meal.

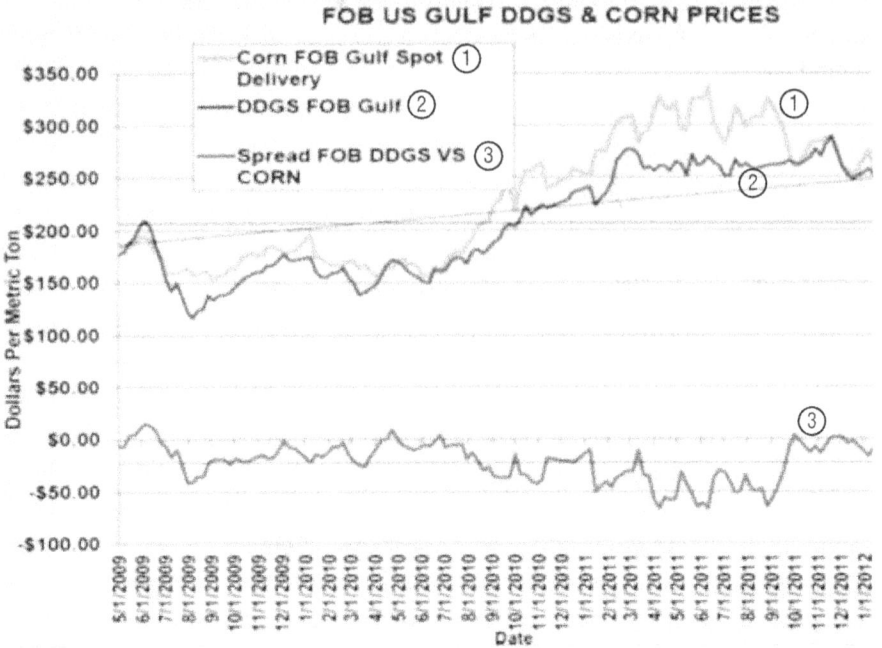

Figure 4 Correlation between USA DDGS and Maize (Corn) prices (Courtesy of US Grains Council)

Bioethanol Europe

Developing only slightly behind the US ethanol industry, the far smaller EU bioethanol industry grew from a need for environmental protection, sustainable development, increased energy security, and the creation of jobs and growth for the European economy. Based upon both the 2003 Biofuels directive and the 2009 Renewable Energy Directive (RED) but also influenced by the Directive on Fuel Quality Standards, the original 2003 directive, since 2011 has been replaced by RED. This introduces a mandatory use of renewable energy in the EU transport sector. Each EU state has issued national renewable energy action plans on how they will achieve their targets by 2020. The plans are broadly road maps showing how each nation intends to include renewable transport fuel up to a level of 10% by 2020. In the UK, the ratio of biodiesel to bioethanol use is approximately 3:2.

In Europe, most commercially produced ethanol is derived from cereal including wheat, maize, barley, triticale and sorghum. In addition ethanol from sugar beet developed as the EU sugar industry was subject to quota reduction as part of the 2006 sugar reform trade agreement. This led to rationalisation of the European sugar industry. A mandated requirement for renewable transport fuel has allowed for surplus sugar quota beet crops to be diverted to fermentation for ethanol. Many European sugar operations will produce ethanol from beet production and a number have also been involved in the development of larger grain to ethanol plants.

With cheaper imports from Brazil and USA as well as high grain prices the economic conditions for ethanol production in Europe have been challenging and over the past 18 months several producers of grain ethanol have reduced or completely halted production. Figure 5 shows how EU production has increased since 2004.

EU ethanol production for fuel
Million litres

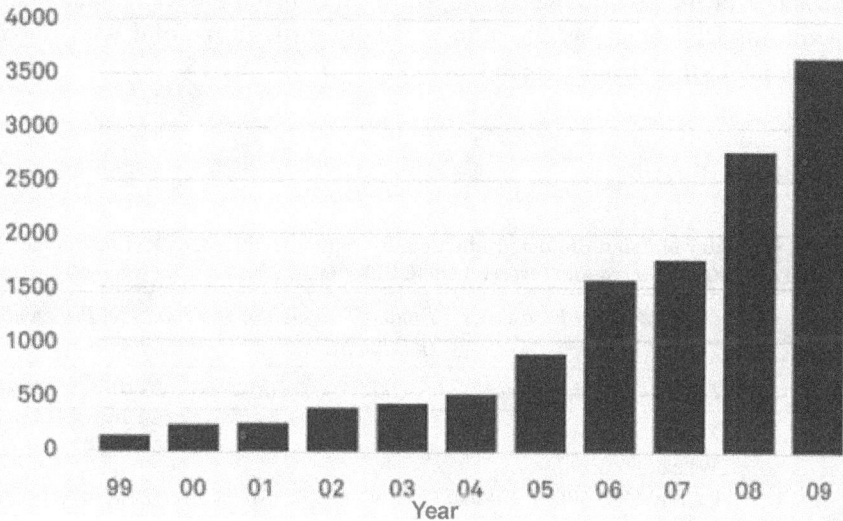

Figure 5 Increase in EU Ethanol production since 1999 (Courtesy of ePURE)

EU biofuel production is mainly in the form of biodiesel (75%). Production of ethanol lags behind and in 2009 was only 10% of that in the US. Further investment in EU ethanol is at present unforthcoming with only 960 million litre of capacity under construction (nearly 50% of which is a single facility, Vivergo Fuels).

The co-product from sugar to ethanol conversion is vinasses and this is mainly for use as a fertiliser. The co-product from grain ethanol is essentially a concentrated form of feed protein usually sold as DDGS but in some cases combining Ethanol with other wet milling processes such as vital gluten removal to produce a dry gluten feed, wheat bran, liquid or moist feed.

The availability of EU origin DDGS has increased since 2005 but volumes are still very modest in comparison with Rape meal or imported Soy Bean, the knowledge of how to use DDGS products across Europe is improving. DDGS has historically been fed to ruminant animals, but more recently has found its way into a selection of mono-gastric diets. The expectation of a 'wave' of new protein in the form of DDGS has potentially been over emphasised. As some of the utilised production capacity results in Vinasses as co-product, the volume of DDGS is actually quite low with production of around 2 million tonnes estimated for 2012. This comes a poor second to the volume of rape meal produced as a co-product to bio diesel production. Other co-products from Bio-ethanol include moist feedstuffs at DMs of around 30% as well as Wheat based syrups at around 24%DM which have found ready on farm markets as well as appeal into Anaerobic Digestion.

During the early period of EU Biofuel DDGS production, a significant percentage was exported from the original producer country. As knowledge and acceptance of the product has improved; local demand has increased. A strong appetite for DDGS in the UK is increasingly difficult to fulfil with imported product due to this strong demand.

Bioethanol in Asia

Table 5. Summary of Asian Biofuel production, by volume and feedstock (Courtesy of OECD:FAO 2008, Mibrant and Overend 2008, Eider et al. 2008)

Country	Currently used Feedstocks		Ethanol Production (million litres)		Biodiesel Production (million litres)	
	Ethanol	*Biodiesel*	*2007*	*2008*	*2007*	*2008*
China	Maize, Wheat, Cassava	Waste Veg Oil	5564	6686	355	355
India	Molasses	Jatropha	2450	2562	45	317
Indonesia	Molasses, Cassava	CPO	177	212	241	753
Malaysia	None	CPO	63	70	217	643
Philippines	Sugarcane	Coconut Oil	62	105	257	211
Thailand	Molasses, Cassava	CPO, Waste Veg Oil	285	408	0	48
Vietnam	Molasses, Cassava	Animal Fat, Used Veg Oil	140	164	0	0
Total			8741	10207	1115	1772

Many Asian countries have set targets and mandates to increase biofuels production but, despite this demand growth, trade tariffs and lack of surplus feedstock production have kept production relatively low in comparison with USA and

Brazil. In Asia, only China is a large scale producer of Ethanol from Grain, with China's contribution to world Biofuel production in 2008 around 3%. The majority of DDGS production is either used internally or exported for use in Japan. The growth in bioethanol production is likely to be far outstripped by the increase in Asian demand for road transport fuel. According to the United States Agency for International Development paper on Biofuels in Asia, large scale production of biofuels is unlikely to make a significant contribution to Asia's future energy demand. Even with rapid up-scaling of first generation biofuel as well as with development and commercialisation of cellulosic ethanol production, biofuel production will potentially account only for 3-14 % of the transport fuel mix.

Bioethanol summary

Development of first generation biofuels has been slower in the UK than much of the rest of Europe, US and Brazil. The most significant change in animal feed raw material availability is the USA market in which a radical transformation has taken place with farmers switching between feeding maize and feeding DDGS. The export market for US maize DDGS worldwide has grown with the exception of the EU and globalisation of commodity prices has allowed for US DDGS to be exported at credible market values rather than sold as a distressed material as was the case in the 1990s and early 2000s.

EU Bioethanol production has grown on a far smaller scale and the extra availability of DDGS and similar co-products has not significantly impacted the overall EU feed raw material market. DDGS producers currently price the product in close correlation to rape seed meal.

Looking back to the early 2000s, there was an expectation that second generation biofuels would have become commercially viable by 2012. A viable cellulosic industry is closer than ever and production of Biobutanol has become a reality in the US but the continued reliance on wheat and maize for ethanol has called into question the reality of achieving the 2020 target of 10% of all road transport fuel to be derived from sustainable/ renewable sources. The RTFO target will be reviewed in 2014 and, as a consequence, we will have a clearer direction on the future development of, and investment in, the biofuels sector.

Biodiesel

Biodiesel is a renewable fuel produced mainly from vegetable oils such as rapeseed oil, sunflower seed oil, soybean oil and palm fruit/kernel oil as well as from used frying oils or animal fats. According to Hamburg based Oil World Journal, in 2008 global production of all oils and fats stood at 160 million tonnes, of which palm oil and palm kernel oil stood at 48 million tonnes (30%) of output, followed by soybean oil at 37 million tonnes (23%) of output.

The EU produces over 50% of global biodiesel mostly from oilseed rape and sunflower as well as some imported soyabean. Production of Biodiesel in the EU has been popular for a number of reasons not least the strong demand platform for such product in the EU but also the relative ease for which biodiesel can used as a pure fuel form or in combination with existing diesel engines in a blend. Biodiesel helps meet emission reduction targets and the oilseed required for production is also seen as an attractive crop as it can be grown on set aside land. Biodiesel production currently uses around 3 million hectares of European land. There are currently around 254 plants in the EU producing around 9.57 million tonnes of biodiesel annually, with Germany the highest producer at 2.86 million tonnes (2010, European Biodiesel Board). However, there exists a large amount of biodiesel production overcapacity with capacity for approximately 22.1 million tonnes of biodiesel production.

Biodiesel production requires a lower level of investment than bio ethanol and many oilseed crush and esterification facilities have been set up in the last 10-12 years. Growth in production of biodiesel in the EU has led to an increase in the availability of rape meal and sunflower meal over recent years.

EU Rapeseed production increased dramatically during the years 2002 to 2010 (ADM 2010). In a typical year a crush of 23 million tonnes of rapeseed will see around 70% used for biodiesel and around 30% for food use. The opportunity for growth in use of rapeseed meal into animal feed in Europe has been far larger than that of DDGS despite the global market for ethanol far outstripping that of biodiesel.

Figure 6 shows the increase in UK rapeseed meal usage in animal feed, reflecting a large increase in usage of the product but not in proportion to the increase in the volume of EU Rapeseed grown. Figure 7.

In summary, biodiesel production is focused in Europe, although US production in 2011 was greater than that of Germany, Europe's biggest producer, and Argentina is increasing biodiesel production from soybean annually. Both US and Argentine production has resulted in significant extra quantities of soybean meal and soya hulls for animal feed, although increased demand has made this increase less apparent. In Asia and Africa, the opportunity for biodiesel is linked to development of new crops such as Jatropha and, as with other crushed oilseeds, the remaining pressed cake can be considered for co-firing or as an animal feed. Less than 5% of palm oil is used in biodiesel but a significant proportion of the South East Asian palm pressed cake and expeller is exported for use as animal feed and for co-firing purposes. Use of palm kernel expeller has increased significantly in Europe.

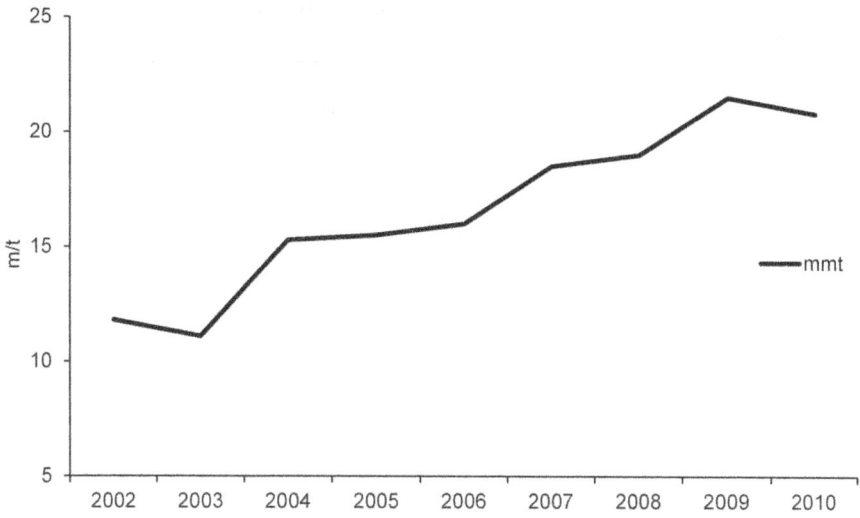

Figure 6 Increase in volume of Rapeseed grown in EU (millions/t) (Courtesy of ADM)

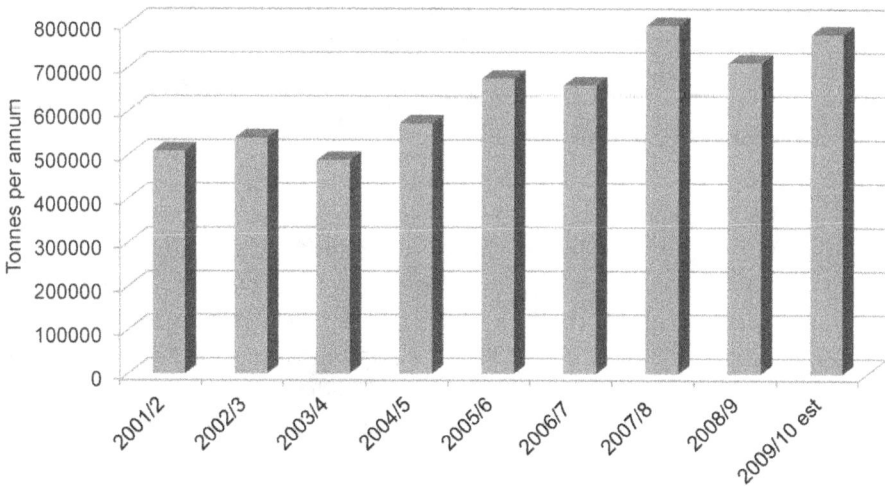

Figure 7 Increase in use of Rapeseed Meal in the UK (Courtesy of ADM)

Table 6. Volumes of Biodiesel by major producer country (Courtesy of European Biodiesel Board)

Production of Biodiesel in 2009 m/litres		%
Germany	2859	16
France	2206	12
US	2060	11
Brazil	1535	9
Argentina	1340	7
Spain	967	5
Italy	830	5
Thailand	610	3
Belgium	468	3
Poland	374	2
Netherlands	364	2
Austria	349	2
China	338	2
Columbia	330	2
S Korea	300	2
Others	2998	17
Total	**17929**	**100%**

Biogas (Anaerobic digestion)

Almost any organic material can be processed through Anaerobic Digestion (AD). Materials with high gas yields are the most attractive. A high gas yield is much sought after for use commercially for conversion to electricity in a low carbon way thus attracting subsidy through ROCS or equivalent certificates or selling to the national grid through feed in tariffs. The original purpose of AD was to utilise waste or to process co-products. The breadth of feedstock has increased with time as the right of combination of ingredients in order to achieve the best and most constant yield are sought.

Aside from biogas, the other outputs of AD are digestate (for use as soil conditioner) and water.

AD Feedstock

The AD will typically utilise biodegradable waste materials but also specially grown energy crops such as maize silage as well as sugar beet, stock feeds and brewing, distilling and sugar industry feed co-products. Fermentation co-products that stimulate rumen bacteria are thought to have a similar positive effect in an AD.

Biomass (Co-Firing)

In autumn 2011, The UK Department for Energy and Climate change issued a consultation document on proposals for levels of banded support under the renewable obligation for the period 2013-2017. Still focused on the 2020 renewable target, the specific objective of the consultation is to support cheapest existing technology such as coal to biomass conversion and co-firing. The government is set to introduce a 1 ROC enhanced co-firing band so that some of the larger coal generators are able to switch partly to biomass. In order to benefit from this support, generators would need to be co-firing at least 15% of their generation. Existing producers are shelving plans to build further dedicated biomass facilities such as the Drax facility in Yorkshire and focus on increasing co-firing renewables with coal in existing facilities.

Supply sources/Feedstock for this type of energy generation include forestry by-products, agricultural residuals such as straw, husks, kernels and perennial energy crops (Myscanthas). Other imported crops such as palm kernel and olive pulp cake are also widely used. The overwhelming majority of co-firing feedstock is currently imported and this looks set to continue. Sustainable sourcing will be part of the audit criteria, but as yet, there is no clarification on how this encompasses utilisation of what might currently be seen as animal feed.

Effect of Biofuels on grain and protein supply

The existing assumption that the emergence of UK bioethanol will result in an abundance of protein feed in the form of DDGS can be expanded to encompass all protein produced globally from processing grain into ethanol as well as high protein oilseed meals. On a local level, the increased demand for grain into Northern England ethanol plants would wipe out any exportable surplus from the UK crop and create an environment of higher grain prices, especially in the North. Regional grain premiums will adjust to extra local demand. With oilseed crush plants in Liverpool and Hull, the North of England and two large ethanol facilities, the availability of mid protein feed in the North of England will be strong.

However, this is a local outlook and the increased availability of all feed proteins on a global scale has been outstripped by increased demand. The US farmer has shown the flexibility to switch between feeding DDGS and maize. It would be hasty to conclude that grain will become more expensive and proteins become cheaper because all feed commodities are increasingly volatile. One thing is fairly certain, the farmer growing grain, soybean or oilseed has an optimistic economic outlook.

Returning to the local outlook, the UK is still hugely reliant on imported proteins as shown in Table 7

Table 7. Annual quantity of Feed Protein used in the UK (HGCA Feediol 2010/2011)

Product	Imports (kt)	Domestic (kt)	Europe (kt)	Usage
Sunflower	354	0	0	354
Rape meal	212	1071	130	1153
Peas and beans		322	205	117
Low pro soya	50			50
UK distillers		300	18	282
EU distillers	153			153
US distillers	134			134
EU gluten	37			37
US gluten	284			284
Mid protein total	1224	1693	353	2564
Soya bean meal	2289	493	68	2714
Total protein market	3513	2186	421	5278

Extra protein produced from UK biofuel can only partly mitigate the effect of an Increase in competition for the UK's share of protein imports.

An obvious effect of stronger price is food price inflation. During the past 30 years in Western Europe, particularly in the UK, the share of income going into food spend has decreased from around 17% in 1987 down to below 10% around 2009.

The initial perception is that food price inflation has been held in check by large retailer competition and a squeeze on producer and processor margins. More recently, as supply lines in general become tighter the seller has been in a stronger position to find a more profitable market. The retailer has passed on higher prices to the consumer. In the UK the % spend on food has increased recently but price inflation, whilst very real, is not likely to cause food riots even with today's austere economic backdrop. However, it is worth noting that UK food inflation (OECD Mar

11) at 6.3%, is three times higher than other G7 nations. 'Global concerns' were stated by the big 4 food retailers.

For a very real food inflation example it is worth looking to China (The Atlantic – Jul 2011). In 2010, inflation in China stood at a high of 6.4%. Within this number, food inflation stood at 14.4% and within that, pork inflation stood at 57%. The Chinese are the second largest consumers of pork per head in the world after Germany. The Chinese pig sector is highly fragmented with numerous small pig farmers highly sensitive to market fluctuations and prices. In the summer of 2009, pork prices were low so farmers slaughtered breeding sows resulting in a dearth of pork and higher prices. A highly volatile feed commodity market for the pig farmer will not have aided a decision based on the longer term outlook.

The examples of the UK and China, whilst very different and slightly away from the main theme, highlight that regardless of biofuel, there exists a rapidly changing world raw material supply and demand outlook, of which biofuels play only a part. The influence of fund speculators who buy into and sell feed commodities is of greater influence on market volatility than a user requiring steady and continuous feedstock supply for biofuel.

Conclusion

Biofuels have been developing globally for nearly 20 years. It is in the past 5 years that world prices have become more volatile. Extra demand for raw materials into biofuel and the extra availability of feed co-product from biofuel (DDGS, rape meal, soya meal, sunflower meal, and soya hulls) may be a driver for further improvement in efficient/targeted nutrition, particularly in ruminant animals, with focus on better feed conversion rates.

The breadth of raw materials feed manufacturers have to choose from may narrow as their appeal outside Feed improves, this encompasses dried, liquid and moist animal feed materials.

In Europe the drive to import fewer protein products will continue as the retailer drives the better utilisation of domestically produced co-products at the expense of imported products. However, a strong reliance on imports of soya bean meal should remain.

The grain farmer will undoubtedly become richer as his customer base widens, and land utilisation will increase alongside improved crop yields. More GM feeds are likely to be accepted into the EU supply chain as Non GM segregation becomes uneconomic.

The increased volatility in feed and grain markets in recent years has co-incided with the emergence of consistent global commodity prices. Whether competing for raw materials for feed or for biofuel the world market has evolved into one with very few regional anomalies and as such the cost of raw material supply into feed around the world looks set to remain globally consistent and transparent.

Bibliography

Associacao Nacional dos Fabricantes de Veiculos Automotores (2010) - Brazilian vehicles sales by fuel type.

Department for Energy and Climate Change (2012) Consultation on proposals for the levels of banded support under the Renewables Obligation for the period 2013-2017 and the Renewables Obligation order Page 58-67.

EPure (2012), EU Ethanol production for fuel www.epure.org

European Biodiesel Board (2010) *European Biodiesel Production*

Fediol (2010) Statistics – Meals – Production, imports, exports and consumption.

Food and Agriculture Organisation (May 2012), *Food Outlook Report.*

Lichts, F.O. (2010) *Industry Statistics 2010. World Fuel Ethanol Production.* Renewable Fuels Association

USDA (2012) US Grains Council, Mar 2012-07-23

9

GLOBAL FOOD SECURITY IN AN ERA OF CLIMATE CHANGE: IMPACT UPON ANIMALS AND THEIR UTILISATION

MARGARET GILL

Aberdeen Centre for Environmental Sustainability, University of Aberdeen, 23 St Machar Drive, AB24 3UU

Introduction

One of the greatest challenges in identifying actions to achieve global food security is how to increase food production with minimal damage to the environment and in particular, with reduced greenhouse gas emissions. This is particularly true for livestock.

The publication of 'Livestock's Long Shadow' (Steinfeld et al., 2006) led to a considerable increase in negative media reports about livestock (Anderson, Gundel and Vanni, 2010) and contributed to calls for people to decrease meat consumption (e.g. Paul McCartney's Meat Free Mondays campaign (http://www.youtube.com/watch?v=34ZlshYwby8) as a means of decreasing greenhouse gas emissions. The number of negative reports appeared to peak in 2009 (Anderson et al., 2010) and the scientific quality of the debate on the web and in scientific papers has improved in recent years. Amongst other seminal publications in 2009 and onwards, FAO published Livestock in the Balance, in 2009 (FAO, 2009), which both highlighted the complexity of the issues facing the livestock sector, and also encouraged a realistic and equitable approach to identifying solutions.

What still receives insufficient attention in that debate, however, is the presentation of data on livestock disaggregated between ruminants and monogastric species, let alone consideration of the pros and cons of different livestock systems. The problem is global, but many of the solutions can only be implemented at the farm level. Feed companies know better than most that ruminants can produce meat and milk without grain, while monogastric species have been bred for fast growth on cereal-based diets. Animal scientists know full well that monogastrics produce relatively low levels of greenhouse gases, yet even within these expert

163

communities, too often we use the generic term 'livestock' rather than take the time and make the effort to consider these very different effects. Feeding more grain to ruminants is unlikely to increase net food production, yet it decreases greenhouse gas emissions, while producing ruminant products from grass makes a very strong net contribution to food production, but produces more greenhouse gases per MJ of product. Decision-makers (from farm to government level) need evidence to evaluate these 'trade-offs'; i.e. the likely impacts on the environment of decisions to improve food production, and the likely impacts on food production of decisions to protect the environment. The animal science community has a key role to play in ensuring the adequacy of that evidence. The risks of not taking action to protect the environment were quantified by Rockstrom et al. (2009) who proposed nine planetary boundaries (of which they quantified seven), the crossing of which could trigger abrupt environmental change.

The aim of this paper is to challenge the animal science/feed communities to inject some more evidence-based science into the debate on the role of livestock in contributing to global food security by presenting more data for livestock species separately, and indeed to quantify the trade-offs between livestock production and the contribution of livestock to crossing at least four of those boundaries (climate change, biogeochemical cycles, biodiversity and land use change). The point is made by looking back in time at firstly global and secondly UK trends in the supply of different livestock products, with a final section on the risks and opportunities for feed supply, but since there have been multiple interpretations of what food security means, the next section sets the context, by considering how food security is measured.

Food security in an inter-connected world

At the Food Summit in 1996, the UN defined food security as:

> *"Food security exists when all people, at all times, have physical and economic access to sufficient, safe and nutritious food to meet their dietary needs and food preferences for an active and healthy life"*

This definition has many facets and thus many different indicators are needed to assess progress, but the target agreed by 189 world leaders in 2000 is contained within the first Millennium Development Goal (http://www.undp.org/content/undp/en/home/mdgoverview.html) namely to:

> *"Reduce by half the proportion of people who suffer from hunger "*

taking 1990 as the baseline and with the target to be achieved by 2015.

In 2000, that looked like an achievable goal as the number of people suffering from severe malnutrition was on a downward trajectory between 1969-71 (893 million) and 1990/92 (842 million), but the number remained close to 840 million in 2000-2002, and the food price spikes of 2007/08 moved the trajectory in a rather different direction. The concept that the world might not be able to feed its growing population made a re-appearance in the media and re-energised the community of scientists involved in food production. The solution to global food security in the 21st century, however, is not just about producing more food, but about understanding the very complex food system which has evolved in recent decades. Global food retail sales were estimated at ~US$ 4 trillion in 2009 by the United States Department for Agriculture (http://www.ers.usda.gov/Briefing/GlobalFoodMarkets/Industry.htm) illustrating that food security is closely tied to global economic health and indeed to the cost of energy. The drivers for the food price spike of 2007/08 were thus stated to include: an increase in energy prices and regulatory changes encouraging the use of crops for biofuel production, in addition to a series of poor wheat harvests in e.g. Australia and a decrease in commodity stocks (Foresight, 2011a).

This recognition of the complexity of the food system and of the potential future risks to food prices from the inter-connections between the environment (including climate change) and food production, led to a number of extensive assessments of the pressures on the global food system, to guide decision-makers on what needs to be done now to ensure future food security (e.g. IAASTD, 2009; INRA and CIRAD, 2009; Foresight, 2011b, etc.). Despite the number of authors involved and the recognition of the complexity of the global food system, Wood et al. (2010) concluded that food production was still the dominant process in the analyses. This is not surprising, given the good documentation of the recent history of substantial growth in agricultural production but, as stated by Wood et al. (2010), it was less helpful in defining the appropriate research questions to deliver the evidence required to feed the projected population of ~9 billion in 2050.

Food security: looking back in time

In some respects, agricultural research has been a success story, since during the period from 1969-71 through to 2005-07, global food supply per person increased by 17% (Table 1). This is remarkable given that global population increased from 3.7 billion to 6.7 billion during the same period. This illustrates the tremendous increase in agricultural production during that time period: slightly below a doubling in both gross cereal production (1.221 to 2.287 billion tonnes) and production of meat + milk (494 to 933 million tonnes).

This increase did not, however, result in food security. In 1990/92 840 million were suffering from severe malnutrition, and after the food price spikes of 2007/08, the number of people suffering from severe malnutrition peaked at over 1 billion in 2009, falling back to 925 million in 2010 (http://www.worldhunger.org/articles/Learn/world%20hunger%20facts%202002.htm).

Table 1 Global food supply in kJ and g protein /capita comparing 1969-71 with 2005-07 (FAOSTAT, 2012 accessed May 2012).

	1969-1971	*2005-2007*
Global food supply kJ/capita	9.93	11.63
Global food supply protein/capita	64.3	76.6

This increase in food production, however, resulted in many negative impacts on the environment (see e.g. Tilman, 1999; Hazell and Wood, 2008), with livestock production attracting particular attention (Steinfeld et al 2006), not least in relation to the production of greenhouse gases. Smith et al. (2007) estimated that globally, agriculture directly accounted for 0.12 of human-induced greenhouse gas emissions but adding in the consequences of changing land uses, fuel and fertiliser costs etc raised this to between 0.17 and 0.32 (Bellarby et al. 2008). Livestock are major contributors to the total for agriculture: 0.09 of the 0.12 direct contribution (Smith et al. 2007) and a total of 0.18 of total anthropogenic emissions estimated by Steinfeld et al. (2006).

Such figures understandably make livestock production a target for greenhouse gas emission reduction, but livestock make a major contribution to food security by providing human edible food from the 3.4 billion ha of grazing land (FAOSTAT, 2012) and are an integral part of some existing ecosystems (e.g. Bignal and McCracken, 1996), which may in turn have an impact on wider environmental health and thereby on the sustaining of crop yields in the longer term. In other words, there is no simple solution as to how best to optimise the contribution of livestock to food security, but rather a need to consider the trade-offs between food production and environmental costs. These trade-offs will differ between species and also between production systems (Gill, Smith and Wilkinson, 2010). Estimation of trade-offs requires a more detailed analysis of the issues, which is where the disaggregation of species (beef, pigs, poultry etc.) data becomes significant.

Historical trends in global supply of livestock products

Livestock have a global asset value of at least US$1.4 trillion (Thornton, 2010) and contribute 0.4 of the global value of agricultural output (FAO 2009). At the global level they contributed ~0.17 of total food energy and 0.39 of total food protein supply in 2007 (FAOSTAT, 2012), compared to 0.15 and 0.34 respectively in 1983 (Delgado, 2005). Approximately 0.6 of the rural poor keep livestock (FAO, 2009a) and ~980,000 rural people suffer from extreme poverty (http://www.ifad.org/rpr2011/). Those contributions, however, do not come without a 'cost', both to the environment (e.g. Steinfeld et al., 2006) and in terms of human health, through transmission of disease (Grace and Jones, 2011). Neither of these risk factors is, however, yet systematically translated into costs of production, and globally the demand for livestock products continues to increase (FAO, 2009). The challenge for the livestock sector is how to manage the risks and opportunities. While recognising evidence of links between the consumption of red and/or processed meat and human health (see e.g. systematic reviews by Sandhu, White and McPherson, 2001 and Santarelli, Pierre and Corpet, 2008), the main focus in this paper is on risks (and research opportunities) associated with pressure on feed resources. In recent years less attention has been paid to the ability of livestock (particularly ruminants) to turn protein which is not edible by humans into high quality human edible protein (Oltjen and Beckett, 1996). Thus this paper focuses on data quoted in terms of protein supply, leading to a final discussion on risks and research needs related to the supply of feed protein.

Animal products (in 2007) supplied 0.39 of total protein supply at a global level, of which 0.45 (0.175 of total protein) was in the form of meat, but this average hides a large geographical diversity, with 47 countries where meat supplied <0.1 of dietary protein and 19 where it supplied >0.4 (Figure 1). Of the top 19 meat eating (per capita) countries, beef provided < 0.25 of the meat protein in 6 and over 0.5 in only one (Argentina), again illustrating the variability between countries and the need to consider national data rather than global averages when looking for ways of decreasing the impact of livestock production on the environment.

These levels of per capita protein supply from meat reflect a steady increase in consumption of meat per capita at a global level (Figure 2), which was originally brought to world attention in the 1990s as part of the International Food Policy Research Institute's (IFPRI) 2020 vision project (Delgado et al., 1999). The consumption (per capita) of milk on the other hand has been relatively stable (Figure 2).

FAO Statistics on rates of growth in meat consumption have been much quoted, but too often it is total meat consumption which is quoted, without observing that the upward trend is being driven by increases in the supply (reflecting demand) of pig and poultry meat per capita, while the supply of beef/capita has decreased by ~25% since its peak in the mid 1970s (Figure 3) and supply of mutton and goat meat has hardly changed. Absolute production has of course increased for all species, but most significantly for pigs and poultry (Table 2)

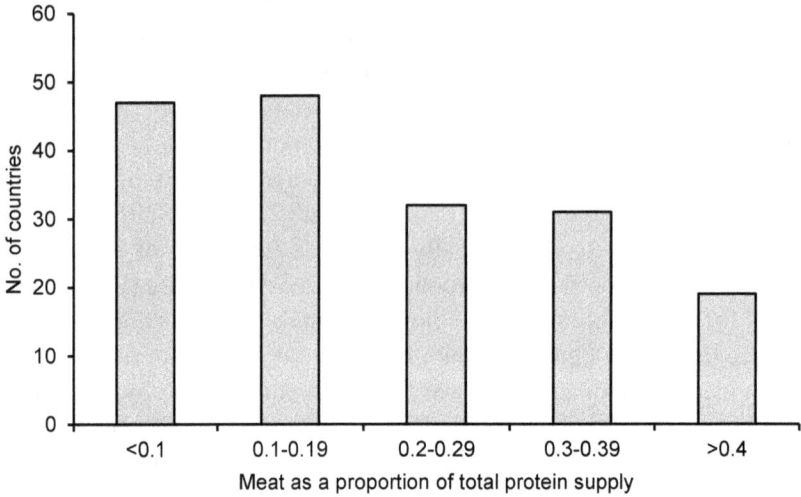

Figure 1 Number of countries (out of total of 177) per category of meat as proportion of total protein supply. (FAOSTAT accessed April and May 2012).

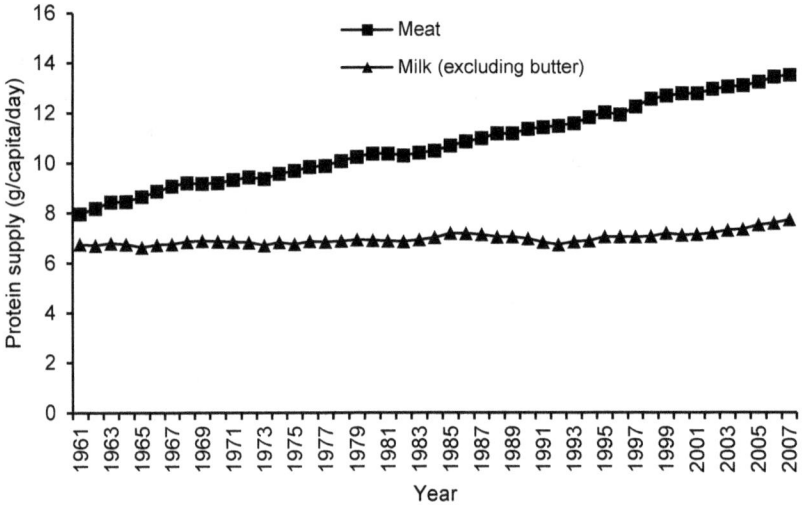

Figure 2 World average supplies of meat and milk (g protein/capita/day) between 1961 and 2007 (FAOSTAT accessed April and May 2012)

This increasing demand for meat from monogastric species (ratio of monogastric meat:ruminant meat has changed from 0.75 in 1961 to 2.0 in 2007) has implications for feed supply, given the greater dependence on grain for feeding monogastric species (compared with ruminants). The CAST report on Animal Agriculture and Global Food Supply published in 1999 gave illustrative diets for beef cattle

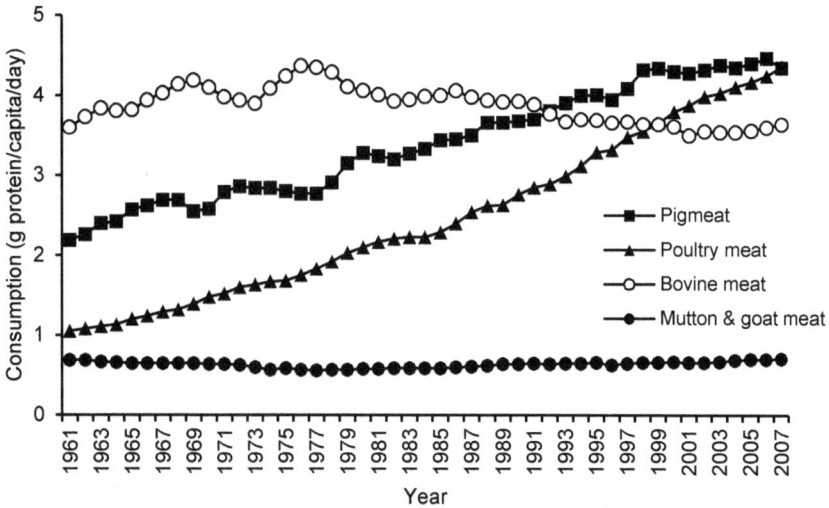

Figure 3 Trends in meat consumption (g protein/capita/day) at a global level between 1961 and 2007 (FAO STAT accessed April and May 2012)

Table 2 Production of meat (million tonnes/yr) from five main species in 1961 and 2007

Species	1961	2007
Cattle meat	27.7	63.3
Mutton and goat	6.0	13.7
Pig meat	24.7	100.0
Poultry meat	9.0	87.9

in the US with significant (47% for California) amounts of components which would not be used for human food, compared to only 18% for pig diets and 32% for broilers. The report also illustrated example components of diets from South Korea, where the use of by-products was considerably higher, resulting in higher efficiencies of both energy and protein use when expressed purely in terms of the efficiency of use of those feed dietary components which could have been used directly by humans for food (Table 3).

What Table 3 shows is the increasing risk of competition with humans for feed components as the trend towards greater consumption of pig and poultry meat continues, with the potential for decreasing dependence if the use of by-products and other non-human edible components of feeds can be increased. The benefits of ruminants in relation to less use of grain need to be balanced, however, against

Table 3 Efficiencies of feed protein use by different species in the US and South Korea (from CAST, 1999)

	USA		South Korea	
	Gross efficiency	*Human edible efficiency*	*Gross efficiency*	*Human edible efficiency*
Beef	0.08	1.19	0.06	6.57
Pigs	0.19	0.29	0.16	0.51
Poultry	0.31	0.62	0.34	1.04

their greater production of the greenhouse gas methane per kg of meat produced (see e.g. Gill et al., 2010). This point will be discussed further in the section on trends within the UK.

The scale of this issue of competition for grain can be seen in terms of the total quantity of compound feed being traded globally, which has risen to 873 million tonnes (Alltech 2012), with China as the main producer of feed at 175.4 million tonnes and the US at 164.92 million tonnes.

Forecasting the future in a time of rapid change is fraught with uncertainty, but the IFPRI IMPACT partial equilibrium model of the agricultural sector was developed to provide insights into long-term changes in supply and demand. Use of this model, together with a suite of other models formed the basis for making future projections for demand and supply in various parts of the food system in 2050 for the International Assessment of Agricultural Knowledge, Science and Technology for Development (IAASTD) that global demand for grain to feed to livestock will account for 553 million tonnes (or 42%) of the projected 1,305 million additional tonnes of grain required by 2050 (Rosegrant, Fernandez and Sinha, 2009). This represents an increase in demand for cereals of 0.7 over figures from 2000.

There is, of course, a considerable degree of uncertainty about any global figures both for what is happening now and even more so about future projections, but it is figures like these which bring pressure on governments to take action to decrease meat consumption, and the livestock sector needs to be in a position from which it can provide evidence to enable trade-offs to be estimated with as much accuracy as possible.

Historical trends in the supply of meat within the UK

Models which operate at the global level are important for highlighting the scale of the problem, but solutions will need to be implemented at farm level, albeit facilitated by national governments. This section therefore considers the equivalent data for the UK.

As with the global trends, the supply of meat per capita in the UK has been increasing (Figure 4) although the significant increases have been confined to the last 2 decades.

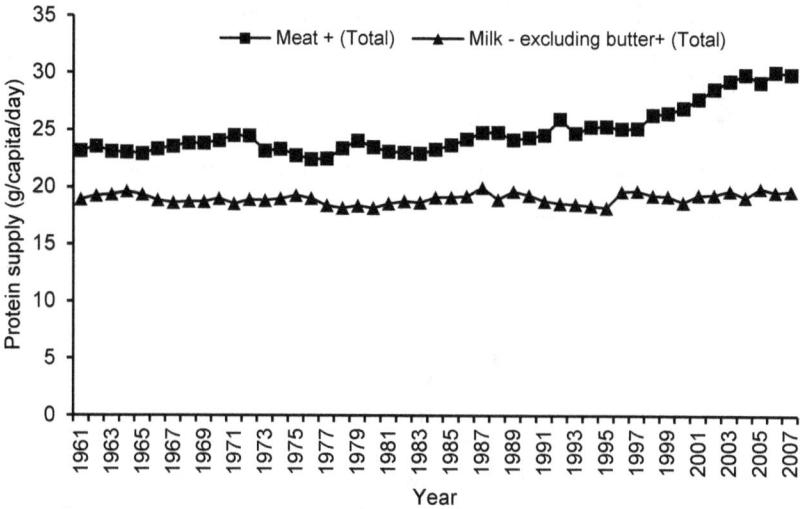

Figure 4 Trends in supply of protein (g/capita/day) as meat and milk in the UK between 1961 and 2007 (FAOSTAT accessed April and May 2012)

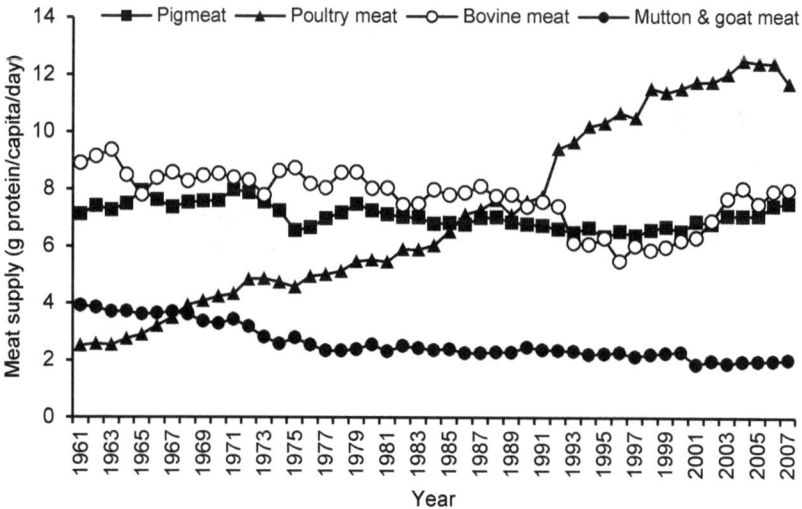

Figure 5 Supply (g protein/capita/day) of meat from cattle, poultry, pigs and sheep and goats in the UK between 1961 and 2007 (FAOSTAT accessed April and May 2012)

Disaggregation of these trends by species (Figure 5) illustrates the increase in supply of poultry meat, as at the global level, but unlike the global trends, there has been relatively little change in the supply of pig meat. Pig meat now (2007) comprises 0.28 of the 3 main meats, with cattle at 0.29. This compares with world average values of 0.35 for pig and poultry meat, and 0.29 for cattle meat.

The CAST report (CAST, 1999) did not estimate efficiencies for UK livestock systems, but Wilkinson (2011) estimated feed conversion ratios for several UK systems using CAST methodology and these have been re-calculated into efficiencies in Table 4.

Table 4 Gross and Human-edible efficiencies of feed protein use for a range of UK livestock systems

	Gross efficiency	*Human-edible efficiency*
Upland beef	0.04	1.09
Cereal beef	0.12	0.33
Pig	0.23	0.36
Poultry	0.33	0.48

This table illustrates that in terms of net food production, upland beef replaces poultry as the most protein efficient system when efficiencies for human edible protein are calculated. The trade-off, however, is increased greenhouse gas emissions. Table 5 (from Gill et al., 2010), shows that although poultry contributed 0.48 of meat production in the UK, their contribution to total greenhouse gas emissions from livestock was only 0.26.

Table 5   Proportional contribution to total meat production and consumption by different livestock species in the UK and their proportional contributions to GHG emissions (from Gill et al., 2010)

Species	*Contribution to Production*	*Contribution to GHG emissions*
Poultry	0.48	0.26
Pigs	0.21	0.16
Cattle	0.22	0.27
Sheep	0.10	0.21

The variation in greenhouse gas emissions per kg product from 18 kg CO_2e/kg human edible protein in product for poultry to 93 for beef and sheep (Gill et al., 2010) therefore needs to be brought into considerations of trade-offs and indeed to trade-offs between environmental impacts and health benefits. Friel et al. (2009)

made a useful contribution to methods for bringing trade-offs to the attention of policy-makers by modelling potential health benefits of different strategies for reducing greenhouse gas emissions from agriculture, but at an aggregated livestock level. What is needed to help inform decision-makers, is models which can look at the trade-offs between the net contributions of different livestock species to food security, to the environment and to health, but these need to be underpinned by evidence.

Feed supply

Another missing part of the evidence required by decision-makers relates to risks to the supply of feed protein. Concern about sources of protein to meet the increasing demand for livestock is not new (see e.g. FAO, 2002 and Defra, 2009), but economic alternatives have not been identified as yet. The Technology Strategy Board (TSB) (http://www.innovateuk.org/content/competition/sustainable-protein-production.ashx) initiated a call for proposals (led by industry with academic partners) seeking to address this issue in two core areas:

1. Increasing the domestic supply of sustainably produced vegetable protein for farmed animals (including land based aquatic and marine based systems)
2. Improving protein and feed conversion efficiency in animal and fish production systems and reducing waste in the food chain to the point of retail sale.

The need for this research may become yet more urgent, however, as data on the vulnerability of the soya crop to climate change becomes available. Recent work (Rose et al., 2012) illustrates the potential for yield decreases in some soya-growing areas in response to temperature rises of even 1.4 °C, with additional indications that these yield drops cannot be compensated for by using adapted varieties.

Figures 6 and 7 illustrate the relatively high dependence of the UK on soya as a protein component of animal feeds. Figure 6 illustrates that it is the primary protein source in compound feeds; Figure 7 illustrates the extent of imports, which started increasing from the early 1980s.

As noted, the TSB is already funding research on increasing the supply of alternative sources of protein; another action which can be taken is to consider the efficiency of protein use. Rankings of efficiencies of use of human edible protein across species and country are shown in Table 6. These rankings illustrate the efficiency of ruminants in terms of protein conversion, followed by poultry and then pigs, but also the differences in the ranking between countries within species. Composition of diets within countries is presumably determined by the

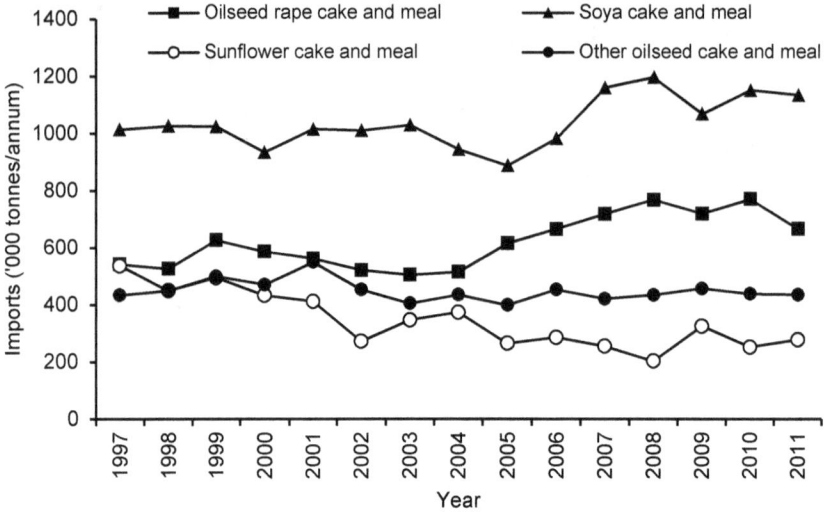

Figure 6 Use ('000 tonnes) of various protein sources in compound animal feeds in the UK by year (Defra, 2012)

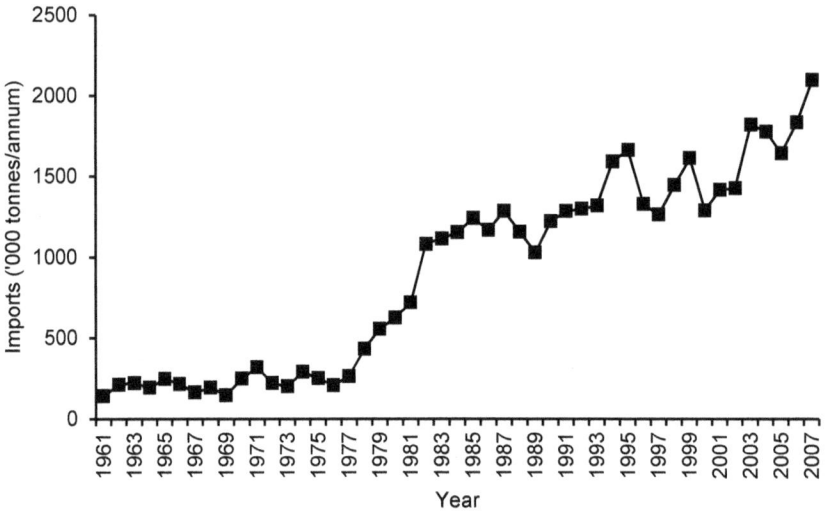

Figure 7 Imports ('000 tonnes) of soyabean cake into the UK from 1970 to 2009 (FAOSTAT, 2012)

economics of production, but the variation illustrates the potential for increasing the efficiency of use of feed protein – another factor which is likely to become of increasing importance in the consideration of trade-offs between food production and negative impacts on the environment.

Table 6 Ranking of efficiency of conversion of human edible feed protein to animal product across 4 countries and 3 species

Country	Species	Human edible efficiency of protein conversion
South Korea	Beef	6.57
Argentina	Beef	6.12
Mexico	Beef	4.39
USA	Beef	1.19
USA	Poultry	1.04
Mexico	Poultry	0.83
Argentina	Poultry	0.69
South Korea	Poultry	0.62
South Korea	Pigs	0.51
USA	Pigs	0.29
Mexico	Pigs	0.21
Argentina	Pigs	0.11

Conclusions

The livestock sector (including along the supply chain and associated industries) makes an important contribution to the economy in many countries as well as providing social benefits in both developed and developing countries. This paper has emphasised the growing urgency for decision-makers to understand the trade-offs between increasing livestock production while minimising negative impacts on the environment, particularly greenhouse gas emissions, and has also highlighted the risk of protein resources becoming limiting. It is likely that at some point, governments may be compelled to include the economic costs of negative environmental effects in the price of agricultural products. To ensure that any such policies are effective and do not inadvertently have an undue negative effect on livestock, there is a need for readily accessible data to estimate these trade-offs.

Analysis of the data presented supports the original proposition that because solutions need to be implemented at farm level, the data need to be considered separately at least in terms of species, but also ideally in terms of type of production system.

There is thus a need for research to look at efficiencies in relation to making the most efficient use of limiting resources, to consider net food production (rather than maximising absolute production) and to estimate environmental impacts at the same time as production outputs.

References

Alltech (2012). Global Feed Summary. http://www.ifif.org/pages/t/ Global+feed+production

Anderson, S., Gundel, S. and Vanni, M. (2010). Evidence of Livestock Sector impacts on the Climate and the wider environment: a UK media survey and a science review. *Working Paper* IIED.

Bellarby J., Foereid, B., Hastings, A. and Smith, P. (2008). *Cool Farming: Climate impacts of agriculture and mitigation potential.* Greenpeace International, Amsterdam, The Netherlands. 43pp.

Bignal, E.M. and McCracken, D.I. (1996). The ecological resources of European farmland. In *The European Environment and CAP Reform: Policies and Proposals for Conservation.* (Ed. M. Whitby). Centre for Agriculture and Biosciences International, Wallingford. pp. 26-42.

CAST [Council for Agricultural Science and Technology] (1999). Animal Agriculture and Global Food Supply. *Task Force Report,* **135,** July 1999, USA.

Defra (2009) http://archive.defra.gov.uk/foodfarm/farmanimal/pigs/task-force/ documents/091207-pig-diet.pdf accessed May 2012.

Defra (2012) http://www.defra.gov.uk/statistics/foodfarm/food/animalfeed/ accessed May 2012.

Delgado, C., Rosegrant, M., Steinfeld, H., Ehui, S. and Courbois, C. (1999). Livestock to 2020. The next food revolution. *Food Agriculture and the Environment discussion paper* No. **28**. International Food Policy Research Institute, Washington DC, Food and Agricultural Organisation, Rome and International Livestock Research Institute, Nairobi.

Delgado, C.L. (2005). Rising demand for meat and milk in developing countries: implications for grasslands-based livestock production. In *Grassland: a Global Resource* (ed. D.A. McGilloway), pp. 29–40. Wageningen Academic Publishers, Wageningen, The Netherlands.

FAO (2004). Protein Sources for the Animal Feed Industry. *Proceedings of Expert Consultation and Workshop* Bangkok 29 April to 3 May 2002.

FAO (2009). *The State of Food and Agriculture: Livestock in the balance.* FAO, Rome.

FAOSTAT (2012). http://faostat.fao.org/site/339/default.aspx

Foresight (2011a). *The Future of Food and Farming. Executive Summary.* The Government Office for Science, London.

Foresight (2011b). *The Future of Food and Farming. Final Project Report.* The Government Office for Science, London.

Friel, S., Dangour, A.D., Garnett, T., Lock, K., Chalabi, Z., Roberts, I., Butler,

A., Butler, C.D., Waage, J., McMichael, A.J. and Haines, A. (2009). Public health benefits of strategies to reduce greenhouse-gas emissions: food and agriculture *Lancet* **374**, 2016–25.

Gill, M., Smith, P. and Wilkinson, J.M. (2010). Mitigating Climate Change: the role of domestic livestock. *Animal,* **4**, 323-333.

Grace, D. and Jones, B. (2011). *Zoonoses (Project 1) Wildlife/domestic livestock interactions.* A final report to the Department for International Development, UK http://www.dfid.gov.uk/r4d/pdf/outputs/livestock/60877-dfid_final25-9-2011.pdf

Hazell, P. and Wood, S. (2008). Drivers of change in global agriculture *Philosophical Transactions of the Royal Society B: Biological Sciences,* **363**, 495-515.

IAASTD (2009). In *Agriculture at a Crossroads Global Report.* (Eds B.D. McIntyre, H.R. Herren, J. Wakhungu and R.T. Watson). Island Press, Washington.

INRA and CIRAD (2009). Agrimonde: Scenarios and Challenges for feeding the World in 2050. http://www.inra.fr/gip_ifrai_eng/activites_programmes_de_l_ifrai/prospective_agrimonde

Oltjen, J.W. and Beckett, J.L. (1996). Role of ruminant livestock in sustainable agricultural systems. *Journal of Animal Science,* **74**, 1406-1409.

Rockström , J., Steffen, W., Noone, K., Persson, A., Chapin, F.S., Lambin , E., Lenton , T.M., Scheffer , M., Folke , C., Schellnhuber, H.J., Nykvist, B., de Wit, C.A., Hughes, T., van der Leeuw, S., Rodhe, H., Sörlin, S., Snyder, P.K., Costanza, R., Svedin, U., Falkenmark, M., Karlberg, L., Corell, R.W., Fabry, V.J., Hansen , J., Walker, B., Liverman, D., Richardson, K., Crutzen, P., and Foley, J. (2009) Planetary Boundaries: exploring the safe Operating Space for Humanity. *Ecology and Society*, **14**, 32.

Rose, G., Osborne, T., Greatrex, H., Hooker, J. and Wheeler, T. (2012). Effects of global climate change on the world's major soybean (Glycine max) and maize (Zea mays) producing regions. *(under review)*

Rosegrant, M.W., Fernandez, M. and Sinha, A. (2009). Looking into the Future for Agriculture and AKST. In *Agriculture at a Crossroads Global Report.* (Eds B.D. McIntyre, H.R. Herren, J. Wakhungu and R.T. Watson). pp 307-376. Island Press, Washington.

Sandhu, M.S., White, I.R. and McPherson, K. (2001). Systematic review of the prospective cohort studies on meat consumption and colorectal cancer risk a meta-analytical approach *Cancer Epidemiology Biomarkers Prevention,* **10**, 439-446.

Santarelli, R.L., Pierre, F. and Corpet, D.E. (2008). Processed meat and colorectal cancer: a review of epidemiologic and experimental evidence. *Nutrition and Cancer*, 60, 131-144.

Smith, P., Martino, D., Cai, Z., Gwary, D., Janzen, H.H., Kumar, P., McCarl, B., Ogle, S., O'Mara, F., Rice, C., Scholes, R.J., Sirotenko, O., Howden, M., McAllister, T., Pan, G., Romanenkov, V., Rose, S., Schneider, U. and Towprayoon, S. (2007). *Agriculture. Chapter 8 of Climate change 2007: Mitigation. Contribution of Working group III to the Fourth Assessment Report of the Intergovernmental Panel on Climate Change* (eds. **B. Metz, O. R. Davidson, P. R. Bosch, R. Dave, L. A. Meyer**), Cambridge University Press, Cambridge, United Kingdom and New York, NY, USA.

Steinfeld, H., Gerber, P., Wassenaar, T., Castel, V., Rosales, M. and de Haan, C. (2006). *Livestock's Long Shadow. Environmental Issues and Options.* Rome, FAO.

Thornton, P.K. (2010). Livestock production: recent trends, future prospects. *Philosphical Transactionsof the Royal Society*, **365** (1554), 2853-2867.

Tilman, D. (1999). Global environmental impacts of agricultural expansion: The need for sustainable and efficient practices. *Proceedings of the National Academy of Sciences, 25,* **96***,* 5995-6000.

Wilkinson, J.M. (2011). Re-defining efficiency of feed use by livestock. *Animal,* **5**, 1014-1022.

Wood, S., Ericksen, P., Stewart, B., Thornton, P. and Anderson, M. (2010). Major international environmental and food assessments: Questions asked and lessons learned. In *Food Security and Global Environmental Change.* (Eds J. Ingram, P. Erickson and D. Liverman). Earthscan, London, Washington.

10

GENOTYPE SELECTION AND MODIFICATION AND THE FUTURE OF LIVESTOCK PRODUCTION

DAVID A. HUME, C. BRUCE. A WHITELAW AND ALAN L. ARCHIBALD
The Roslin Institute and Royal (Dick) School of Veterinary Studies, University of Edinburgh, Roslin EH25 9PS, Scotland, UK.

Abstract

The challenge for the next 50 years is to increase the productivity of major livestock species to address the food needs of the world, whilst at the same time minimising the environmental impact. We present an update of our optimistic view of the ways in which this challenge can be met. The completion of genome sequences, and high-density analytical tools to map genetic markers, allows for whole-genome selection programs based on linkage disequilibrium for a wide spectrum of traits simultaneously. High throughput sequencing and functional genomics are rapidly progressing towards genuinely predictive biology. Based upon these advances it will be possible to redefine genetic prediction based on allele sharing, rather than pedigree relationships and to make breeding value predictions early in the life of the potential sires. Selection will be applied to a much wider range of traits, including those that are directed towards environmental or adaptive outcomes. In parallel, reproductive technologies will continue to advance to allow acceleration of genetic selection, probably including recombination *in vitro*. Transgenesis and/or mutagenesis will be applied to introduce new genetic variation or desired phenotypes. Traditional livestock systems will continue to evolve towards more intensive integrated farming modes that control inputs and outputs to minimise the impact and improve efficiency. The challenges of the next 50 years can certainly be met, but only if governments, charities and industry reverse the long-term disinvestment in agriculture research.

179

Food Security – the challenge

Although population growth in the developed nations has reached a plateau, no slowdown is predicted in the developing world until about 2050. The UN recognises that to meet the global food demand will require that we nearly double our current agricultural output from the same amount of, or less, agricultural land. As fossil fuels stocks continue to decline, there is additional pressure on land to supply not only our needs for food, but also for energy and chemical feedstock. The global challenge is to develop sustainable systems to meet these demands each year from one year's worth of sunshine. Others, including members of the UK Government Office for Science's Foresight Project on Global Food and Farming Futures have ably summarised the Food Security challenge (Godfray et al., 2010).

Here we address the animal sector of the agrifood industry, noting past successes in delivering improved productivity to meet demand and the drivers of future demand. This is an update of a previous submission to the UK Foresight Review (Hume et al., 2010). We offer our predictions of the means by which future demand for animal products can be met through a combination of continuing incremental improvements in productivity and the adoption of new technologies with the potential to deliver step changes in productivity.

The demand for animal products

There are many cultures, or individuals within cultures, who live relatively healthy lives consuming relatively little or no animal protein and many would argue that the challenge of feeding the human population would best be met by reducing livestock production. Livestock themselves consume energy derived from plants that might otherwise be consumed directly by humans; although pigs, poultry and cultivated fish are the fastest growing sectors of livestock production, ruminant animals remain important. Small ruminants and poultry provide the major sources of animal protein to the poorest farmers, and increasing their productivity is a key route to escape from poverty. In traditional pasture grazing, ruminants consume feed that would not be available to humans. This will certainly become more important as more land becomes marginal for arable agriculture in the face of climate change, and as populations the world over reduce their dependence on staple crops and diversify their diets.

The demand for animal protein will certainly continue to grow over the next 20 years, especially in developing countries as they become more affluent. There is little likelihood that vegan diets will be acceptable or prevalent in the medium term, and the dairy and poultry (egg) sectors, which provide acceptable animal protein sources to vegetarians, especially the poultry sector, are currently highly dependent upon grain. It would be unwise to build strategies for achieving food security upon assumptions of altruistic or government advised changes in eating behaviour. Efforts to encourage changes in eating habits on health grounds and hence in terms of self-interest have been largely unsuccessful as the obesity epidemic testifies. Modest decreases in meat consumption in some developed countries will be more than outweighed by growth in demand in emerging economies and the developing world. Aside from the widespread and growing preference of affluent humans for animal protein, there is also the argument that not all land (or sea) is appropriate for the effective production of plants that can be consumed by humans.

The needs will vary between societies. The better off, often referred to as Western, will look to food not only as nutrition, but also to contribute to a healthy and long life. The Developing countries, where population numbers are still increasing, will look to agriculture as the primary source of essential food and also as a source of export income. Thus, we need to plan for increased production of animal products. In the face of climate change, and competing demands on resources, the challenge will be to meet this demand for animal products whilst at the same time reducing the overall impact. In essence we need more and healthier animals, that make better use of foodstuffs while reducing the impact of waste products.

This ambitious agricultural landscape will require continued advances of traditional methods and approaches, such as husbandry and genetics, and the broad up-take of biotechnological solutions.

Past successes

In the past 40+ years, there have been major productivity gains in dairy cattle, pigs and poultry (Table 1, Van den Steen et al., 2005). Perhaps surprisingly, given how much has been said about the environmental impact of livestock production (Steinfeld et al., 2006) there have also been significant reductions in the greenhouse gas emissions and global warming potential per tonne of animal product (Table 2.) These gains have been achieved through a combination of genetic improvement and better husbandry, nutrition and disease control. The dairy, pig and poultry sectors are highly structured with a small number of international companies controlling large proportions of the breeding and production. The sheep, goat and beef cattle sectors are less highly structured and for these species together with others (e.g. buffalo, deer, llama, alpaca, camel) there remains considerable scope for improvements in productivity. By contrast to land-based agriculture, we are at early stage in fish domestication, and there are likely to be potential productivity and feed efficiency gains to be had.

Table 1: Improvements in livestock productivity over the past 40-50 years

| Species | Trait | *Indicative Performance* | | |
		1960s	*Present (2005)*	*% Change*
Pig	Pigs weaned/sow/year	14	21	50
	Lean meat %	40	55	37
	Feed conversion ratio (FCR)	3.0	2.2	27
	Kg lean meat/ton feed	85	170	100
Broiler chicken	Days until 2 kg is reached	100	40	60
	Feed conversion ratio	3.0	1.7	43
Layer hen	Eggs per year	230	300	30
	Eggs/ton feed	5000	9000	80
Dairy cow	Kg milk/cow/lactation	6000	10000	67

Modified from van der Steen et al. (2005)

Table 2: % change in greenhouse gas emissions and global warming potential achieved through genetic improvement (1988-2007)

	CH_4	NH_3	N_2O	GWP_{100}
Chickens – layers	-30	-36	-29	-25
Chickens – broilers	-20	10	-23	-23
Pigs	-17	-18	-14	-15
Cattle – dairy	-25	-17	-30	-16
Cattle – beef	0	0	0	0
Sheep	-1	0	0	-1

Sources: Project for Defra by Genesis Faraday Partnership and Cranfield University (AC0204),

Animal agriculture

The future changes to agriculture will probably take three forms. First, to meet the current growing demand, a rapid and sustainable increase in overall animal protein production will occur over the next 10 years. Secondly, alternative uses of farm livestock and poultry will be developed, and thirdly, completely new approaches to food production will be implemented. The UK science-base is well placed to make significant contributions to all three phases.

Within an overarching aim of improving the sustainability of animal production systems, including minimising their environmental footprint there are three objectives that need to be addressed:

- To maximise the number of productive offspring per breeding male and female

- To maximise the efficiency of converting feed (or solar energy) and water into useful animal products

- To minimise waste and losses through infectious and metabolic disease and stress

The scientific disciplines in biological sciences that are relevant to the research required to address these objectives include genetics, immunology, nutrition, physiology, and reproductive biology. Cross-disciplinary working with scientists with skills in mathematics, physics and computing science will be required for effective research. Whilst the UK animal science base has strengths in genetics, genomics and disease research, including immunology, there is a shortage of skills and expertise in whole animal biology, including physiology, reproductive biology and nutrition.

Some of the major targets for the future of livestock production are to:

- Maximise the number of offspring produced by each female animal that are also fit for purpose

- Minimise losses of production due to environmental variables including disease and stress from other animals, production systems or climate change

- Maximise the welfare of the animals (at least in Western agriculture)

- Maximise the efficiency of energy utilisation in the generation of animal protein

- Minimise wastage of animal protein at every stage of production and utilisation

- Minimise the impact of livestock production on the environment in terms of both inputs and outputs.

- Add value to livestock by producing desirable outcomes in addition to food.

The ways that we envisage these objectives being achieved are:

1) Maximise the number of offspring produced by each female animal that are also fit for purpose

There are three challenges – to increase total number of animals (in a global arena), to maximise development of appropriate phenotypes, and to optimise sex bias to reflect animal usage.

Improved efficiency of animals will involve continued selection, based upon genome-wide selection using complete sequencing of genomes (Green, 2009; Meuwissen et al., 2001; Hill, 2010). The generation of all of our major breeds of livestock has involved a significant degree of inbreeding to fix desired traits. In standard production schemes of most major livestock, selected pedigree lines with desired traits are intercrossed to generate hybrid vigor or heterosis. Optimisation of cross-bred performance is one of the main challenges facing the livestock industry and one of the major routes to increasing productivity. Heterosis, and its undesirable cousin, inbreeding suppression, are generally attributed to the presence within the genome of significant numbers of deleterious mutations (Charlesworth and Wills, 2009). The presence of such mutations in humans has been confirmed in the 1000 Genomes Project, which has confirmed that most individuals carry hundreds of deleterious alleles that would generate serious genetic disease as homozygotes. The presence of these alleles at relatively high frequency in humans has been attributed to the massive population explosion and the comparative absence of selection (Keinan and Clark, 2012). The same condition might apply to the major livestock species which have expanded alongside the human population, but the effective population size is constrained by selective breeding. Nevertheless, high throughput sequencing of chicken and pig genomes supports the view that each animal carries a substantial genetic load (unpublished observations). The combination of massively high throughput genome sequencing, and improved functional genome annotation, means that we can envisage the identification of seriously deleterious mutations in individual animals and targeted breeding to eliminate the carriers. Combining genetics with gene expression analysis (so-called genetical genomics) reveals that important allelic variants that impact on production traits regulate the level of expression of genes as well as their protein-coding capacity (Cabrera et al., 2012). Amongst other gains, molecular selection to eliminate deleterious mutations could produce an increase in the number of viable progeny and their postnatal survival (in mammals) or hatchability (in birds) due to a reduction of the number of developmental lethals.

Identification of breeding value of high genetic merit sires will become more and more efficient as total genome sequencing is coupled with much more sophisticated progeny testing and tracking. In all major livestock, cloning of productive animals will also become possible and cheap, and will require careful management to ensure that there is sufficient variation in populations to mitigate catastrophic loss in a pandemic. Advances in systems biology, and knowledge from analysis of genotype-phenotype relationships will make such selection less empirical. Total genetic merit indices, which integrate genomic markers with multiple traits to maximise multiple desirable traits simultaneously (Green, 2009; Coleman et al., 2009) will gain greater and greater predictive power.

Such genetic/genomic technologies will be applied to a number of issues that currently constrain livestock productivity. They will permit improved selection for new fecundity genes that will increase the numbers of offspring, especially in pigs, sheep and other production animals of more relevance to the developing world. An area of increasing importance is the link between maternal nutrition and stress and the productivity and fertility of offspring. The literature in this area has emphasised effects on human disease and anxiety, but there is also evidence for effects of both prenatal and postnatal stress on reproductive performance in pigs (Ashworth et al., 2011). Available evidence indicates this has an epigenetic basis, and in future it will be possible to mitigate the effects of maternal stress in the offspring through genetic selection for genes expressed in the mother, and through possible nutritional or other manipulation in the offspring (Vo and Hardy, 2012).

Fertility is a significant issue for both the dairy and meat chicken industries. In the former, fertility has been declining by 1% per annum for several decades. If the decline in fertility associated with increases in milk yield arose entirely from a causal linkage between effects on milk yield and fertility, the effects would not be separated even by precision breeding. But there is already reason to suggest that this is not the case, and fertility loss can be reversed, through genome-wide selection on multiple traits, without completely compromising milk production (Coleman et al., 2009). Genetic gains will probably not compensate entirely for the fact that loss of body condition in animals that efficiently partition energy intake into milk rather than body maintenance renders them less fit to breed. The investment in the milking animal is significant – feeding from birth to puberty, through pregnancy and lactation. Solutions may be based upon deciding whether multiple lactations are required to secure an adequate return on this investment or whether an artificially prolonged single lactation could represent a better return.

In the broiler chicken and turkey sectors fertility is also a constraint on productivity - which necessitates nutrient deprivation of broiler layers to achieve reasonable levels of egg production. This is a significant welfare issue; broiler breeders show clear evidence of physiological stress as well as an increased incidence of abnormal behaviours; they are essentially chronically hungry (Mench, 2002). We anticipate that application of multiparameter genome-wide selection will be able to address this issue, allowing broiler layers themselves to contribute to meat production, and to increase their effective egg production. This will generate very substantial increases in overall productivity as well as addressing current welfare concerns.

At least some of the gain in productivity of animals such as poultry has been at the expense of other losses; for example through osteoporosis and ascites in layers and broilers respectively. It is already known that some of these issues have a genetic basis that is amenable to further manipulation (Dunn et al., 2007). We also anticipate that growing understanding of the avian and mammalian livestock immune systems will reveal a link between production traits and immune status that could lead to a compromise between the two, to obviate the potential trade-off between improved disease resistance and lowered production.

It is unlikely that existing genetic variation will continue to generate the rate of gain obtained in the past. We consider it very likely that genetically-modified animals will be required and that they will be accepted. Transgenic Atlantic salmon expressing either the antifreeze protein of winter flounder, or the Chinook salmon growth hormone gene, are already on the way to the table, albeit with considerable opposition from environmental groups. Transgenesis to generate desired traits will certainly be possible, and is likely to be acceptable if the benefits to the consumer in terms of cost, health, animal welfare or environment are clear. Alternatives that may be acceptable more rapidly will also involve targeted or untargeted mutagenesis with new technologies such as zinc finger nucleases and TALENs (Li et al., 2010. Le Provost et al., 2010) followed by conventional breeding and selection. This could circumvent the consumer objection to genetically-modified animals, in that the introduced mutations would be indistinguishable from those occurring naturally, and the animals will be no more genetically-modified than the large majority of food crops. For example, in the case of control of ovulation in chickens and dairy cattle, increased knowledge of the control of ovulation will permit rational mutagenesis to improve fertility/fecundity and circumvent the fertility/production compromise. It will probably be possible to introduce into cattle, pigs, goats or indeed other sheep breeds, genetic variants that are known to improve fertility/fecundity in sheep (Souza et al., 2004).

Sorting of sperm for the purpose of preselection of sex has been possible for some 20 years (de Graaf et al., 2009). In the short to medium term, understanding of the molecular basis of sex determination and technologies for sex selection will permit sex biased production of offspring, ensuring that most beef cattle, meat sheep, pigs and broiler chickens born are male (and in the case of pigs, do not have boar taint), whilst layer chickens and dairy cattle are female. This change alone will generate increases in the overall efficiency of the livestock industries that will take several of the steps needed to address increased demand. Such selection will also increase the availability of multipurpose animals (e.g. dairy cattle with useful beef production).

We are also entering a new era with regard to assisted reproduction through our increasing understanding of developmental biology underpinning an ever increasing technical ability to isolate and culture stem cells. For example, recent advances in the cultivation and genetic modification of primordial germ cells in chickens offer new avenues for preservation and recovery of desired genotypes (Macdonald et al., 2012). Similarly, the successful isolation and cultivation of spermatogonial stem cells, already available in rodents, to cattle offer new routes to genetic manipulation (Oatley, 2010). Initially these technologies can be simply applied to maximise healthy birth rates of animals with existing desired traits. Looking over a 5-10 year window, with the advances in embryonic stem (ES) cells and induced pluripotent stem cell (iPS) technology that are currently underway (Martins-Taylor and Xu, 2010), combined with controlled stem cell differentiation to produce germ cells *in vitro* (Aflatoonian and Moore, 2006), we envisage that *in vitro* sexual recombination will become feasible as a new way of generating genetic diversity. The easier stage, the production of male gametes *in vitro* combined with genome-wide selection, will massively accelerate the rate at which desirable traits could be propagated into livestock populations through artificial insemination. This is especially important in cattle and sheep, which have long generation times and small offspring number.

2) Minimise losses of production due to environmental variables including disease, stress and nutrition

It is already clear that animals vary in natural susceptibility to pathogens. Furthermore, as our climate changes, redistributing temperatures around the globe, livestock will be exposed to diseases and pests that have previously been geographically restricted and to which they have no intrinsic resistance. There are also clear genetic impacts on response to stress and aggressive behaviours. The availability of all the major livestock genomes has revealed that each species has an idiosyncratic immune system, and it is the genes and variants that are species specific that also contribute most to variation within a species. Comparative genomics and genetics will give major insights into the molecular basis of disease susceptibility that will permit rationale selection.

Combinations of transgenesis and selective breeding will reduce these impacts. We can anticipate that major endemic diseases, as well as new diseases, will be mitigated by selection of resistant animals or by genetic modification. For example, the recent demonstration of transgenic resistance to avian flu in chickens has the potential to mitigate the massive impact of this disease (Lyall et al, 2011). Arguably, the zoonotic potential of highly-pathogenic influenza could influence public acceptance of the technology. The Roslin Institute is involved in efforts to generate trypanosome resistance in cattle, which would greatly reduce a major burden on beef and dairy production in East Africa. Similarly, we and others have shown that resistance to bovine TB has a heritable component, and we believe that breeding for resistance will form a substantial part of the strategy for eradication of tuberculosis in the UK (Brotherstone et al., 2010) and of other major disease burdens in other countries. It does need to be recognised that, given the low fertility and long generation times of large livestock, the transmission of desirable disease-resistance traits into national herds will take many years unless we can apply assisted reproductive technologies mentioned above to transmit through the male germ line. In the meantime, major advances in vaccine technologies, based upon knowledge of species-specific immune biology and including novel ideas like transgenic vaccinating plants, will likely reduce the impact of endemic diseases.

3) Maximise the welfare of the animals

The goals of animal genetic improvement are firmly grounded in the paradigm of animal production, which naturally refers to concepts of efficiency, productivity, and quality. However, too often ignored in public discourse is the fact that sustainability and animal welfare are also central considerations in this paradigm. It is an inescapable principle that the maximization of productivity cannot be accomplished without minimizing the levels of animal stress. Furthermore, the definition of efficiency (product per unit input) requires sustainability.

Welfare priorities differ between societies and geographical areas. Compromises to animal well- being or sustainability may be more or less unacceptable to different cultures. For example, live animal exports remain an issue for countries such as Australia. Although many welfare issues are directly addressed through improved control of disease and genetic selection for behaviour traits (such as reduced aggression), aspects of husbandry and farming practices in many cases will need to change. Gaining a greater understanding of the underlying mechanisms regulating behaviour in animals is essential to fully address the welfare agenda. There are ethical arguments for improving the environments in which animals are kept rather than selecting genotypes that can cope with and remain productive in adverse production environments. However, it is worth remembering that selection for behaviours such as docility and herdability has already occurred, and was essential to the domestication of animals including cattle and pigs which are potentially dangerous large animals. In concert, there must be recognition by society that some degree of compromise between welfare aspirations and production demands may have to be reached.

An important advance that will occur will be the development of rational, quantifiable measurements of welfare to replace anthropomorphic and emotive measures favoured by some welfare advocates. It may well be that both animal welfare, and environmental impact, are best served by initiatives such as the so-called "battery" dairy for 8000 cows proposed in Lincolnshire, despite the fact that the proposal in question was abandoned due to concerns about the concentration of environmental contamination. Such intensive production facilities could release arable land, and as in the examples of the >30,000-cow Fair Oaks Farm near Chicago in the US, will eventually be sited close to, or even within, urban environments.

4) Maximise the efficiency of energy utilisation in the generation of animal protein

By contrast to the productivity gains in poultry and birds, ruminants have lagged behind. There is a clear opportunity as evidenced by genetic data in beef cattle breeds (Crowley et al., 2009), that continued selection can improve feed conversion and any other trait of interest. Selection will be applied to animals to optimise their adaptation to particular feeds or environments. There are many successful precedents for selection of animals to deal with specific environments. In the US, the beefmaster cattle, derived from admixture of Hereford, Shorthorn and Brahman cattle were heavily selected on what has become known as the Six Essentials - Weight, Conformation, Milking Ability, Fertility, Hardiness and Disposition. Similarly, in Australia, the Droughtmaster was selected for parasite resistance, heat tolerance, environmental adaptation, high fertility, calving ease, docility, excellent meat quality. With the increasing sophistication of genomics, we will revisit such selection processes to generate new "purpose-built" breeds. For example, Hayes et al., (2009) recently examined the sensitivity of milk production to environmental conditions (weather) and thereby demonstrated the feasibility of selecting dairy peak sires whose daughters would be most productive at low levels of feeding. As discussed above, we will also be in a position to understand the mechanism, and maximise the benefits, of heterosis (hybrid vigour) in defined intercrosses, which are the mainstay of meat production in pigs, sheep and cattle.

An alternative approach to feed efficiency is already available, in the form of additives and treatments, such as growth promoting steroid and protein hormones. There has been considerable opposition to such treatments as unnatural, and concerns about residues in animal products, especially in the EU. We envisage that there will be rational, evidence-based research into the level of such residues and the cost-benefit. We consider it likely that, as with GMOs, the use of what might be called pharmacological approaches to improved production, such as steroids in finishing of beef cattle, and growth-promoting peptides such as growth hormone in dairy cattle and pigs, will be shown to be acceptable and safe to both the animals and humans who consume their meat, and there will be new alternative treatments identified that optimise performance.

Broadly speaking, other solutions to efficiency will involve improvement of production systems, feedstocks, animals, and in the case of ruminants, microflora. Current use of grains and cereals (produced from quality arable land) to feed animals is especially inefficient and probably unsustainable. It competes with alternative uses including biofuels and direct nutrition of humans. But the alternative of conventional grass feeding does not allow intensive animal production. We envisage the creation of new plant varieties that optimise the nutritional value attainable from more marginal land. These will include salt and drought-resistant varieties that can help to reverse desertification (especially in the face of climate change). New feeds may include genetically modified plants with increased protein or carbohydrate content, or improved digestibility (for example by reducing the cellulose content). It may also include the creation of food from unconventional sources of carbon that would otherwise be wasted , such as woodpulp or fresh or saltwater algae. New feedstuffs will also address environmental impacts, as in the case of phytase feeding to pigs (which could be addressed in a genetically modified plant). We consider it likely that new feedstuffs will be designed to reduce greenhouse gas emission by ruminants (alongside manipulation of the microflora).

A significant environmental issue in the case of ruminants is greenhouse gas production. Future breeding strategies for cattle will need to consider this output (Boichard and Brochard, 2012). One way of increasing productivity in dairy cattle is to increase survival and longevity to reduce replacement needs and the number of nonproductive animals. New technologies will allow the mitigation of methane emission through direct monitoring of rumen gas production, capture and manipulation of the gut microorganisms to reduce methane production (e.g. methanophiles). This, in turn, will increase effective conversion of plant carbon, at worst directly into CO_2, and at best, into energy available to the animal. On the host side, there is little doubt that the rumen microbiota and the host coevolve and it is already known that animals that are more efficient produce less methane (Zhou et al., 2010). We therefore envisage mutation and selection for animals that have substantially reduced methane production by virtue of both further improvements in food conversion efficiency by the host and altered rumen environment.

5) Minimise wastage of animal protein at every stage of production and utilisation

Much of what has been described above addresses this issue. Specifically we will continue to optimise feed conversion, as described above, and optimise bioprocessing steps in food production. In many countries, animal (and human) waste is used as fertiliser, although there remain concerns about food safety as a consequence. Higher intensity farming practices/systems will allow more efficient collection of waste, and alternative uses of waste products, such as options for use as inputs for farmed microbial production systems and/or biogas production.

Concerns about food safety and the BSE crisis have understandably inhibited previous procedures for capturing and recycling animal and food waste, such as feeding of swill to pigs or supplementing animal feed with rendered animal material. Beyond changes in behaviour of the food industry, retailers and the general public to reduce food wastage, imaginative yet safe systems are required to recycle biological material wasted / discarded throughout the food chain from farm to fork.

6) Minimise the impact of livestock production on the environment in terms of both inputs and outputs.

The so-called "long shadow" of livestock production, comprising land degradation, climate change and air pollution, water shortage and pollution and loss of diversity, has been reviewed in detail in an FAO Report in 2006 (Steinfeld et al., 2006). This area is somewhat outside our expertise. Clearly, as the relative cost of meat escalates with demand, small scale production will become more economically viable, and there will be a return to mixed farms in which waste from broad acre crops is available as feed for animal production. We anticipate that there will be a move towards completely new production systems; for example vertical farms (www.verticalfarm.com) within cities and within multistorey buildings, with solar capture and aeroponic or hydroponic plant growth, water recycled through the system. Such systems will also capture and recycle animal effluent liquids, solids, gases and even body heat and will address climate change indirectly by permitting grazing land to be returned to forest. A challenge for the future will be to identify and adapt animals to completely different artificial production environments, with implications of welfare and productivity. As discussed above, such "evolution" is clearly possible; we might, for example, consider that smaller animals (small deer, goats, or mini-pigs) are more cost-effective and efficient.

7) Add value to livestock by producing desirable outcomes in addition to food.

The production of value-added protein products such as biopharmaceuticals in milk and eggs is clearly already feasible. We can envisage a new generation of nutriceuticals, and oral-acting vaccines, that may be appropriate for both human and other animal consumption. The possibility of generating animals (using GMO, mutation and selection or novel feedstuffs) that have improved nutritional value (for example pigs with increased amounts of omega-3-fatty acids) is already upon us (Rothschild and Plastow, 2008), and will likely be adopted more widely as the relative value of such products becomes more apparent to consumers. We can also envisage the modification of wool in sheep to produce fibres of greater value, and possible production of desired biotechnology products in offal meats that are currently not used other than for rendering as animal feed.

Conclusion

Agricultural science has been enormously successful in providing an inexpensive supply of high-quality and safe foods to developed and developing nations. These advances have largely come from the implementation of technologies which focus on efficient production and distribution systems, as well as the selective breeding and genetic improvement of cultured plants and animals. The global demand for animal products is also substantially growing, driven by a combination of population growth, urbanization, and rising incomes.

Animal products contain concentrated sources of protein with amino acid compositions that complement those of cereal and other vegetable proteins. They also contribute to human intakes of calcium, iron, zinc and several B group vitamins. In developing countries where diets are based on cereals or bulky root crops, eggs, meat and milk are critical for supplying energy in the form of fats. In addition, animal-derived foods contain compounds that actively promote long-term health. We predict the demand for animal protein will continue to grow over the next 20 years. We also predict that the ever-increasing sophistication of animal genetics will continue to contribute to future agriculture and, although largely shunned to-date, animal biotechnologies can and will provide many of the solutions for tomorrow's agriculture.

What will constrain these efforts is investment. Large animal research is expensive. Over the past 20 years, there has been systematic underinvestment in the sector by governments all over the world, and expertise and infrastructure has declined (Green, 2009). This is not a sector that can be left to industry investment. The applications of genomic selection require accurate phenotype determination from large numbers of animals. The profit margins for farming livestock at the individual farmer (or animal) level are small. Animals and genes cannot (and probably should not) be patented, so there is little room for very large industry players in the sector. Even in the poultry and pig breeding industries, where there is consolidation of the sector, the global players are dwarves compared to pharmaceutical companies. We are confident that the sustainable gains in productivity of livestock can be achieved within the next 20 years. They will only be achieved if governments recognise that the required research is "public good", and reenter and reengage with the livestock research sector with substantial investment.

References

Aflatoonian, B. and Moore, H. (2006) Germ cells from mouse and human embryonic stem cells. *Reproduction*, **132**, 699-707.

Ashworth C.J., Hogg, C.O., Hoeks, C.W., Donald, R.D., Duncan, W.C., Lawrence, A.B. and Rutherford, K.M. (2011) Prenatal social stress and postnatal pain affect the developing pig reproductive axis. *Reproduction*, **142**, 907-914.

Boichard. D. and Brochard, M. (2012) New phenotypes for new breeding goals in dairy cattle. *Animal*, **6**, 544-50.

Brotherstone, S., White, I.M., Coffey, M., Downs, S.H., Mitchell, A.P., Clifton-Hadley, R.S., More, S.J., Good, M. and Woolliams, J.A. (2010) Evidence of genetic resistance of cattle to infection with Mycobacterium bovis. *J. Dairy Sci.* **93**, 1234-42.

Cabrera, C.P., Dunn, I.C., Fell, M., Wilson, P.W., Burt, D.W., Waddington, D., Talbot, R., Hocking, P.M., Law, A., Knott, S., Haley, C.S. and de Koning, D.J. (2012) Complex traits analysis of chicken growth using genetical genomics. *Anim. Genet.* **43**, 163-171.

Coleman, J., Pierce, K.M., Berry, D.P., Brennan, A. and Horan, B. (2009) The influence of genetic selection and feed system on the reproductive performance of spring-calving dairy cows within future pasture-based production systems. *J. Dairy Sci.* **92**, 5258-69.

Charlesworth,, D. and Wills, J.H. (2009) The genetics of inbreeding depression. *Nature Reviews Genetics*, **10**, 783-796.

Crowley, J.J., McGee, M., Kenny, D.A., Crews, D.H. Jr, Evans, R.D. and Berry, D.P. (2010) Phenotypic and genetic parameters for different measures of feed efficiency in different breeds of Irish performance-tested beef bulls. *J. Anim Sci.* **88**, 885-94.

de Graaf, S.P., Beilby, K.H., Underwood, S.L., Evans, G. and Maxwell, W.M. (2009) Sperm sexing in sheep and cattle: the exception and the rule. *Theriogenology*, **71**, 89-97.

Dunn, I.C., Fleming, R.H., McCormack, H.A., Morrice, D., Burt, D.W., Preisinger, R. and Whitehead, C.C. (2007) A QTL for osteoporosis detected in an F2 population derived from White Leghorn chicken lines divergently selected for bone index. *Animal Genetics*, **38**, 45-49.

Godfray, H.C.J., Beddington, J.R., Crute, I.R., Haddad, L., Lawrence, D., Muir, J.F., Pretty, J., Robinson, S., Thomas, S.M. and Toulmin, C. (2010) Food Security: The challenge of feeding 9 billion people. *Science*, **327**, 812-818.

Green, R.D. (2009) Future needs in animal breeding and genetics. *J. Dairy Sci.* **87**, 793-800.

Hayes, B.J., Bowman, P., Chamberlain, A.J., Savin, K., van Tassell, C.P., Sonstegard, T.S. and Goddard, M.E. (2009) A validated genome wide association study to breed cattle adapted to an environment altered by climate change. *PLOS ONE* **4**, e6676.

Hill, W.G. (2010) Understanding and using quantitative genetic variation. *Philosophical Transactions of the Royal Society B. Biological Sciences*, **365**, 73-85.

Hume, D.A., Whitelaw, C.B.A. and Archibald, A.L. (2011) The future of animal production-Improving productivity and sustainability. Foresight Review. *J. Agric. Sci.* **149**, 9-16.

Keinan, A. and Clark, A.G. (2012) Recent explosive human population growth has resulted in an excess of rare genetic variants. *Science*, **336**, 740-743.

Le Provost, F., Lillico, S., Passet, B., Young, R., Whitelaw, B. and Vilotte, J.L. (2010) Zinc finger-nuclease technology heralds a new era in mammalian transgenesis. *Trends Biotechnol.* **28**, 134-41.

Li, T., Huang, S., Zhao, X., Wright, D.A., Carpenter, S., Spalding, M.H., Weeks, D.P. and Yang, B. (2011) Modularly assembled designer TAL effector nucleases for targeted gene knockout and gene replacement in eukaryotes. *Nucleic Acids Res.* **39**, 6315-25.

Lyall, J., Irvine, R.M., Sherman, A., McKinley, T.J., Núñez, A., Purdie, A., Outtrim, L., Brown, I.H., Rolleston-Smith, G., Sang, H. and Tiley, L. (2011) Suppression of avian influenza transmission in genetically modified chickens. *Science*, **331**, 223-6.

MacDonald, J., Taylor, L., Sherman, A., Kawakami, K., Takahashi, Y., Sang, H.M. and McGrew, M.J. (2012) Efficient genetic modification and germ-line transmission of primordial germ cells using piggyBac and Tol2 transposons. *Proc. Natl. Acad. Sci. USA.* 2012 May 14.

Martins-Taylor, K. and Xu, R.H. (2010) Determinants of pluripotency: from avian, rodents to primates. *J. Cell Biochem.* **109**, 16-25.

Mench, J.A. (2009) Broiler Breeders: feed restriction and welfare. *World Poultry Science J.* **58**, 23-29.

Meuwissen, T.H.E., Hayes, B.J. and Goddard, M.E., (2001) Prediction of total genetic value using genome-wide dense marker maps. *Genetics*, **157**, 1819-29.

Oatley, J.M. (2010) Spermatogonial stem cell biology in the bull: development of isolation, culture, and transplantation methodologies and their potential impacts on cattle production. *Soc. Reprod. Fertil. Suppl.* **67**, 133-43.

Rothschild, M.F. and Plastow, G.S. (2008) Impact of genomics on animal agriculture and opportunities for animal health. *Trends Biotechnol.* **26**, 21-25.

Souza, C.J., González-Bulnes, A., Campbell, B.K., McNeilly, A.S. and Baird, D.T. (2004) Mechanisms of action of the principal prolific genes and their application to sheep production. *Reprod. Fertil. Dev.* **16**, 395-401.

Steinfeld, H., Gerber, P., Wassenaar, T., Castel, V., Rosales, M. and de Haan, C. (2006) Livestock's Long Shadow. Environmental Issues and Options. FAO Report. ftp://ftp.fao.org/docrep/fao/010/A0701E/A0701E00.pdf

van der Steen, H.A.M., Prall, G.F.W. and Plastow G.S. (2005) Application of genomics to the pork industry. *J. Anim. Sci.* **83**, E1-E8.

Vo, T. and Hardy, D.B. (2012) Molecular mechanisms underlying fetal programming of adult disease. *J. Cell Commun. Signal.* May 24 Epub.

Zhou, M., Hernandez-Sanabria, E. and Guan, L.L. (2009) Assessment of the microbial ecology of ruminal methanogens in cattle with different feed efficiencies. *Appl. Environ. Microbiol.* **75**, 6524-33.

11

GENETIC SELECTION OF POULTRY BASED ON DIGESTIVE CAPACITY – IMPACT ON GUT MICROBIOTA

I. GABRIEL, B. KONSAK, S. MIGNON-GRASTEAU

INRA UR 83, Avian Poultry Research, Nouzilly 37380, France

Introduction

The genetic selection of animals has always searched to improve the growth performance of animals and feed efficiency, and this trait will remain the main objectives of genetic selection. Feed efficiency can be improved by selecting for growth, feed conversion ratio (FCR) or feed intake, which are heritable (Pym, 1990). As digestive efficiency is one of the components of feed efficiency, its improvement contributes to the global aim of optimization of feed efficiency, and therefore can be used for genetic selection (Mignon-Grasteau et al., 2004). This capacity to digest feed is all the more important now that more and more unconventional feedstuffs with variable or low digestibility values will be used for animal feeding instead of conventional feedstuffs such as wheat, maize and soya to decrease competition for crop vegetal resources between man and animal. Moreover in Europe, the use of local feedstuffs is needed to decrease the dependence on soya as a protein source, as it mainly comes from importation. Although nutritional means such as feed additives (enzymes, phytobiotics . . .) can be used to adapt animals to these new feedstuffs, genetic selection can also be used to improve adaptation of animals (Dockès et al., 2011). However, the genetic selection performed up until now on feed efficiency has led to chickens with non optimal digestive efficiency, as shown by their lower apparent metabolisable energy corrected for nitrogen retention (AMEn) compared to slow growth rate lines (Carré et al., 2008). Indeed, high growth rate commercial chickens, Ross PM3 broilers, exhibited a 2-9% lower AMEn than a chicken line with median growth rate but selected on AMEn.

Moreover, nowadays, sustainability of poultry breeding needs to include in addition to economic objectives, environmental and sociological objectives. Regarding preservation of the environment, an increased digestive efficiency means less animal wastes and manure. Regarding social demands, an increase in digestibility would lead to an improved animal health and welfare, through a decreased nutrient content in the intestine and a lower microbiota development or a better equilibrium between favorable and unfavorable bacteria. Indeed, it has been shown that the undigested compounds are involved in dysbacteriosis (Klis and Lensing, 2007), or the occurrence of necrotic enteritis due to certain *Clostridium perfringens* strains (Timbermont et al., 2011), or coccidiosis (Crévieu-Gabriel and Naciri, 2001). Moreover, the undigested dietary compounds increase the quantity of fermentation substrates in the litter and the frequency of pododermatitis (Shepherd and Fairchild, 2010).

To answer to these needs, at the Poultry Research Unit of INRA, a divergent selection program began in 2002 using AMEn as the criterion for digestive efficiency (Mignon-Grateau et al., 2004). Contrarily to diets based on maize and soyabean meal, a diet containing a high level of wheat (336 g/kg) allowed a rather high difference in metabolisable energy between chicken lines (Pym et al., 1984). Indeed, wheat diets were often observed to result in low digestibilities when compared with maize diets and to lead to high variability between birds (Choct et al., 1999; Carré et al., 2002). These problems of wheat digestion largely depend on wheat samples, those with high viscosity and hardness resulting in lowest digestibilities (Carré et al., 2002). The program of divergent selection was thus performed by using a high concentration (525 g/kg) of high viscosity wheat due to its richness in arabinoxylan and a medium hardness value (Rialto cultivar, Carré et al., 2002, Mignon-Grasteau et al., 2004). Moreover, a high fat concentration with high vegetal oil added (60-80 g/kg) instead of 10-20 g/kg as usually done for such median growing lines, was used to increase differences between birds, due to the difficulty of young birds to digest lipids. The two lines were named D+ (high digester) and D- (low digester) and have been selected on AMEn during 8 generations, and reproduced without selection for 2 additional generations. Heritability of AMEn estimated on the first, second and eighth generations was high (0.30 to 0.38, Mignon-Grasteau et al., 2004; de Verdal et al., 2011b).

These divergent lines now represent a unique model to study the physiological limiting factors of digestion. The interest in using such genetic lines, instead of alternative approaches such as knockout animals or polymorphism genotyping, lies in the fact that a hierarchy in genetic determinants can be proposed. Estimation of the genetic parameters makes it possible to establish how selection impacts on the phenotype, as the morphology of the gut organs, and offers the opportunity to anticipate any undesirable effects of AMEn selection, before its introduction in selection schemes. Genetic correlations can also be used as a tool to propose selection criteria related to the objective of selection but easier to measure than the trait itself. Finally, a quantitative trait locus analysis is currently undertaken on a classical F2 cross between these 2 lines which, combined with the phenotypic differences observed between D+ and D- birds, will help to propose a list of candidate genes for selection.

This selection has been performed on AMEn used as the criteria for digestive efficiency. Animal digestive capacity corresponds to its capacity to extract compounds from the diet by hydrolyzing macromolecules to absorbable molecules and absorb them, with its enzymatic / absorbent system, and also with the help or competition of its digestive microbiota. Several recent studies showed the essential role of host microbiota, particularly digestive microbiota in the physiology of the host, not only for digestive tract function, but also for the whole host physiology. Moreover as the host and its digestive commensal microbiota co-evolve after their first contact, a high individual variability in digestive microbiota is observed (Zhu et al., 2002; Gabriel et al, 2007; Torok et al, 2008). Thus several studies have shown that digestive microbiota depends on animal genetics. For example, in humans, microflora are much more similar between homozygous twins than between unrelated persons or heterozygous twins (Van de Merwe et al., 1983; Stewart and Chadwick, 2005; Zoetendal et al., 2004; Dicksved et al., 2008). Differences in digestive microbiota according to animal genetics has also been observed in other mammals (Toivanen et al., 2001; Gulati et al., 2012), and also in birds such as the chicken (Lumpkins et al., 2010). It can be expected that genetic selection on a trait that has a direct effect on the biotope of digestive microbiota, that is digestive area, has an impact on the microbiota. However, due to the numerous effects of digestive microbiota on the host, the relationship between host and microbiota is probably not only a change of microbiota due to a change in its biotope, but also the establishment of a new balance between the host, its capacity to hydrolyze dietary compounds and its microbiota (Hooper et al., 2002). We thus analyzed digestive microbiota of D+ and D- lines, that have been divergently selected based on AMEn, to understand the relationships between the microbiota and digestive efficiency.

In this chapter, after a review of current knowledge on digestive microbiota in chicken and its effect on the host, the phenotypic characteristics of the D+ and D- lines known at the present time will be presented. These characteristics concern their digestive values as well as the consequences on their zootechnical performances, and digestive tract. In the last part of this chapter, data obtained recently on the digestive microbiota will be presented, as well as further work needed to increase knowledge on relationships between digestive microbiota and digestive capacity of chicken.

Digestive microbiota in poultry and effects on its host

HISTORY OF STUDIES OF THE MICROBIOTA

Several studies on digestive microbiota in poultry were performed between 1970 and 1980 both on conventional and germ-free birds, to study the effect of presence or absence of microbiota. Moreover, other studies were performed by using high doses of antibiotics or probiotics, showing the effects of modifications of digestive microbiota . With the announcement of the ban on antimicrobial growth promoters in animal feed toward the end of the XX century, a new development of studies appeared that investigated the digestive microbiota of rearing animal such as poultry, and mainly focused on means to control it. Thus several reviews have been performed on digestive microbiota description and its role that we will sum up subsequently (Fuller, 1984; Furuse and Okumura, 1994; Mead, 1997; Vispo and Karasov, 1997; Apajalahti et al., 2004; Gabriel et al., 2006; Rehman et al., 2007; Dibner et al., 2008).

Until recently, one of the main problems with studying microbiota, was the availability of appropriate methods to explore it. Indeed a large majority of species cannot be easily cultivated (70-90%). Thanks to the development of new independent approaches to culture in microbial ecology (particularly for environmental microbiota and for digestive microbiota in human due to implication in health), new tools became available and have been used to study digestive microbiota of livestock.

The most commonly used methods at the present time are qualitative methods such as fingerprint techniques such as gradient gel electrophoresis with denaturing compounds or temperature, or terminal restriction fragment length polymorphism analysis, or capillary electrophoresis single strand conformation polymorphism, and quantitative methods, such as fluorescent *in situ* hybridization or quantitative PCR (Inglis et al., 2012).

QUANTITY AND DIVERSITY OF THE MICROBIOTA OF CHICKEN ALONG THE GASTROINTESTINAL TRACT

Briefly, at hatch, the digestive tract of the chicken contains a relatively low number of bacteria, although not sterile as shown by detectable bacteria in embryo from 16 d, with about 100 colony forming units (CFU) / g in caeca and yolk sac in embryo at 18 d, and 10^6 CFU / g and 10^4 CFU / g in caeca and yolk sac respectively 3 h after hatch (Binek et al., 2000; Kizerwetter et al., 2008; Pedroso, 2009; de

Oliveira et al., 2010). Further development of digestive microbiota depends on the environment of the eggs at hatching, and rearing environment following hatch.

To be able to grow in a given part of the digestive tract, microorganisms need substrates and have to multiply at a sufficiently fast rate to compensate for elimination by several mechanisms such as antimicrobial substances and predators (e.g. other bacteria and bacteriophage), digestive transit, and cell and mucus renewal. This explains why microbiota can vary to a large extent among the different parts of the gastrointestinal tract.

In the chicken, the major sites of bacterial localization are the crop and the caeca, and to a lesser extent the small intestine. For example Guardia et al. (2011) determined that the total bacterial load was 5.5×10^{11}, 5.3×10^{10} and 7.4×10^{12} copies of 16S rDNA/g[1] of fresh samples in the crop, the terminal ileum and the caeca respectively.

The crop is considered as the inoculum of the following digestive tract, with the dominant group being *Lactobacillus* (Fuller, 1984; Gong et al., 2007; Guardia et al., 2011). The proventriculus and the gizzard, due to their low pH lead to a fall in bacterial population. In the duodenum, conditions are not favorable to bacterial development for several reasons: high oxygen pressure due to villi movement leading to exchange of oxygen between blood vessels and digestive content, high concentration in antimicrobial compounds such as digestive enzymes and bile salts, reflux movement from jejunum to gizzard leading to a fast modification of the biotope. In the following small intestine, the environment becomes more favorable to bacterial growth thanks to lower oxygen pressure, and lower digestive enzyme and bile acids concentrations, the latter being reabsorbed by the host and degraded by microbiota. Due to these changes along the small intestine, microbiota evolved between the upper part (duodenum-jejunum) to the lower part of the small intestine (Torok et al., 2008). However, the dominant bacteria are *Lactobacillus* (Fuller, 1984; Lu et al., 2003; Guardia et al., 2011).

In the caeca, the biotope is the most favorable for bacterial growth for several reasons. Firstly, oxygen pressure is lower due to lack of villi and reduced mobility limiting the exchange with the intestinal wall and the thick mucus layers. Secondly, this biotope is relatively stable, due to the low renewal of the digestive content. Indeed, the continuous entrance of substrates are mixed with already present digesta and the caeca are emptied only 1 to 2 times per day (Clench, 1999). The substrates are composed of fine particles of digesta and urinary compounds rich in uric acid backflowed from the cloaca, that can be used by several bacterial

---

1 Expression of results: copies of ADNr16S due to the reference used for the assay, knowing that the number of copies of ADNr16S varies greatly according to bacteria species (Lee et al., 2009; Rastogi et al., 2009). It varies from 1 to 15, with for the most important bacterial groups in digestive tract of chicken : 4 to 6 for *Lactobacillus*, 3 to 15 (average 9) for *Clostridium*, 5 to 7 for *Bacteroides*, 7 for *E.coli*.

species (Mead, 1997). Thus in these digestive contents, it has been evaluated that 50% of the biomass would be of bacterial origin (Clench, 1999). In contrast to the crop and the small intestine, the bacterial composition of the caeca is more diverse, and the major group is *Clostridium* (Lu et al, 2003; Guardia et al., 2011; Moore et al, 2011).

This digestive microbiota can be located in the lumen or at the mucosal surface or in the mucus layer(s). The luminal microbiota depends on available nutrients, transit rate and the presence of antibacterial compounds. It can be considered that this microbiota acts mainly as an aid for starch hydrolysis in the crop (Szylit et al., 1980; Champs et al., 1981)). In the small intestine, bacteria are considered as competitors of the host, due to their high metabolic potential with high hydrolystic activity In the caeca, digestive microbiota allows the production of short chain fatty acids (SCFA) from undigested compounds. The mucosal microbiota in the crop, has been described as adhesive to the mucosa developing several cell layers (Fuller 1984). Mucosal microbiota, in the small intestine of chicken, would be adherent to the epithelial cells (Yamauchi et al, 1990; Pearson et al., 1992), or localized in the single mucus layer (Johansson et al., 2011). In the lower part of the digestive tract, in the caeca, digestive microbiota have been described to form a 200 cells deep layer (Fuller, 1984), or may be localized in the upper layer of mucus near the intestinal content, and not in the lower layer of mucus (Johansson et al., 2011). This mucosal microbiota depends on available substrates coming from the mucosa such as desquamated cells or mucins, and molecules coming from the digestive contents diffusing into the protein matrix of mucus. It also depends on bacteria adhesins (Juge et al., 2012), specific adhesive sites on the mucus or mucosa, on mucus or cell renewal rates, on antibacterial substances such as secretory antibodies or peptides as defensins, or expression of innate immune receptors, contributing to the innate immune system of the digestive tract (Salzman et al., 2010; van Dijk et al., 2008; Hooper and Macpherson, 2010; Crhanova et al., 2011). These bacteria are particularly important from a physiological point of view, due to their narrow contact with the host and their function in the control of pathogens, modulation of digestive mucosal immunity, and their effect on digestive epithelium cells. However, in the chicken, this mucosal microbiota, different from the luminal microbiota, from the first works of Fuller (1984) has been relatively little studied compared to the studies on digestive contents (Zhu et al 2002; Collado and Sanz, 2007; Gong et al., 2007; Guardia et al., 2009; Moore et al., 2011; Malmuthuge et al., 2012).

The bacterial community present in the digestive tract shows a high phylogenetic complexity, particularly in the caeca. Apajalahti et al. (2004) found 640 different species, and more recent studies using 16S rRNA metagenomic pyrosequencing showed as much as 783 operational taxonomic units or OTU (Danzeisen et al., 2011; Moore et al., 2011; Nordentoft et al., 2011).

This bacterial community can be modified by several factors such as the first inoculum (Gulati et al., 2012), dietary components (Mathlouti et al., 2002; Apajalahti et al., 2004) or diet structure (Williams et al., 2008; Amerah et al., 2009) or feed additives such as antibiotic growth promotors (Danzeisen et al., 2011) or alternatives to antibiotic growth promotors such as organic acids, prebiotic, probiotic, vegetal compounds, enzymes, clay, charcoal ... (Gabriel et al., 2006; Yang and Choct, 2009; Huyghebaert et al., 2011; Bedford and Cowieson, 2012), or by stress (Suzuki et al., 1989), the nervous system (Lyte et al., 2010), rearing environment (Putskam et al., 2005; Gong et al., 2008; Guardia et al., 2011) and host genetic as indicated previously.

The phylogenetic complexity of digestive microbiota, and its high number of genes as shown by recent analyses of functional gene content using pyrosequencing in chicken (Qu et al., 2008; Danzeisen et al., 2011), derives from the intermediate of numerous metabolites and/or the direct action of bacteria on numerous physiological processes on the host, that can be beneficial or deleterious.

EFFECTS OF THE DIGESTIVE MICROBIOTA ON THE HOST

Digestive microbiota can be considered as an organ in the digestive tract that uses nutrients and metabolites, recognizes and synthesizes neuroendocrine hormones, interfaces with the nervous system that innervates the gastrointestinal tract, and as digestive epithelium products cell biomass (Lyte, 2010). As indicated previously, the digestive microbiota and the host have co-evolved after their first contact, and are considered as a supraorganism with numerous cross-talk between microbial and host cells (Lederberg, 2000). They seem to be more than mutually tolerant, and to be in a mutualistic relationship when equilibrium is reached.

Thus, the digestive microbiota has an effect on its live environment, the digestive tract. It contributes to the development, morphology and functionality of the digestive tract (Coates 1980, Furuse and Okumura 1994; Bäcked et al., 2005), stimulates mucin production and uses them as substrate, and it may modify intestinal transit.

These effects have consequences for animal digestion of carbohydrates, lipids, and proteins. Whereas Szylit et al. (1980) and Champs et al. (1981) showed that the microbiota is involved in starch digestion by bacterial hydrolysis in the crop, it acts mainly as competitor of the host in the small intestine. However, microbiota may have a positive effect by releasing nutrients that may be absorbed by the host in the small intestine or caeca, the latter also being able to absorb carbohydrates and amino acids (Moreto and Planas 1989), although the extent and benefit for the host of this activity is not known. Moreover fermentation of undigested compounds, mainly in the caeca, and bacterial metabolism of uric acid, allows producing SCFA, that can be absorbed by the digestive epithelium (Mead, 1997). It may represent 3-4% of energy supply or even 3 times more, but more studies are needed to determine the true involvement of digestive microbiota in energy supply (Jozefiak et al., 2004). Ammonia may also be absorbed and converted to non essential amino acids, although the biological importance is not known (Vispo and Karasov, 1997). Thus, for lipids, in young chicken of 3 weeks, microbiota led to a decrease of 2 points of apparent faecal digestibility for vegetal oil and 10 points for animal fat (Boyd and Edwards, 1967, Kussaibati et al., 1982b). Digestibility of saturated fatty acids, such as palmitic and stearic acids are highly decreased, whereas digestibility of unsaturated fatty acids, such as oleic and linoleic acids is not modified by microbiota (Boyd and Edwards, 1967). This is due to deconjugation of bile salts by some bacterial species, such as *Lactobacillus* (Kim and Lee, 2005). However the change in faecal digestibility may be due in part to endogenous lipids and bacterial biomass. For protein digestibility, effect of microbiota may depend on sensitivity to hydrolysis of proteins, bacteria being able to hydrolyse some resistant proteins for enzyme host (Salter 1973; Salter and Fulford, 1974; Kussaibati et al., 1982a). Concerning starch digestibility, no effect of microbiota was observed with maize starch by Kussaibati et al. (1982a). Due to the effect of digestive microbiota on nutrient digestibility, it can have an effect on metabolisable energy, positive or negative, (Kussaibati et al., 1982b; Furuse and Okumura, 1994). Moreover, for diets rich in soluble non-starch polysaccharides, leading to increased viscosity of digestive contents, microbiota is considered to be involved in the negative effect observed on digestion (Bedford and Cowieson, 2012), although according to Maisonnier et al. (2003) it is not the main factor. It can also not be ruled out that if chickens have access to litter it may allow them to practice coprophagy that may allow them to benefit from the bacterial cell composition as proteins or vitamins, although the quantitative importance of this phenomenon is not known.

The commensal microbiota is implicated in digestive health of animals. It contributes to the protection against harmful microorganisms (barrier effect) and stimulates the immune system (Ismail and Hooper, 2005; Sharma et al., 2010), leaving the host in a permanent inflammatory states (Klasing et al., 1991). Digestive microbiota contribute to production of toxic substances and conversely to detoxification of some compounds.

The digestive microbiota can also influence extra-digestive physiology of the host. Indeed, commensal bacteria by their metabolites or constituents, or even themselves, that pass through the digestive epithelium, have effects on the animal metabolism for example fattening (Bäcked et al., 2004; Cani et al., 2007), or on the central nervous system with effects on behavior (Lyte, 2010; Diamond et al., 2011).

These effects of microbiota lead to an increase of protein synthesis in the liver (metabolism and detoxification of bacterial products) and in the intestine (organ with high turnover) of +25% and + 45% respectively, corresponding to an increase of total protein synthesis of 6-8% (Muramatsu et al., 1987). Energy requirement is also increased by microbiota (Furuse and Okumura, 1994). Digestive microbiota may also contribute to mineral and vitamin nutrition (Gabriel et al., 2006).

Moreover the bacterial activity has consequences on non digestive pathologies, and thus animal welfare, such as conjunctivitis and respiratory problems due to irritant compounds products released by bacterial fermentation in the litter material (Thomke and Elwinger, 1998). These fermentations also have consequences on contact dermatitis (Shepherd and Fairchild, 2010) or pathogen development in the litter. All these effects have consequences on animal production, as well as on growth performance and product quality.

Globally, the digestive microbiota represents a cost for the animal, due to the competition with the host enzymes in the small intestine, and due to the stimulation of the immune system, and thus maintenance metabolic cost. However the digestive microbiota provides a protection against harmful microorganisms by the barrier effect and stimulation of immune system, is involved in starch hydrolysis in the crop, and allows energy recovery from compounds undigested by the host enzymatic system in the caeca. It may allow the animal to be more adaptable to environmental changes, as suggested by changes with environmental factors such as dietary composition or rearing conditions (Vispo and Karasov, 1997), thus improving its robustness. The balance state between the genetics of the host, dietary compounds and the digestive microbiota, has consequences for the host phenotype at the digestive level, and also at the animal scale.

In conclusion, from a nutritional point of view, the optimal microbiota would be one that allows for conversion of non digestible feed compounds and endogenous products (such as mucus and desquamated cells) by the host, to absorbable compounds such as SCFA. From a point of view of global host physiology, optimal microbiota would be one that converts unused digestive compounds by the host to absorbable energetic compounds and also allows for the best beneficial /harmful ratio for optimal host physiological function, as immunity stimulation to protect the host against harmful microorganisms but not too high inflammation, or optimal lipid metabolism.

Experimental model of birds selected on AMEn and consequences for digestive microbiota

The divergent D+ and D- lines allow determination of the limiting factors in digestive efficiency in the conditions of the selection, with a high content of wheat as the cereal source, a cultivar rich in arabinoxylan, and a high content of lipids, to maximize differences between individuals. The lines were selected on their AMEn at 3 weeks of age. This age was chosen because it represents a key period in gastrointestinal tract development. In order to maintain performances at a common level between lines, body weight was constrained among both lines.

DIGESTIVE CAPACITY AND DIGESTIVE TRACT OF D+ AND D- LINES

D+ and D- birds were characterized for several parameters on a large number of birds, as well as on digestive efficiency parameters, zootechnical parameters and organ size of the digestive tract in the upper and middle part (Mignon-Grasteau et al., 2004; de Verdal et al., 2010b, 2011b). Moreover, several studies were performed to study more deeply some parameters of their digestive physiology.

Due to their mode of selection, D+ birds showed low variability in their digestive capacities as they are near to the upper limit of possible values, whereas on the contrary D- birds showed high variability (Mignon-Grasteau et al., 2010; de Verdal et al., 2011b). This characteristic is also observed for other parameters studied in these two divergent lines as digestive organ size.

The difference between the two lines evolved with successive generations. Therefore, from the first generation of selection, a significant difference in digestive capacity (AMEn, lipid, starch and protein digestibility) was observed, and the differences increased with selection. It was accompanied by differences in anatomy of the digestive tract especially in relative weight of gizzard observed as soon as the first generation (Mignon-Grasteau et al., 2004; Péron et al., 2006), whereas a difference in small intestine relative weight was observed only from the 5th generation (Garcia et al., 2007; de Verdal et al., 2011b).

AMEn and faecal digestibility

Apparent metabolisable energy

The AMEn at 3 weeks of age showed a higher value of +13.2% between D+ and D- birds at the 2nd generation (Mignon-Grasteau et al., 2004), and +33.5% at the 8th generation (de Verdal et al., 2011b), showing the increased divergence in this selected character. At 8 weeks of age, this difference between the lines disappeared for the 2nd generation (Carré et al., 2005), whereas it persisted for the 9th generation (de Verdal et al., 2010b). Thus the results observed at 3 weeks of age would still hold for the whole production cycle.

However, the results are highly diet-dependent. Although D+ chickens showed a small variation in AMEn between maize and wheat (2.9%), D- chickens displayed a high AMEn variation (10.3%) (Carré et al., 2008). Thus D- birds showed higher difficulties to adapt to a wheat diet, compared to D+ birds. Moreover D- chickens showed a limited capacity to digest an easily digestible diet, as shown by their lower AMEn than D+ chickens with a maize diet (-5.2%).

Other feed x genotype interactions have been observed between these lines. For example, a soft wheat cultivar compared to a hard one resulted in an AMEn improvement in D+ birds (+6.1%) but not in D- birds (Péron et al., 2006). A fine particle diet with maize as cereal source resulted in digestion improvement only in the D+ birds (+2.2%), whereas a deterioration was observed in the D- birds (-2.5%) (Rougière et al., 2009).

Heritability of AMEn is also diet-dependent. It has been estimated in different experiments between 0.30 and 0.38 when birds were fed with wheat, and only 0.15 when they were fed with maize (Mignon-Grasteau et al., 2004, 2010a; de Verdal et al., 2011b). The strong positive genetic correlations estimated between these traits recorded in both diet treatments (0.73 to 0.88) however showed that selecting on these traits with wheat diets would improve performance both on wheat and maize diets.

Excreta digestibilities

As D+ birds fed with wheat diets were characterized at the 5th generation by a higher AMEn than D- birds (+36.5%), the D+ birds were characterized by higher faecal digestibilities of lipids, starch, and proteins, with a highest difference observed for lipid (+58.0%), intermediate for starch (+39.3%), and lowest although significant for protein (+13.3%) (Carré et al., 2007). However with a maize diet, at the 6th generation, differences between lines were lower as well as for AMEn (+6.4%), and for digestibility, the higher difference was observed for protein digestibility (+9.1%) followed by lipid digestibility (+5.6%), and the lowest difference although significant was for starch digestibility (+1.3%) (Rougière et al., 2009). Thus the limiting factors for the D- birds digestibility were dependent on the cereal source.

Heritabilities of faecal digestibility of lipids, starch and proteins for the 8th first generations were 0.25 to 0.29 (Mignon-Grasteau et al., 2010a). Genetic correlations between AMEn and faecal lipid, starch and protein digestibilities were 0.80 to 0.91 (Mignon-Grasteau et al., 2004, 2010a). As for AMEn, heritability was much lower when birds were fed with maize (0.04 to 0.09), except for starch that presented equivalent levels of heritability with both diets.

Besides the improved digestive efficiency, selection on AMEn shows a positive effect on total animal wastes, composed of undigested compounds and metabolic wastes. Thus D+ birds showed a 34.9% lower nitrogen and a 19.0% lower phosphorus excretion relative to nitrogen and phosphorus intake (de Verdal et al., 2011c). Moreover the ratio of nitrogen to phosphorus in excreta was lowered by -20.3% in D+ chickens which implies that losses of nitrogen after excretion have to be more limited in D+ than in D- birds (-15% vs -35%) in order to produce a manure equilibrated for fertilization (Mignon-Grasteau et al., 2010b). Indeed heritability of nitrogen excreted / nitrogen intake, phosphorus excreted / phosphorus intake and nitrogen excreted / phosphorus excreted is moderate, 0.29, 0.22 and 0.18 respectively, and the genetic correlations between AMEn and these 3 traits are highly negative, -0.99, -0.64, and -0.84, respectively.

Bird performance

D+ birds were also characterized at the 8th generation by lower feed intake from 17 to 23 d (-21.5%) than D- birds, improved feed efficiency (+58.0%), higher weight gain (WG) (+13.7%) and higher body weight at 23 d (+14.5%) (de Verdal et al., 2011b). The lower feed intake and lower FCR of D+ birds compared to D- birds was observed from the 2nd generation, -11.4% and -25.6% respectively, whereas no significant effect was observed on WG (Mignon-Grasteau et al., 2004). At 8 weeks, age at which birds reached the market weight, the difference in body weight completely disappeared (de Verdal et al., 2010b).

The higher feed intake of D- birds was explained as an attempt to compensate for their poor feed efficiency and thus the lack of energy obtained from the diet (Carré et al., 2008). Differences between lines for feed efficiency, at the 9th generation, were observed to be significantly different from 7 to 21 d and 21 to 53 d when birds reached the market age, but not from 4 to 7 d (de Verdal et al., 2010b). Differences in feed intake were observed to be significantly different from 4 to 7 d.

Heritability of zootechnical performance showed a moderate to high value at the 8th generation, ranging from 0.21 for FCR, 0.30 for WG and 0.47 for feed intake (De Verdal et al., 2011b), near to those obtained at the 2nd generation, with 0.27-0.32 for FCR, 0.31-0.35 for WG and 0.47 for FI (Mignon-Grasteau et al., 2004). These results are consistent with the high genetic correlations estimated between FCR and AMEn, which ranged between -0.77 and -0.99, and with the low correlations between AMEn and body weight at 3 weeks of age (0.10 to 0.24, Mignon-Grasteau et al., 2004; de Verdal et al., 2011b).

Moreover, it is noteworthy that D+ and D- lines showed different behaviours towards a new environment and diet (Pelhaitre et al., 2012).

Digestive tract anatomy and physiology

Studies on characterization of these lines showed anatomical and physiological differences in all the parts of the digestive system which together have major complementary roles. Analysis of covariance with feed intake as covariate showed that the quantity of feed passing through the gastrointestinal tract cannot be the only cause of difference between the lines (de Verdal et al., 2011b).

Upper part of the digestive tract: crop and stomach

The crop

Digestion of feed in chicken begins in the crop where diet is humidified and is mixed with some enzymes coming from digestive reflux, feed ingredients and microbiota (Duke, 1986 ; Denbow, 1999). Bacterial amylase coming mainly from *Lactobacillus* species has been implicated in starch hydrolysis (Szylit et al., 1980; Champs et al., 1983).

For the D+ and D- lines, observation of crop showed no difference in relative weight at 3 weeks of age or in pH of its content at 7, 21 or 53 d (de Verdal et al, 2011ab). A trend for a higher retention time of fine particles (+88%) in D+ birds was observed at 9 d of age, but only numerically higher at 29 d (+ 43%) with a maize diet (Rougière et Carré, 2010). Differences may be more important with wheat diet, as shown by higher difference in digestive efficiency. Although the absence of line effect on the relative weight of the crop, heritability estimates of this trait for the animal of the 8th generation at 23 d showed a moderate value (0.21).

The proventriculus-gizzard complex

In birds, the stomach is composed of two parts: the proventriculus or glandular part where hydrochloric acid and pepsinogen are produced; and the gizzard or muscular part, where digesta are ground by muscular contractions. Particles are directed through the pylorus to the small intestine as they reach a critical size of about 0.5-1.5 mm (Ferrando et al.,1987). The pylorus is not a sphincter as it allows reflux from the duodenum to the gizzard. This organ is more developed when diet includes coarse particles as whole cereals (Gabriel et al., 2003; Svihus, 2011). Chemical and enzymatic hydrolysis of proteins occurs in the gizzard thanks to the low pH and pepsin, which is active within a large range of pH in the chicken (Crévieu-Gabriel et al., 1999). It allows hydrolysis of the major dietary proteins as well as of the surrounding protein matrix of starch granules in wheat with high hardness value. The mechanical action of the gizzard allows cell wall breakdown and particle size reduction of dietary components, leading to an increased area for improved contact between enzymes and substrates.

It is in this compartment that the differences between D+ and D- birds are the most striking. The relative weights of the proventriculus and gizzard are higher in D+ birds than D- birds, +21.9% and +34% respectively, at 3 weeks of age at the 8th generation (de Verdal et al., 2011b). However a great variability is observed in the proventriculus weight of D+ birds due to the presence of enlarged proventriculus in some families of D+ birds (Rougière and Carré, 2010; de Verdal et al., 2011b), as observed with ground diet contrary to whole cereal diet (O'Dell et al., 1959; Gabriel et al., 2003; Taylor and Jones, 2004). This difference is absent at hatch and appear after contact with the feed as soon as 7 d, reach a maximum at 3 weeks of age and disappear at 8 weeks with wheat diet (Péron et al., 2006; Garcia et al., 2007; de Verdal et al., 2010b). When fed with a maize diet, the difference was considerably reduced but persisted from 9 to 63 d (Rougière and Carré, 2010).

Evolution of gizzard weight with selection on AMEn is consistent both with its high heritability (0.53) and its positive genetic correlation with AMEn (0.43; de Verdal et al., 2011b). Proventriculus weight was also positively correlated with AMEn (0.59) and with gizzard weight (0.26-0.81; Rance et al., 2002, de Verdal et al., 2011b), which explains its evolution in these lines, despite its poor heritability (0.09).

At the 8th generation, pH of gizzard content was lower in D+ birds than in D- birds at 3 weeks of age (de Verdal et al., personal communication). Pepsin activity in the proventriculus tissue was observed to be higher in D+ birds when expressed as per animal body weight (Péron et al., 2007), however the pepsin activity in digestive content is not known.

The isthmus area between the proventriculus and the gizzard showed a 4 times larger lumen and a 1.4 larger total area of this region for D+ than for D- birds (N. Rideau, personal communication.). This is the region where are located the interstitial cells of Cajal, the pacemaker of gizzard contraction (Reynhout and Duke, 1999). In D- birds, the isthmus mucosa has a more oval shape, is more twisted, and its muscular part is more developed than in D+ birds.

A higher mean retention time was observed in the stomach of D+ than in D- chickens at 9 and 29 d with a maize diet (Rougière and Carré, 2010). This may improve nutrient accessibility in D+ birds by increasing time for grinding and enzymatic activity. For D- birds, the lower mean retention time can be explained by a failure in the gizzard relaxation process of these birds during resting periods (no access to diet or light) (Rougière et al., 2012). According to Rougière and Carré (2010), the mean retention time in the proventriculus-gizzard system was a major factor associated with genotype differences between the D+ and D- genetic lines.

These studies with D+ and D- lines bring new knowledge related to digestive physiology, concerning the role of gizzard. For a long time, the importance of gizzard in the optimal digestion of proteins and lipids in the chicken has been recognized, by showing decrease of digestion in gizzardectomized chicken especially with coarse particles (Fritz et al., 1936). Several studies showed that a greater development of the gizzard is related to improved digestibility (Hetland and Svihus, 2001; Ravindran et al., 2006). In D+ and D- lines, the individual relative weights of the gastric compartment were found to be strongly positively linked to retention times

(Rougière and Carré, 2010). This is in agreement with the observation that a longer gizzard mean retention time (adjusted to a mean body weight) is associated with a heavier gizzard in Leghorn than in broiler chickens (Shires et al., 1987). Moreover, a significant positive relationship was observed in D+ and D- lines between the retention time of fine feed particles in the proventriculus-gizzard system and the digestive efficiency assessed by measured AMEn / calculated AMEn or by faecal digestibility of proteins (Rougière and Carré, 2010). Thus gastric retention time was proposed as a major limiting factor for digestive efficiency in chickens. Furthermore, retention time in the stomach of D+ and D- lines was modified by the introduction of fibre in the diet, but with a different effect according to line: fibre decrease transit time in D+ birds, and increase it in D- birds (Rougière and Carré, 2010). According to these results, it has been hypothesized that the critical size controlling gastric emptying depends on rheologic properties of feed particles of the diet, but also on genetic factors. However retention time seems not to be the only major limiting factor as decreased retention time with fibre in D+ birds led to decreased AMEn and protein digestibility, but in D- birds, the increased retention time with fibre led to increased protein digestibility, but decreased AMEn.

Middle part of the digestive tract: the small intestine

The small intestine is the site of hydrolysis of feed compounds by pancreatic and intestinal enzymes with the help of bile acids for lipids. The intestinal surface area is highly developed in order to increase the contact between its epithelium and components in the digestive tract, and to allow for final hydrolysis and absorption by enterocytes.

The higher feed intake of D- birds contributes to higher intestinal content in these birds (+54%, Garcia et al., 2007). This higher intestinal content may in part be responsible for the higher development of intestinal segment tissue to cope with higher digesta quantities to process. However, statistical analysis that included feed intake as a covariate showed that it is not the only factor responsible for the difference in the digestive tract (de Verdal et al., 2011b). According to Rougière and Carré (2010); the intestine enlargement observed in D- compared to D+ birds was probably an adaptive process trying to counteract the low digestive efficiency in D- birds in the upper part of the digestive tract. It can also be an adaptation of D- birds compensating for their higher sensitivity to the negative effect of viscosity of arabinoxylan on absorption (Garcia et al., 2007). This higher development is facilitated by the availability of space in the rib cage due to lower stomach development in these birds.

The contrast in development between the upper and middle part of the digestive tract is consistent with the moderate negative genetic correlation between gizzard weight and jejunum density (-0.56) (de Verdal et al., 2011b). This is in agreement with results showing lower development of gizzard and higher development of small intestine with ground wheat instead of whole wheat inclusion (Gabriel et al., 2003), or with a diet with fine instead of coarse particles (Nir et al., 1994). The difference in small intestine between D+ and D- lines appeared later than those of the gizzard, being not observed at hatching and 7d, but detected at 9 d with maize diet, and persisted until 53 and 63 d with wheat or maize diet, although the difference between lines was considerably reduced at the end of the rearing period (de Verdal et al., 2010ab; Rougière and Carré, 2010). This delay in divergence in the upper and lower part of the gastrointestinal tract is consistent with the hypothesis that the small intestine grows in response to the functional efficiency of the gizzard. One can assume that the difference in small intestine size is not due to a delay in development of the digestive tract at the beginning of life, as observed with delay in feed accessibility to young chicken (Noy and Uni, 2010), as the yolk sac relative weight is not significantly different between the two lines at hatch (de Verdal et al., 2010a), and none were empty (de Verdal, personal communication).

This higher relative intestinal weight in D- birds at 3 weeks of age concerns each of the three segments, although less pronounced in duodenum (+15%) than in jejunum (+37%) and ileum (+40%) (de Verdal et al., 2011b). This discrepancy between the 3 segments could be due to the fact that the absorption process predominates in the jejunum and ileum (Denbow, 1999). This higher relative weight is due to increased length (+3%, +6% and +4%, for duodenum, jejunum and ileum respectively) but mainly to increased density (weight to length ratio) (+12%, +30% and + 31%, for duodenum, jejunum and ileum respectively). Heritability estimates of intestinal traits for birds in the 8th generation at 23 d showed high values for weight, length and density of these 3 small intestinal segments (from 0.28 to 0.50) (de Verdal et al., 2011b). High positive genetic correlations were observed between the weight of the duodenum, the jejunum and the ileum (0.62 to 0.88), as observed by Rance et al. (2002). This implies a parallel evolution of the 3 intestinal segments.

The increased density of intestinal segments may be explained in part by changes observed at the microstructure of the intestine. Indeed, D- chickens have higher villi height in the jejunum, greater villus area and crypts size in the three intestinal segments (de Verdal et al., 2010a). Moreover, the tunica muscularis is thicker in the three intestinal segments of D- birds that may be due to higher intestinal content to move along the intestine (de Verdal et al., 2010a).

The higher villi area of D- birds may suggest a higher potential of membrane hydrolysis and absorption in their intestine. Moreover, in the jejunum, they may have a higher efficiency as higher villi may mean more mature enterocytes, as enterocytes mature when moving up the villi. Although increased development in absorptive surface in the intestine was observed, D- birds are not able to compensate for their lower proventriculus-gizzard functionality, as shown by their lower total tract digestibility of starch, proteins and lipids. This may be due to a lower digestive functionality of epithelium. This may also be due to a lower accessibility of nutrients in the small intestine of D- chickens. This may be in part due to a limitation in absorption capacity, as shown by the pronounced effect of xylanase in a wheat diet on conjugated bile salts in D- birds supplemented with antibiotics, as viscosity primarily acts on absorption (Garcia et al., 2007).

The higher development of crypt size in D- birds, may indicate a more intense cell production, necessary for higher villi development. No difference between lines was observed for the villus height / crypt depth ratio, showing a similar balance between membrane hydrolysis / absorptive potential and cell turnover in the two chicken lines.

More goblet cells per villus were observed in D- birds in jejunum and ileum, which may lead to higher mucin secretion (de Verdal et al., 2010a). This may be due to higher need to protect the epithelium due to heavier digesta content or protection against microorganisms (Forstner and Forstner, 1994; Laboisse et al., 1996; Johansson et al., 2011). Other mechanisms of innate immune system may be stimulated, such as lymphocyte cells, and contribute to higher density of intestinal tissues of D- birds in jejunum and ileum. This higher mucin production may lead to higher endogenous wastes, as these glycoproteins are difficult to hydrolyze, and may thus contribute to lower apparent protein digestibility of the D- birds. Moreover if this increase mucin production leads to a thicker mucus layer, although a higher number of goblet cell does not necessarily lead to a thicker mucus layer, it may restrict nutrient absorption (Iiboshi et al., 1996), contributing to lower digestibility. This may explain the high negative genetic correlation observed between AMEn and small intestinal weight segments, jejunum (-0.67) and ileum (-0.77) (de Verdal et al., 2011b).

All these modifications at the intestinal level might lead to a higher maintenance cost for D- birds as the intestinal epithelium has a high turn-over, and mucin production represents an energy cost, and this may contribute to the lower feed efficiency of the D- birds.

D+ birds fed with a maize diet had a higher relative weight of the pancreas (+15%), which was positively associated with the gizzard weight (Rougière and Carré, 2010). It suggests a common pathway for regulation of growth of the pancreas and gizzard. However, with a wheat diet, difference lower relative weight of pancreas (-16%) was observed in D+ birds (Péron et al., 2007). In the latter study, proteolytic activity in this organ expressed per body weight, was lower in D+ birds when wheat was of low hardness value, but without a difference when wheat was of high hardness value. No data is available in regards to digestive enzymatic activities in intestinal contents.

Digestive contents of D+ and D- lines showed some differences in their composition in terms of pH and bile salts. pH of the intestinal content showed no difference between lines at 7 d, but was higher for D+ birds in duodenum and ileum at 21 d and in ileum at 53 d (de Verdal, personal communication), which is the opposite to what was observed in the gizzard content, as was observed with whole wheat feeding (Gabriel et al., 2003).

Intestinal contents of D+ birds showed more conjugated bile acids and total bile acids (Garcia et al., 2007). This may be due to higher synthesis or lower degradation by digestive microbiota (Garcia et al., 2007) and probably explains partly the difference in lipid digestibility between the lines. However, supplementing diet with xylanase and antibiotics together from 8 d of age did not suppress the difference in lipid digestibility between lines despite similar bile acid levels. This means that this difference in digestion efficiency between lines could not be explained only in terms of bile salts. Other limiting factors should exist in D- birds that relate to the secretion of digestive enzymes or absorption capacities (Rougière et al., 2010).

No difference in transit time was observed between the lines when fed a maize/soyabean diet (Rougière and Carré, 2010). However, with wheat the results may be different.

Besides the composition in small intestine in terms of pH and bile acids that differed between the two lines, starch, protein and lipid content are probably not the same, as suggested by the differences in faecal digestibility between the two lines, and the different gap between digestibility of starch, proteins and lipids of the two lines with larger difference for lipids, intermediate for starch and lowest for proteins with wheat diet as characterized at the 5th generation (Carré et al., 2007). Thus, undigested compounds of D+ birds are lower and may be relatively more concentrated in protein, and conversely undigested compounds of D- birds are more important and may be far more concentrated in starch. It must however be taken into account that the undigested components measured at the faecal level, as performed until now for the evaluation of digestibility in the D+ and D- lines, are only an approximation of components at the end of the small intestine. Indeed it does not take into account further bacterial metabolic modifications. Indeed bacteria use the undigested components in the lower digestive tract with additional urinary products as substrates leading to bacterial biomass, with a specific composition[2] and bacterial products as SCFA. Despite these microbial metabolic activities, a difference between composition of small intestinal content of the two lines can still be presumed, due to the relative low modification of microbiota in birds compared to mammals, although not negligible, as assessed

---

2   About 50-70% of crude protein, 8-10% lipids and 20-25% saccharides with structural and exo-polysaccharides and nucleic acids, but with variability according to species

by its relatively low contribution in excreta, estimated to be 11% of dry matter and 25% of protein in chickens (Parsons et al., 1982).

Contrary to these differences in chemical composition of intestinal content, and despite differences in gizzard development in the two lines, distribution of particle size in the digestive contents of the ileum of the two lines after feeding a diet with wheat of high or low hardness values, showed no significant difference (Péron et al., 2007).

Lower part of the digestive tract: Caeca/colon

The lower part of the digestive tract has been less studied in the D+ and D- lines than the upper and middle part, as it is widely accepted that in birds, major digestive processes occur in the upper and middle parts, with the lower part being relatively small compared to that of mammals.

The caeca are two blind sacs at the end of the small intestine. Villi present in the proximal area of caeca act as filters allowing entrance of only liquids and small particles of the digesta. Moreover urine can backflow from the cloaca. Caeca are the site of reabsorption of water and electrolytes, immune cell production, and the major site of bacterial fermentation in chicken and may contribute to energy extracted from the feed by the host-microbiota association, thanks to reabsorption of bacterial metabolites.

Although less studied, some data are available about the caeca of D+ and D- birds. At the 8th generation, at 3 weeks of age, higher digestive contents were observed in the caeca in D+ birds (+80%; H. de Verdal, personal communication) and at 4 weeks of age with maize / soya diet a higher relative tissue weight (+29%; Rougière and Carré, 2010). Moreover higher transit time was observed in D+ birds (x2; Rougière and Carré, 2010). Thus at 3 weeks of age, caecal functions appeared more developed in D+ than in D- birds, which may contribute to higher energy extracted from the diet, and thus higher AMEn.

Moreover, as explained previously for small intestinal composition, one can expect that the differences in composition of caecal contents in terms of starch, proteins and lipids between D+ and D- birds are similar to the difference in composition of excreta, despite modification by bacterial metabolism as explained before, and filtration of digesta at the caecal entrance. Thus contents may be relatively rich in protein for D+ birds and conversely relatively rich in starch for D- birds. Moreover, concerning the caeca, urinary compounds composed mainly of uric acid are present, and may be more concentrated in D+ than D- birds (De Verdal et al., 2011c).

Concerning the colon, also named rectum in birds, it has a short size, lower than caeca, and lower retention time. It may be implied in water and electrolyte reabsorption as well as SCFA and other bacterial metabolites, in a lower extent than the caeca. This digestive part has been little studied in birds due to its low size, and has not been studied in D+ and D- lines.

All the changes observed in the digestive tract morphology and physiology lead to a change in terms of available substrates and digestive environment such as pH, those parameters being implied in digestive microbiota development.

CONSEQUENCES OF SELECTION ON AMEn ON DIGESTIVE MICROBIOTA

Digestive microbiota of D+ and D- birds

Digestive microbiota of the two divergent chicken lines was studied in birds from the 10th generation, in two digestive segments, the small intestine, more precisely the terminal ileum and the caeca. For these studies, birds were reared on litter for the first days of life, and placed in individual cages after 10 days of life, as in other works on these lines for AMEn determination. The analyses showed clear differences between microbiota of the two lines in both the digestive contents and in the mucosa.

In the ileum contents, no significant difference in total bacteria load per gram of fresh weight was shown with a mean value of 4.28×10^{10} copies of 16S rDNA/g (Konsak et al., 2012). As small intestine content is 50% more important in D- birds (Garcia et al., 2007), the total bacterial biomass in the small intestine is expected to be higher in D- birds. Comparison of bacterial fingerprint, which provides an overview of the major bacteria, showed variability between animals of the same line was slightly higher in D+ birds (Gabriel et al., 2011; Konsak et al., 2011). Moreover, statistical analysis of the fingerprints of the two bird lines showed significant difference between the two lines. More precisely, identification of specific bacteria showed a higher amount of a strain of a long segmented filamentous organism in D+ birds, belonging to cluster I of *Clostridium*, and a strain of *L. crispatus* in D- birds (Konsak et al., unpublished data). Moreover, quantitative analysis of the main bacterial groups found in the digestive tract of chickens (*Lactobacillus* and *Clostridium* genus, for the main phylum Firmicutes, *E. coli* species for the phylum Proteobacteria, and *Bacteroides* for the phylum Bacteroidetes) of this microbiota, showed difference (Konsak et al., 2012). Thus, D+ chickens showed a higher amount of *C. coccoides* and D- chickens a higher amount of *E. coli*.

In the caeca contents, as in the ileum contents, no significant difference in total bacteria load per gram of fresh weight was shown with mean value of 4.36×10^{11}

copies of 16S rDNA/g (Konsak et al., 2012). As caecal content is 80% higher in D+ birds (H. de Verdal, personal communication), the total bacterial biomass in this organ is expected to be higher in D+ birds compared to D- birds, and clearly higher than those of their small intestine, in contrast to D- birds that may have a similar or slightly higher bacterial load in the small intestine than in their caeca. Conversely to the ileum content, variability between microbiota of animals of the same line was lower in D+ birds (Gabriel et al., 2011; Konsak et al., 2011). Moreover, a high difference between the fingerprints of the two bird lines was observed, and a higher relative amount of an *E. coli* strain was found in D- birds (Konsak et al., unpublished data). Moreover, quantitative analysis of the main bacterial groups showed in D+ birds more *C. leptum* group, and in D- birds more *Lactobacillus*, and particularly *L. salivarius*, a dominant lactic acid bacteria in the broiler digestive tract (Engberg et al., 2000; Souza et al., 2007; Gong et al., 2007), and more *E. coli* (Konsak et al., 2012).

In the ileal mucosa, no difference in total bacteria load per tissue between lines was observed in the distal part of ileum with 2.49×10^9 copies of 16S rDNA/ segment (Konsak et al., 2012). However, the concentration in the mucus layer may be different. Indeed, higher digestive content and higher tissue weight implied higher mucosa area. Moreover, a higher number of goblet cells in villi in D- birds may lead to a higher mucus layer thickness. Thus a lower bacterial concentration in mucus matrix may be assumed. Quantitative analysis of the main bacterial groups of the digestive tract of chicken, showed in D- birds, more *L. salivarius* (Konsak et al., 2012).

In the caecal mucosa, no difference in total bacteria load per tissue between lines was observed with 7.66×10^9 copies of 16S rDNA/segment (Konsak et al., 2012). However, as this tissue is more developed in D+ birds, mucosal area is higher. Moreover, as explained previously, bacterial load is expected to be higher, which may lead to higher thickness of the mucus layer(s) to protect the epithelium. In consequence, the bacterial density in the mucus layer may be lower in D+ birds. As in the caecal content, a high difference between fingerprints of the two bird lines was observed, and a higher relative amount of an *E. coli* strain in D+ birds, and a *L. salivarius* strain in D- birds (Gabriel et al., 2011; Konsak et al., 2011; Konsak et al., unpublished data). In this mucosa, quantitative analysis of the main bacterial groups, showed more total *Lactobacillus*, as well as *L. salivarius* and *L. crispatus* in D- birds (Konsak et al., 2012).

To go further in the characterization of the digestive microbiota, by quantification of the main bacterial groups, a study was performed on a F2 cross between D+ and D- lines and on a high number of birds (144 animals) with high range of AMEn (from 7.6 to 16.1 MJ/kg) (Gabriel et al., unpublished data). The study was focused on one of the more discriminant biotope observed previously, caecal content (Gabriel et al., 2011). Significant relationships were observed between a faecal nutrient component, starch content and the concentrations of caecal bacteria, *Lactobacillus* and ratio between *Lactobacillus* and *Clostridium*. A higher starch content is thus associated with a higher development of *Lactobacillus*, especially *L. crispatus* and *L. salivarius*, and with higher ratios of *L. crispatus* to *C. leptum* and of *L. salivarius* to *C. leptum*, and conversely with a low ratio of *C. leptum* to *Lactobacillus*. Significant heritability estimates were observed for bacterial numbers, or higher for bacterial ratios. Thus heritability ranged between 0.11 and 0.14 for the genus *Lactobacillus*, and more precisely with *L. salivarius*. Higher heritability estimates were obtained (h^2 close to 0.20) for the ratios of *L. salivarius* to *C. leptum* and of *C. leptum* to *C. coccoides*. The highest heritability was estimated for the ratio of *C. coccoides* to *Lactobacillus* (h^2=0.34). These estimates imply that the development of microbiota is partly controlled by the genetics of the host. These results obtained on F2 cross of divergent genetic lines confirmed previous studies in mammals as well as in chickens that proposed that digestive microbiota may be dependent on host genetics. For future studies, it would also be interesting to evaluate the importance of genetics of the host on microbiota development under different diets, as other studies showed that chicken microbiota development was affected by the diet.

Are the differences of microbiota only the consequence of digestive biotope modification?

The differences in digestive microbiota between the two lines of chickens selected on digestive capacity may be partly due to the consequence of change of biotopes of the digestive segments due to differences in digestive physiology and intestinal contents.

As indicated previously the inoculum of middle and lower parts of the digestive tract is the microbiota of the crop. At present, no statistical difference between the two lines was observed at the level of this organ, except a trend to a higher retention time in D+ birds at 9 d but not at 29 days with maize diet (Rougière and Carré, 2010). The microbiota of this organ has not been studied until now.

Going down to the following segments of the digestive tract, microbiota undergoes the acidic pH of the stomach. As mentioned previously, in D+ birds, the contents have a lower pH and a higher retention time, leading to more deleterious conditions for bacterial survival in these birds. After this chemical selection of bacteria, leading to high reduction of their number, some of them persist due to development of acid survival systems (Jensen et al., 2012; Hong et al., 2012a; Ramos-Morales, 2012).

In the small intestinal contents, conditions of bacterial growth became more appropriate, especially towards the distal part. Microbiota development depends on environmental conditions, digestive transit, presence of inhibitors, growth factors, predators, and available substrates (from exogenous and endogenous origins).

As stated previously, these environmental conditions are not the same in the small intestine of D+ and D- birds. In D+ birds, pH was higher than in D-birds, which may affect bacterial balance. In D- birds, if the higher quantity of goblet cells in villi leads to a thicker mucus layer, it may have a negative effect on oxygen diffusion from blood vessels (Saldena et al., 2000) leading to lower oxygen concentration in digestive content, and thus on bacterial balance according to their sensitivity to oxygen. Substances such as bile acids can inhibit bacterial growth. In D+ birds, these acids contents are higher, which gives them higher power to control microbiota growth in the small intestine.

Apart from the environmental conditions in the small intestine that differ between the two lines, available substrates are probably not the same. Firstly, due to the difference in digestibility between the two lines, substrates are present in higher amounts in D- birds. Secondly, as the differences in digestibility efficiency between lines are larger for lipids, intermediate for starch and lowest for proteins as characterized at the 5th generation by Carré et al. (2007), relative quantities of these compounds in the small intestine are probably different as explained previously. According to the concentration of these substrates, some bacteria groups are more adapted, according to their enzymatic equipment. Thus, as the intestinal content of D+ birds may be well balanced with relatively high concentration in proteins, this may explain the higher content in *Clostridium* able to use various substrates according to species and strains (Fonty and Chaucheyras-Durand, 2008). On the contrary, as the intestinal content of D- birds may be more concentrated in starch, which is favorable to *Lactobacillus,* and may explain the higher load of *L. crispatus*.

In addition to changes in proteins, saccharides and lipids composition of small intestinal content, the origin of these compounds and thus their susceptibility to hydrolysis may vary. They are composed of undigested dietary components and components produced by the host. The former depend on diet composition, and are composed of undigested dietary proteins, starch and lipids, and dietary fibre mainly coming from plant polysaccharides such as arabinoxylan of wheat. Components produced by the host are mucus, mainly mucin (glycoprotein with low sensitivity to hydrolysis, Carlstedt et al., 1993), desquamated cells from the digestive tract and dead bacterial cells. This second source of substrates represents an important source of proteins. It depends on mucus production and rate of cell turnover in the digestive tract (animal and microbial cells). In the case of D- birds, this part may represent a higher amount than in D+ birds as suggested by the higher number of goblet cells in villi of these birds and their higher crypt depth.

In the caeca, as for intestinal content, D+ birds may have a relative well balanced composition although richer in proteins, and may have higher content of uric acid, whereas D- birds may have a relative high starch concentration. In the D+ chickens that are subjected to lower fermentation in the small intestine compared to D- birds, one can suppose that undigested digesta are composed essentially of components undigestible by the host enzymes such as non-starch polysaccharides and endogenous proteins, and may favour fermentation by certain bacteria, which could explain the higher development of caeca in D+ birds. As for the ileum, the caecal content composition may explain the preferential development of *Clostridium* in D+ birds and *Lactobacillus* in D- birds.

For the bacteria of the mucosa, present in the mucus layer(s), no difference in total load was observed between the two lines, as well as in the small intestine and in the caeca. However, as explained previously, a lower concentration in mucus matrix of the small intestine of D- birds, and of the caeca of D+ birds may be assumed. These differences may be due to modification of the composition of the major component of mucus, mucin. And yet, these glycoproteins represent binding sites for bacteria. Moreover mucin is a substrate for bacteria, as well as desquamated cells and molecules able to pass through the mucous gel. Quantity of desquamated cells may be changed if cell turn-over is affected by selection as suggested by higher crypt depth in the small intestine of D- birds. The reachable molecules in the mucus may be modified due to changes in animal digestion as well as bacterial fermentations in the digestive lumen. This may explain the higher development of *Lactobacillus* in the digestive mucosa of D- birds compared to D+ birds. Moreover changes in digestive physiology may lead to changes in physicochemical parameters, such as pH or redox potential, in the mucin matrix. It can also not be ruled out that AMEn selection may have led to selection on antimicrobial peptides as defensins, as the genetic of the host is implied in the level of gene expression of these peptides (Hong et al., 2012b). However, we do not have such information about the D+ and D- lines.

We thus saw that the differences between the D+ and D- lines in digestive efficiency, anatomy and histology of the digestive tract compartments may explain some of the differences in composition of their microbiota. Reciprocally, the digestive microbiota, as indicated at the beginning of this paper, has numerous effects on the digestive tract, and also on the whole physiology of its host and can thus influence digestive and feed efficiency of the host.

Effect of digestive microbiota of the D+ D- lines on the host

The contribution of digestive microbiota in the difference between D+ and D- lines was shown by the different effect of a high dose of antibiotic from 8 d of age in the diet of these chickens, with higher effects in D- than D+ birds on AMEn and growth performance (Garcia et al., 2007). The higher bacterial load in the small intestine of D- birds may be responsible for the lower pH of small intestinal contents and may lead to fermentation of diet compounds instead of host digestion causing a diversion of nutrients to the bacteria to the detriment of the host. Thus an inverse relationship between small intestinal bacterial density and growth efficiency has been shown (Apajalahti et al., 2004). On the contrary, in the D+ birds, high fermentative activity in the caeca of undigestible compounds by the host, may lead to higher energy extracted from the diet.

The bacteria may be responsible for the higher epithelium development of the small intestine of D- birds as certain strains have an effect on epithelial cells. It may also be an adaptation of the host to compete with bacteria for the use of dietary compounds. However, the microbiota may increase the integrity of the epithelium through upregulation of cross-bridging proteins (Hooper et *al.*, 2001), and thus decrease intestinal absorption as in birds, paracellular absorption is an important way of nutrient absorption (Caviedes-Vidal et al., 2007). Moreover, the effect of microbiota on intestine could also pass through a stimulation of the intestinal immune system, which is the most important immune system of the body. As presented before higher level of bacteria in the small intestine of D- birds compared to D+ birds may be responsible in part to the higher goblets cells in villi of the D- chickens, as they can stimulate mucin production (Sakata and Setoyam 1995), contributing to innate intestinal immune system. This increased bacterial load may also lead to inflammation and increase expression of antimicrobial peptides as defensins (Menendez and Brett Finlay, 2007). Thus digestive microbiota may contribute to the higher relative weight and density of the small intestine of D- birds.

This high development of bacteria may lead to higher amounts of harmful products that need to be detoxified and may contribute to higher liver relative weight in D- birds (+2.6%; de Verdal et al., 2011b). Moreover the low level of bile acids in the small intestine of D- birds may be in part due to their deconjugation by bacteria such as *Lactobacillus* (Maisonnier et al., 2003; Kim and Lee, 2005), which are present in large quantity in these birds. Consistently with this hypothesis, the beneficial effects of high dose of antibiotics on conjugated bile acids content is higher in D- than in D+ line (+109% and +36% respectively), and consequently improved lipid digestibility and AMEn more in D- birds (+35% and +14%) than in D+ birds (+5.7% and +2.6%, Garcia et al., 2007). Indeed although *Lactobacillus* genus is more often seen as beneficial bacteria, some species and strains can also have negative effects (Guban et al., 2006). Our results obtained on D+ and D- lines, are in agreement with results obtained by Moore et al (2011) with commercial broiler chickens of high and low AMEn (12 birds of the quarter higher and 12 birds quarter lower of a group of animals; +3.5%) showing more *Lactobacillus* in jejunum mucosa of low AMEn birds. This deconjugation of bile acids by microbiota may also contribute to the higher liver weight of D- birds due to extra synthesis of these compounds. Moreover it cannot be excluded that the basal endotoxemia due to commensal bacteria leads to modification of hepatic metabolism with consequence on bile acid synthesis (Beno et al., 2003; Cani et al, 2007). All these extra-syntheses in D- birds may contribute to a lower feed efficiency.

Conversely, even if *E. coli* is often seen as deleterious bacteria, which may be the case for the detected strain in the caeca content of D- birds, the one detected in D+ birds caecal mucosa may have beneficial effects as some *E. coli* strains are used as probiotics (Zschüttig et al., 2012).

In the same manner as for *E. coli*, some species and strains of *Clostridium*, more frequent in D+ bird digestive tract, can have positive effects, despite this bacterial group often being associated with negative effects. This is for example the case of the long segmented filamentous bacteria present in a higher amount in D+ bird ileum content. This bacteria belongs to cluster I of *Clostridium* and is a common inhabitant of intestinal mucosa in mammals and birds such as the chicken (Snel et al., 1995) and was also found in jejunum contents of chickens (Lu et al., 2003). It is implicated in the development of the intestinal immune system, intestinal motility, and the development of intestinal epithelial cells. *C. coccoides* and *C. leptum* are also in higher number in the digestive tract of D+ birds. These bacteria are considered beneficial as they produce SCFA, such as butyrate contributing to the maintenance of intestinal health (Scheppach, 1994; Eeckhaut et al, 2011). In the chicken, the *C. leptum* group is mainly represented by bacteria *Faecalibacterium* that has several beneficial effects on intestinal tract health (Bjerrum et al., 2006, Lund et al., 2010). By their fermentative products such as SCFA they may contribute to energy from the diet for the host. Thus, by using the F2 cross between D+ and D- lines, links between AMEn and caecal digestive microbiota were observed. High AMEn was associated with low amounts of *E. coli* expressed in absolute values, and also in relative values compared to all other bacterial groups (*Lactobacillus*, *L. salivarius*, *L. crispatus*, *C. coccoides*, *C. leptum*). On the contrary, a low AMEn was associated with high amounts of *E. coli* expressed in absolute, and high amounts of *E. coli* relative to *Clostridium*. These low AMEn are also associated with high amounts of *L. salivarius* expressed in absolute, and a higher proportion of *L. salivarius* compared to *Lactobacillus* groups and *Clostridium* groups (*C. coccoides* and *C. leptum*). The observation of associations between caecal microbiota and AMEn with the F2 cross between D+ and D- lines corroborates the results of Torok et al. (2011), obtained with birds of a commercial line, showing correlations between fingerprint of digestive microbiota of ileum and caeca contents and AMEn. These results obtained with D+ and D- lines also confirm results obtained by Moore et al. (2011) by using high and low FCR broiler commercial chickens showing more *Clostridium* in caecal contents of high AMEn birds. Moreover, this F2 cross of D+ and D- lines shows that a significant amount of variability in AMEn can be explained by some components of caecal microbiota. Thus, *L. salivarius* number can explain significantly 9% of this variability, with a negative effect. Similarly the bacterial ratio of Log *L.*

salivarius to Log *C. leptum* explains a greater part of the variability (13%), with a negative effect.

It cannot be excluded that the microbiota of D+ is responsible for a decrease in viscosity of the small intestinal contents as some bacterial strains of the digestive tract of the chicken can hydrolyze non-starch polysaccharides (Mead, 1997; Beckmann et al, 2006). However at the present day, no data on intestinal viscosity of D+ and D- lines are available.

Besides the effect of different microbiota of D+ and D- lines on the digestive tract, it may be responsible for effects out of the digestive tract. It can thus be hypothesized that the different behaviour of D+ and D- lines (Pelhaitre et al., 2012) may in part be explained by their different digestive microbiota due to the effect of microbiota on behaviour (Lyte, 2010; Diamond et al., 2011).

Results on digestive microbiota of D+ and D- lines showed that, more than the absolute quantity of bacteria of each group, it is the equilibrium between the different bacterial groups that plays a role in digestive efficiency. Indeed, ratios of different bacteria groups affected more AMEn than quantity of each group, and the ratios were also more controlled by the host, as shown by their higher heritability. This can be explained by the fact that the effect of microbiota is not due to a group of bacteria, but to their interactions. Indeed, as indicated previously in this paper, digestive microbiota is a complex equilibrium between numerous species and even bacterial strains. More precisely, it is the combination of their activity that lead to the global effect of microbiota. Indeed, it is not the presence of the bacterial species that is important for the effect of microbiota, but the activities of all of these bacteria in this complex ecosystem.

Conclusion

The higher digestive efficiency of D+ birds compared to D- birds, fed with a wheat-based diet, appears to be linked to their digestive physiology, while D- birds are limited in their capacity, but also to their high adaptability to specific components of wheat, as shown by the diet-dependent differences between lines.

In D+ birds, the higher development of the proventriculus-gizzard complex leading to higher retention time and thus lower pH, leads to higher digestion in this upper part of the digestive tract, and has been proposed as the major factor responsible for the higher digestive efficiency of D+ birds. This high digestibility in the upper part of the digestive tract may lead to easily digestible compounds in the small intestine, that may be quickly hydrolyzed by bird digestive enzymes and absorbed, leading to a low amount of available substrates for digestive microbiota, with a composition relatively equilibrated although high in protein, and may explain the relative importance of *Clostridium*. In the last part of the digestive tract, the caeca, main components may be composed of dietary molecules not hydrolysable by enzymes of the host, as well as endogenous components difficult to hydrolyze. These substrates may be responsible for the development of caecal bacteria, rich in *Clostridium* that may product SCFA that may increase energy extracted from the diet for the host. In summary, in D+ birds, the digestion and maintenance metabolic cost of the digestive tract may be optimized along the different parts of the digestive tract, with action of the host physiology and enzymes in the upper and middle part, and digestive microbiota in the lower part, leading to minimal wastes.

On the contrary in the D- birds, the under-development of their gizzard, due to failure in the gizzard relaxation process, leads to a lower retention time and a higher pH in the proventriculus-gizzard complex, and seems to be responsible for a part of their lower digestive functionality. It may also be responsible for a different selection of digestive microbiota. Indeed, this smaller proventriculus-gizzard complex development may lead to lower efficiency of gizzard bacterial filter, and thus a greater bacterial load passing in the small intestine. Moreover a higher amount of undigested compounds, probably rich in starch gives a high amount of substrate for bacterial growth, and favor *Lactobacillus* development. The low digestibility in the upper part of the digestive tract may be responsible for the more developed intestine, passing through an increase of epithelium area to try to cope with high undigested compounds, and increase muscle layer to move the higher amount of digestive content. The high bacterial load may be responsible for the higher stimulation of innate digestive immune system by increasing the number of goblet cells, suggesting increased mucus production. These changes in microbiota may be responsible for the lower lipid digestibility, and thus AMEn, due in part to bile acid deconjugation. These modifications in the upper and middle part of the digestive tract may lead to modification also in the lower part, with lower fermentative activity in the caeca with different bacterial composition probably due to a change in available substrates, and this may have an effect on energy recovery in this organ. To cope with this low digestive efficiency, D- birds increase their feed intake, contributing to increased amount of digestive content and with consequences for bacterial growth.

Moreover, contrary to D- birds, D+ birds appeared to be more able to adapt to a diet of low quality such as a diet rich on non-starch polysaccharides of wheat as shown by their lower decrease in AMEn than D- birds fed with wheat of high viscosity. They may have developed a mechanism to be less sensitive to deleterious effects of these hydrosoluble polysaccharides on intestinal viscosity.

However further knowledge in physiology of D+ and D- lines is needed to test these mechanistic biological hypotheses. For example, more information is needed on the motricity and regulation of the gastric emptying as this organ seems to explain an important part of the difference between lines. Moreover, more knowledge is required at the intestinal level. Differences in anatomy of the small intestine have been described, but its digestive functionality is not known, as well as its consequences on digestive efficiency at the end of the small intestine. This knowledge would allow to determine the physiological limiting factors of digestion in order to suggest means to alleviate them. For genetic selection, it may allow to determine how this selection impacts on the phenotype and anticipate any undesirable effects before its introduction in selection schemes. Moreover, it may help to propose a list of candidate genes.

It is also important to know if D+ birds that have been selected by feeding wheat of high viscosity value, are able to adapt to other feedstuffs with other limiting factors in their digestibility. It will also be important to describe these birds in an environment closer to the production environment (on litter with animal groups, not in individual cage), as it would probably affect performances but also microbiota development, among others due to possibility of coprophagy, and then relationships between host, microbiota and digestive performances.

Regarding microbiota, it is important to know when the differences in microbiota composition between D+ and D- lines appear during the development of the birds. Moreover, a more extensive characterization is needed, as minor groups may also largely affect physiology of the host. This characterization may concern as well as the small intestine and the caeca, but also the crop. In addition, the functionality of the microbiota has to be studied, especially regarding to its consequences on the host digestive tract functionality, but also development of digestive immune function that is implied in digestive disease resistance, and consequently on global immune system.

Although relationships have been observed between bacterial groups and AMEn, the results were obtained in specific conditions (wheat diet, cage rearing). Moreover these links do not implied a causality link between these bacterial groups and phenotype such as AMEn, the phenotype being a balance between genotype, environment as diet and rearing conditions, and functionality of the digestive microbiota. Further works are thus needed to determine the involvement of digestive microbiota in digestive efficiency, measured by AMEn.

References

Amerah, A. M., Ravindran, V., and Lentle, R. G. (2009). Influence of insoluble fibre and whole wheat inclusion on the performance, digestive tract development and ileal microbiota profile of broiler chickens. *British Poultry Science*, **50**, 366-375.

Apajalahti, J., Kettunen, A., and Graham, H. (2004). Characteristics of the gastrointestinal microbial communities, with special reference to the chicken. *World's Poultry Science Journal*, **60**, 223-232.

Bäckhed, F., Ding, H., Wang, T., Hooper, L. V., Koh, G. Y., Nagy, A., Semenkovich, C. F., and Gordon, J. I. (2004). The gut microbiota as an environmental factor that regulates fat storage. *Proceedings of the National Academy of Sciences of the United States of America*, **101**, 15718-15723.

Bäckhed, F., Ley, R. E., Sonnenburg, J. L., Peterson, D. A., and Gordon, J. I. (2005). Host-bacterial mutualism in the human intestine. *Science*, **307**, 1915-1920.

Beckmann, L., Simon, O., and Vahjen, W. (2006). Isolation and identification of mixed linked beta -glucan degrading bacteria in the intestine of broiler chickens and partial characterization of respective 1,3-1,4- beta -glucanase activities. *Journal of Basic Microbiology*, **46**, 175-185.

Bedford, M. R., and Cowieson, A. J. (2012). Exogenous enzymes and their effects on intestinal microbiology. *Animal Feed Science and Technology*, **173**, 76-85.

Beno, D. W., Uhing, M. R., Jiyamapa-Serna, V. A., Goto, M., Chen, Y., Vasan, A., Deriy, L. V., and Kimura, R. E. (2003). Differential induction of hepatic dysfunction after intraportal and intravenous challenge with endotoxin and Staphylococcal enterotoxin B. *Shock*, **19**, 352-357.

Binek, M., Borzemska, W., Pisarski, R., Blaszczak, B., Kosowska, G., Malec, H., and Karpinska, E. (2000). Evaluation of the efficacy of feed providing on development of gastrointestinal microflora of newly hatched broiler chickens. *Archiv für Geflügelkunde*, **64**, 147-151.

Bjerrum, L., Engberg, R. M., Leser, T. D., Jensen, B. B., Finster, K., and Pedersen, K. (2006). Microbial community composition of the ileum and cecum of broiler chickens as revealed by molecular and culture-based techniques. *Poultry Science*, **85**, 1151-1164.

Boyd, F. M., and Edwards, H. M. (1967). Fat absorption by germ-free chicks. *Poultry Science*, **46**, 1481-1483.

Cani, P. D., Amar, J., Iglesias, M. A., Poggi, M., Knauf, C., Bastelica, D., Neyrinck, A. M., Fava, F., Tuohy, K. M., Chabo, C., Waget, A., Delmee, E., Cousin, B., Sulpice, T., Chamontin, B., Ferrieres, J., Tanti, J.-F., Gibson, G. R., Casteilla, L., Delzenne, N. M., Alessi, M. C., and Burcelin, R. (2007). Metabolic endotoxemia initiates obesity and insulin resistance. *Diabetes*, **56**, 1761-1772.

Carlstedt, I., Herrman, A., Karlsson, H., Sheehan, J., Fransson, L. A., and Hansson, G. C. (1993). Characterization of two different glycosylated domains from the insoluble mucin complex of rat small intestine. *Journal of Biological Chemistry*, **268**, 18771-18781.

Carré, B. (2002). Carbohydrate chemistry of the feedstuffs used for poultry. In

Poultry feedstuffs : supply, composition and nutritive value - 2002, pp 39-56. Edited by J. M. McNab and K. N. Boorman.CABI Publishing, Wallingford (UK).

Carré, B., Mignon-Grasteau, S., Svihus, B., Péron, A., Bastianelli, D., Gomez, J., Besnard, J., and Sellier, N. (2005). Nutritional effects of feed form, and wheat compared to maize, in the D+ and D- chicken lines selected for divergent digestion capacity. In *15th European Symposium on Poultry Nutrition – 2005,* pp 42-44. Edited by World Poultry Science Association, Budapest (Hungary).

Carré, B., Mignon-Grasteau, S., Péron, A., Juin, H., and Bastianelli, D. (2007). Wheat value: improvements by feed technology, plant breeding and animal genetics. *World's Poultry Science Journal,* **63,** 585-596.

Carré, B., Mignon-Grasteau, S., and Juin, H. (2008). Breeding for feed efficiency and adaptation to feed in poultry. *World's Poultry Science Journal,* **64,** 377-390.

Caviedes-Vidal, E., McWhorter, T. J., Lavin, S. R., Chediack, J. G., Tracy, C. R., and Karasov, W. H. (2007). The digestive adaptation of flying vertebrates: High intestinal paracellular absorption compensates for smaller guts. *Proceedings of the National Academy of Sciences of the United States of America,* **104,** 19132-19137.

Champ, M., Szylit, O., and Gallant, D. J. (1981). The influence of microflora on the breakdown of maize starch granules in the digestive tract of chicken. *Poultry Science,* **60,** 179-187.

Choct, M., Hughes, R. J., and Bedford, M. R. (1999). Effects of a xylanase on individual bird variation, starch digestion throughout the intestine, and ileal and caecal volatile fatty acid production in chickens fed wheat. *British Poultry Science,* **40,** 419-422.

Clench, M. H. (1999). The avian cecum: update and motility review. *Journal of Experimental Zoology,* **283,** 441-447.

Coates, M. E. (1980). The gut microflora and growth. In *Growth in animals – 1980,* pp 175-188. Edited by T. L. J. Lawrence. Butterworths, London (UK).

Collado, M. C., and Sanz, Y. (2007). Characterization of the gastrointestinal mucosa-associated microbiota of pigs and chickens using culture-based and molecular methodologies. *Journal of Food Protection,* **70,** 2799-2804.

Crévieu-Gabriel, I., Gomez, J., Caffin, J. P., and Carré, B. (1999). Comparison of pig and chicken pepsins for protein hydrolysis. *Reproduction Nutrition Development,* **39,** 443-454.

Crévieu-Gabriel, I., and Naciri, M. (2001). Dietary effect on chicken coccidiosis. *INRA Productions Animales,* **14,** 231-246.

Crhanova, M., Hradecka, H., Faldynova, M., Matulova, M., Havlickova, H.,

Sisak, F., and Rychlik, I. (2011). Immune response of chicken gut to natural colonization by gut microflora and to Salmonella enterica serovar enteritidis infection. *Infection and Immunity*, **79**, 2755-2763.

Danzeisen, J. L., Kim, H. B., Isaacson, R. E., Tu, Z. J., and Johnson, T. J. (2011). Modulations of the chicken cecal microbiome and metagenome in response to anticoccidial and growth promoter treatment. *PLoS One*, **6**, e27949.

Denbow, D. M. (1999). Gastrointestinal anatomy and physiology. In *Sturkie's Avian Physiology -1999*, pp 299-325. Edited by P. D. Sturkie. Academic Press, San Diego (USA).

De Oliveira, J. E., Scott, T. A., van der Vossen, J. M. B. M., Ouwens, A. M. T., Hangoor, E., and Montijn, R. C. (2010). Establishing beneficial bacteria in the gut of chickens prior to hatching. In *2nd TNO Beneficial Microbes Conference - 2010*, pp 44. Noordwijkerhout (the Netherland).

de Verdal, H., Mignon-Grasteau, S., Jeulin, C., Le Bihan-Duval, E., Leconte, M., Mallet, S., Martin, C., and Narcy, A. (2010a). Digestive tract measurements and histological adaptation in broiler lines divergently selected for digestive efficiency. *Poultry Science*, **89**, 1955-1961.

de Verdal, H., Narcy, A., Le Bihan-Duval, E., and Mignon-Grasteau, S. (2010b). Excretion and gastro-intestinal tract development in chickens divergently selected on their capacity of digestion. In *XIIIth European Poultry Conference – 2010*, 6 pages, Tours (France).

de Verdal, H. (2011a). Genetic selection in view of limiting excretion in chickens. Thesis, 327 pages. Univ. Tours, François Rabelais (France).

de Verdal, H., Narcy, A., Bastianelli, D., Chapuis, H., Même, N., Urvoix, S., Le Bihan-Duval, E., and Mignon-Grasteau, S. (2011b). Improving the efficiency of feed utilization in poultry by selection. 1. Genetic parameters of anatomy of the gastro-intestinal tract and digestive efficiency. *BMC Genetics*, **12**, DOI: 10.1186/1471-2156-12-59.

de Verdal, H., Narcy, A., Bastianelli, D., Chapuis, H., Même, N., Urvoix, S., Le Bihan-Duval, E., and Mignon-Grasteau, S. (2011c). Improving the efficiency of feed utilization in poultry by selection. 2. Genetic parameters of excretion traits and correlations with anatomy of the gastro-intestinal tract and digestive efficiency. *BMC Genetics*, **12**, DOI: 10.1186/1471-2156-12-71.

de Verdal, H., Narcy, A., Chapuis, H., Bastianelli, D., Même, N., Le Bihan-Duval, E., and Mignon-Grasteau, S. (2011d). Genetic selection in view of limiting excretion in chickens. In *Journées de la Recherches Avicoles* - 2011, pp 212-216. Tours (France).

Diamond, B., Huerta, P. T., Tracey, K., and Volpe, B. T. (2011). It takes guts to grow a brain : Increasing evidence of the important role of the intestinal microflora in neuro- and immune-modulatory functions during development and adulthood. *Bioessays*, **33**, 588-591.

Dibner, J. J., Richards, J. D., and Knight, C. D. (2008). Microbial imprinting in gut development and health. *Journal of Applied Poultry Research*, **17**, 174-188..

Dicksved, J., Halfvarson, J., Rosenquist, M., Jarnerot, G., Tysk, C., Apajalahti, J., Engstrand, L., and Jansson, J. K. (2008). Molecular analysis of the gut microbiota of identical twins with Crohn's disease. *ISME Journal*, **2**, 716-727.

Dijk, A. v (2008). Avian defensins. *Veterinary Immunology and Immunopathology*, **124**, 1-18.

Dockès, A. C., Magdelaine, P., Daridan, D., Guillaumin, A., Remondet, M., Selmi, A., Gilbert, H., Mignon-Grasteau, S., and Phocas, F. (2011). Farming and breeding goals for sustainable animal breeding - views and expectations of stakeholders from the production chains and the general public. *INRA Productions Animales*, **24**, 285-296.

Duke, G. E. (1986). Alimentary canal : secretion and digestion, special digestive functions, and absorption. In *Avian Physiology – 1986*, pp 289-302. Edited by P. D. Sturkie. Springer Verlag, New york (USA).

Eeckhaut, V., Van Immerseel, F., Croubels, S., De Baere, S., Haesebrouck, F., Ducatelle, R., Louis, P., and Vandamme, P. (2011). Butyrate production in phylogenetically diverse Firmicutes isolated from the chicken caecum. *Microbial Biotechnology*, **4**, 503-512.

Engberg, R. M., Hedemann, M. S., Leser, T. D., and Jensen, B. B. (2000). Effect of zinc bactracin and salinomycin on intestinal microflora and performance of broilers. *Poultry Science*, **79**, 1311-1319.

Ferrando, C., Vergara, P., Jimenez, M., and Gonalons, E. (1987). Study of the rate of passage of food with chromium-mordanted plant-cells in chickens (*Gallus-Gallus*). *Quarterly Journal of Experimental Physiology and Cognate Medical Sciences*, **72**, 251-259.

Fonty, G., and Chaucheyras-Durand, F. (2008). *Digestive ecosystems*, 311 pages. Edited by J.P. Larpent. Lavoisier, Paris (France).

Forstner, J. F., and Forstner, G. G. (1994). Gastrointestinal mucus. In *Physiology of the gastrointestinal tract – 1994*, pp 1255-1283. Edited by L.R. Johnson. Raven Press, New York (USA).

Freestone, P. P., Sandrini, S. M., Haigh, R. D., and Lyte, M. (2008). Microbial endocrinology: how stress influences susceptibility to infection. *Trends in Microbiology*, **16**, 55-64.

Fritz, J. C., Burrowsandh, W. H., and Titus, H. W. (1936). Comparison of digestibility in gizzardectomized and normal fowls. *Poultry Science*, **15**, 239-243.

Fuller, R. (1984). Microbial activity in the alimentary tract of birds. *Proceedings of the Nutrition Society*, **43**, 55-61.

Furuse, M., and Okumura, J. (1994). Nutritional and physiological characteristics in germ-free chickens. *Comparative Biochemistry and Physiology*, **109A**, 547-556.

Gabriel, I., Mallet, S., and Leconte, M. (2003). Differences in the digestive tract characteristics of broiler chickens fed on complete pelleted diet or whole wheat added to pelleted protein concentrate. *British Poultry Science*, **44**, 283-290.

Gabriel, I., Lessire, M., Mallet, S., and Guillot, J. F. (2006). Microflora of the digestive tract: critical factors and consequences for poultry. *World's Poultry Science Journal*, **62**, 499-511.

Gabriel, I., Leconte, M., Guillon, J., Rideaud, P., Moreau-Vauzelle, C., and Dupont, C. (2007). Individual variability in the digestive flora of the broiler chicken analysed by molecular fingerprint. In *16ᵗʰ European Symposium on Poultry Nutrition – 2007*, pp 305-308 Strasbourg (France).

Gabriel, I., Guardia, S., Konsak, B., Leconte, M., Rideaud, P., Moreau-Vauzelle, C., Dupont, C., and Mignon-Grasteau, S. (2011). Comparison of chicken digestive microbiota selected on their metabolizable energy. In *9emes Journees de la Recherche Avicole - 2011*, pp 760-764, Tours (France).

Garcia, V., Gomez, J., Mignon-Grasteau, S., Sellier, N., and Carré, B. (2007). Effect of xylanase and antibiotic supplementations on the nutritional utilisation of a wheat diet in growing chicks from genetic D+ and D- lines selected for divergent digestion efficiency. *Animal*, **1**, 1435-1442.

Gong, J., Si, W., Forster, R. J., Huang, R., Yu, H., Yin, Y., Yang, C., and Han, Y. (2007). 16S rRNA gene-based analysis of mucosa-associated bacterial community and phylogeny in the chicken gastrointestinal tracts: from crops to ceca. *FEMS Microbiology Ecology*, **59**, 147-157.

Gong, J., Yu, H., Liu, T., Gill, J. J., Chambers, J. R., Wheatcroft, R., and Sabour, P. M. (2008). Effects of zinc bacitracin, bird age and access to range on bacterial microbiota in the ileum and caeca of broiler chickens. *Journal of Applied Microbiology*, **104**, 1372-1382.

Guban, J., Korver, D. R., Allison, G. E., and Tannock, G. W. (2006). Relationship of dietary antimicrobial drug administration with broiler performance, decreased population levels of *Lactobacillus salivarius*, and reduced bile salt deconjugation in the ileum of broiler chickens. *Poultry Science*, **85**, 2186-2194.

Guardia, S., Furet, J. P., Recoquillay, F., Juin, H., Lessire, M., Leconte, M., Rideaud, P., Moreau-Vauzelle, C., Dupont, C., Guillot, J.F., and Gabriel, I. (2009). A comparison of two methods to extract bacterial DNA of the digestive tract. In *6ᵗʰ International Symposium of Anaerobic Microbiology - 2009*, pp 39-40. Liblice (Czech republic).

Guardia, S., Konsak, B., Juin, H., Lessire, M., Rideaud, P., Moreau-Vauzelle, C.,

Dupont, C., Guillot, J. F., and Gabriel, I. (2011). Effects of stocking density on growth performance and digestive microbiota of broiler chickens. *Poultry Science*, **90**, 1878-1889.

Gulati, A. S., Shanahan, M. T., Arthur, J. C., Grossniklaus, E., von Furstenberg, R. J., Kreuk, L., Henning, S. J., Jobin, C., and Sartor, R. B. (2012). Mouse background strain profoundly influences Paneth cell function and intestinal microbial composition. *PLoS One*, **7**, e32403.

Hetland, H., and Svihus, B. (2001). Effect of oat hulls on performance, gut capacity and feed passage time in broiler chickens. *British Poultry Science*, **42**, 354-361.

Hong, W., Wu, Y. E., Fu, X., and Chang, Z. (2012a). Chaperone-dependent mechanisms for acid resistance in enteric bacteria. *Trends in Microbiology*, **20**, 30-39.

Hong, Y. H., Song, W., Lee, S. H., and Lillehoj, H. S. (2012b). Differential gene expression profiles of -defensins in the crop, intestine, and spleen using a necrotic enteritis model in 2 commercial broiler chicken lines. *Poultry Science*, **91**, 1081-1088.

Hooper, L. V., Wong, M. H., Thelin, A., Hansson, L., Falk, P. G., and Gordon, J. I. (2001). Molecular analysis of commensal host-microbial relationships in the intestine. *Science*, **291**, 881-884.

Hooper, L. V., Midtvedt, T., and Gordon, J. I. (2002). How host-microbial interactions shape the nutrient environment of the mammalian intestine. *Annual Review of Nutrition*, **22**, 283-307.

Hooper, L. V., and Macpherson, A. J. (2010). Immune adaptations that maintain homeostasis with the intestinal microbiota. *Nature Reviews Immunology*, **10**, 159-169.

Huyghebaert, G., Ducatelle, R., and Van Immerseel, F. (2011). An update on alternatives to antimicrobial growth promoters for broilers. *Veterinary Journal*, **187**, 182-188.

Iiboshi, Y., Nezu, R., Cui, L., Chen, K., Khan, J., Yoshida, H., Sando, K., Kamata, S., Takagi, Y., and Okada, A. (1996). Adhesive mucous gel layer and mucus release as intestinal barrier in rats. *Journal of Parenteral and Enteral Nutrition*, **20**, 98-104.

Inglis, G. D., Thomas, M. C., Thomas, D. K., Kalmokoff, M. L., Brooks, S. P., and Selinger, L. B. (2012). Molecular methods to measure intestinal bacteria: a review. *Journal of AOAC International*, **95**, 5-23.

Ismail, A. S., and Hooper, L. V. (2005). Epithelial cells and their neighbors. IV. Bacterial contributions to intestinal epithelial barrier integrity. *American Journal of Physiology - Gastrointestinal and Liver Physiology*, **289**, G779-784.

Jensen, H., Grimmer, S., Naterstad, K., and Axelsson, L. (2012). In vitro testing of commercial and potential probiotic lactic acid bacteria. *International Journal of Food Microbiology*, **153**, 216-222.

Johansson, M. E., Ambort, D., Pelaseyed, T., Schütte, A., Gustafsson, J. K., Ermund, A., Subramani, D. B., Holmén-Larsson, J. M., Thomsson, K. A., Bergström, J. H., van der Post, S., Rodriguez-Piñeiro, A. M., Sjövall, H., Bäckström, M., and Hansson, G. C. (2011). Composition and functional role of the mucus layers in the intestine. *Cellular and Molecular Life Sciences*, **68**, 3635-3641.

Juge, N. (2012). Microbial adhesins to gastrointestinal mucus. *Trends in Microbiology*, **20**, 30-39.

Jozefiak, D., Rutkowski, A., and Martin, S. A. (2004). Carbohydrate fermentation in the avian ceca: a review. *Animal Feed Science and Technology*, **113**, 1-15.

Kim, G. B., and Lee, B. H. (2005). Biochemical and molecular insights into bile salt hydrolase in the gastrointestinal microflora - A review. *Asian-Australasian Journal of Animal Sciences*, **18**, 1505-1512.

Kizerwetter-Swida, M., and Binek, M. (2008). Bacterial microflora of the chicken embryos and newly hatched chicken. *Journal of Animal and Feed Sciences*, **17**, 224-232.

Klasing, K. C., Johnstone, B. J., and Benson, B. N. (1991). Implications of an immune response on growth and nutrient requirements of chicks. In *Recent Advances in Animal Nutrition – 1991*, pp 135-146. Edited by W. Haresign and D. J. A. Cole. Butterworth-Heinemann Ltd, Oxford (UK).

Klis, J. D. v. d., and Lensing, M. (2007). Wet litter problems relate to host-microbiota interactions. *World Poultry*, **23**, 20-22.

Konsak, B., Guardia, S., Leconte, M., Moreau-Vauzelle, C., Dupont, C., Mignon-Grasteau, S., and Gabriel, I. (2011). Comparison of the digestive microbiota between two divergent lines of chickens selected based on digestive capacity. In *7ᵗʰ International Symposium of Anaerobic Microbiology - 2011*, pp 17. Smolenice (Slovakia).

Konsak, B., Guardia, S., Leconte, M., Moreau-Vauzelle, C., Dupont, C., Doré, J., Levenez, F., Mignon-Grasteau, S., and Gabriel, I. (2012). Comparison of the digestive microbiota between two divergent lines of chickens selected based on apparent metabolisable energy. In *8ᵗʰ INRA-Rowett Symposium on Gut Microbiology - 2012*, Clermont-Ferrand (France).

Kussaibati, R., Guillaume, J., and Leclercq, B. (1982a). The effect of gut microflora on the digestibility of starch and proteins in young chicks. *Annales de Zootechnie*, **31**, 483-488.

Kussaibati, R., Guillaume, J., Leclercq, B., and Lafont, J. P. (1982b). Effect of the intestinal microflora and added bile salts on the metabolisable energy and digestibility of saturated fats in the chicken. *Archiv für Geflügelkunde*,

46, 42-46.

Laboisse, C., Jarry, A., Branka, J. E., Merlin, D., Bou-Hanna, C., and Vallette, G. (1996). Recent aspects of the regulation of intestinal mucus secretion. *Proceedings of the Nutrition Society*, **55**, 259-264.

Lartigue, G. d., Barbier de la Serre, C., Espero, E., Lee, J., and Raybould, H. E. (2011). Diet-induced obesity leads to the development of leptin resistance in vagal afferent neurons. *American Journal of Physiology. Endocrinology and Metabolism*, **301**, E187-195.

Lederberg, J. (2000). Infectious history. *Science*, **288**, 287–293.

Lee, Z. M. P., Bussema III, C., and Schmidt, T. M. (2009). rrnDB: documenting the number of rRNA and tRNA genes in bacteria and archaea. *Nucleic Acids Research*, **37**, D489-D493.

Lu, J., Idris, U., Harmon, B., Hofacre, C., Maurer, J., and Lee, M. D. (2003). Diversity and succession of the intestinal bacterial community of the maturing broiler chicken. *Applied Environmental Microbiology*, **69**, 6816-6824.

Lumpkins, B. S., Batal, A. B., and Lee, M. D. (2010). Evaluation of the bacterial community and intestinal development of different genetic lines of chickens. *Poultry Science*, **89**, 1614-1621.

Lund, M., Bjerrum, L., and Pedersen, K. (2010). Quantification of *Faecalibacterium prausnitzii*- and *Subdoligranulum variabile*-like bacteria in the cecum of chickens by real-time PCR. *Poultry Science*, **89**, 1217-1224.

Lyte, M. (2010). The microbial organ in the gut as a driver of homeostasis and disease. *Medical Hypotheses*, **74**, 634-638.

Maisonnier, S., Gomez, J., Bree, A., Berri, C., Baeza, E., and Carré, B. (2003). Effects of microflora status, dietary bile salts and guar gum on lipid digestibility, intestinal bile salts and histo-morphology, in broiler chickens. *Poultry Science*, **82**, 805-814.

Malmuthuge, N., Li, M., Chen, Y., Fries, P., Griebel, P. J., Baurhoo, B., Zhao, X., and Guan, L. L. (2012). Distinct commensal bacteria associated with ingesta and mucosal epithelium in the gastrointestinal tracts of calves and chickens. *FEMS Microbiology Ecology*, **79**, 337-347.

Mathlouthi, N., Mallet, S., Saulnier, L., Quemener, B., and Larbier, M. (2002). Effects of xylanase and b-glucanase addition on performance, nutrient digestibility, and physico-chemical conditions in the small intestine contents and caecal microflora of broiler chickens fed a wheat and barley-based diet. *Animal Research*, **51**, 395-406.

Mead, G. C. (1997). Bacteria in the intestinal tract of birds. In *Gastrointestinal Microbiology: Gastrointestinal Microbes and Host Interactions – 1997*, pp 216-240. Edited by R. I. Mackie, B. A. White and R. E. Isaacson. Vol. 2,

Chapman Hall, Microbiology Series, NewYork (USA).

Menendez, A., and Brett Finlay, B. (2007). Defensins in the immunology of bacterial infections. *Current Opinion in Immunology*, **19**, 385-391.

Merwe, J. P. v d, Stegeman, J. H., and Hazenberg, M. P. (1983). The resident faecal flora is determined by genetic characteristics of the host. Implications for Crohn's disease? *Antonie Van Leeuwenhoek*, **49**, 119-124.

Mignon-Grasteau, S., Muley, N., Bastianelli, D., Gomez, J., Péron, A., Sellier, N., Millet, N., Besnard, J., Hallouis, J. M., and Carré, B. (2004). Heritability of digestibilities and divergent selection for digestion ability in growing chicks fed a wheat diet. *Poultry Science*, **83**, 860-867.

Mignon-Grasteau, S., Juin, H., Sellier, N., Bastianelli, D., Gomez, J., and Carré, B. (2010a). Genetic Parameters of Wheat- or Corn-based Diets in Chickens. In *9th World Congres of Applied Livestock Production – 2010*, 4 pages . Leipzig (Germany).

Mignon-Grasteau, S., Bourblanc, M., Carré, B., Dourmad, J. Y., Gilbert, H., Juin, H., Noblet, J., and Phocas, F. (2010b). Reducing manure in poultry and pig productions by selection. *INRA Productions Animales*, 23, 415-426.

Moore, R. J., Stanley, D., Konsak, B. M., Haring, V. R., Hughes, R. J., Geier, M. S., and Crowley, T. M. (2011). Correlations between variable broiler performance and gene expression and microflora in the gut. In *Proceedings of the 22nd Annual Australian Poultry Science Symposium – 2011*, pp 9-16. Sydney, New South Wales (Australia).

Moreto, M., and Planas, J. M. (1989). Sugar and amino acid transport properties of the chicken caeca. *Journal of Experimental Zoology*, **sup 3**, 111-116.

Muramatsu, T., Nakajima, S., and Okumura, J. (1994). Modification of energy metabolism by the presence of the gut microflora in the chicken. *British Journal of Nutrition*, **71**, 709-717.

Nir, I., Hillel, R., Shefet, G., and Nitsan, Z. (1994). Effect of grain particle size on performance. 2. Grain texture interactions. *Poultry Science*, **73**, 781-791.

Nordentoft, S., Molbak, L., Bjerrum, L., De Vylder, J., Van Immerseel, F., and Pedersen, K. (2011). The influence of the cage system and colonisation of *Salmonella Enteritidis* on the microbial gut flora of laying hens studied by T-RFLP and 454 pyrosequencing. *BMC Microbiology*, **11**, DOI 10.1186/1471-2180-11-187.

Noy, Y., and Uni, Z. (2010). Early nutritional strategies. *World's Poultry Science Journal*, **66**, 639-646.

O'Dell, B. L., Newberne, P. M., and Savage, J. E. (1959). An abnormality of the proventriculus caused by feed texture. *Poultry Science*, **38**, 296-301.

Parsons, C. M., Potter, L. M., Brown, R. D. J., Wilkins, T. D., and Bliss, B. A. (1982). Microbial contribution to dry matter and amino acid content of poultry excreta. *Poultry Science*, **61**, 925-932..

Pearson, G. R., McNulty, M. S., McCracken, R. M., and Curran, W. (1992). Scanning electron microscopic observations of segmented filamentous bacteria in the small intestine of domestic fowl. *Veterinary Record*, **111**, 365-366.

Pedroso, A. A. (2009). Which came first: the egg or its microbia ? *The Poultry Informed Professional, University of Georgia*, **Issue 107**, July/August 2009, 1-5.

Pelhaitre, A., Mignon-Grasteau, S., and Bertin, A. (2012). Selection for wheat digestibility affects emotionality and feeding behaviours in broiler chicks. *Applied Animal Behaviour Science*, **139**, 114-122.

Péron, A., Gomez, J., Mignon-Grasteau, S., Sellier, N., Besnard, J., Derouet, M., Juin, H., and Carré, B. (2006). Effects of wheat quality on digestion differ between the D+ and D- chicken lines selected for divergent digestion capacity. *Poultry Science*, **85**, 462-469.

Putskam, M., Vizzier-Thaxton, Y., Dozier, W. A., Thaxton, J. P., Roush, W. B., Branton, S. L., Morgan, G. W., Miles, D. M., and Lott, B. D. (2005). Evaluation of stocking density on intestinal microflora of broilers. *Poultry Science*, **84**, 108.

Pym, R. A. E., Nicholls, P. J., Thomson, E., Choice, A., and Farrell, D. J. (1984). Energy and nitrogen-metabolism of broilers selected over 10 generations for increased growth-rate, food-consumption and conversion of food to gain. *British Poultry Science*, **25**, 529-539.

Pym, R. A. E. (1990). Nutritional genetics. In *Poultry Breeding and Genetics - 1990*, pp 847-876. Edited by R. D. Crawford. Elsevier edition, Amsterdam (The Netherlands).

Qu, A., Brulc, J. M., Wilson, M. K., Law, B. F., Theoret, J. R., Joens, L. A., Konkel, M. E., Angly, F., Dinsdale, E. A., Edwards, R. A., Nelson, K. E., and White, B. A. (2008). Comparative metagenomics reveals host specific metavirulomes and horizontal gene transfer elements in the chicken cecum microbiome. *PLoS One*, **3**, e2945.

Ramos-Morales, F. (2012). Acidic pH: Enemy or ally for enteric bacteria? *Virulence*, **3**, 103-106.

Rance, K. A., McEntee, G. M., and McDevitt, R. M. (2002). Genetic and phenotypic relationships between and within support and demand tissues in a single line of broiler chicken. *British Poultry Science*, **43**, 518-527.

Rastogi, R., Wu, M., DasGupta, I., and Fox, G. E. (2009). Visualization of ribosomal RNA operon copy number distribution. *BMC Microbiology*, **9**, doi: 10.1186/1471-2180-9-208.

Ravindran, V., Wu, Y. B., Thomas, D. G., and Morel, P. C. H. (2006). Influence of whole wheat feeding on the development of gastrointestinal tract and performance of broiler chickens. *Australian Journal of Agricultural Research*, **57**, 21-26.

Rehman, H. U., Vahjen, W., Awad, W. A., and Zentek, J. (2007). Indigenous bacteria and bacterial metabolic products in the gastrointestinal tract of broiler chickens. *Archives of Animal Nutrition*, **5**, 319-335.

Reynhout, J. K., and Duke, G. E. (1999). Identification of interstitial cells of Cajal in the digestive tract of turkeys (Meleagris gallopavo). *Journal of Experimental Zoology*, **283**, 426-440.

Rougière, N., Gomez, J., Mignon-Grasteau, S., and Carré, B. (2009). Effects of diet particle size on digestive parameters in D(+) and D(-) genetic chicken lines selected for divergent digestion efficiency. *Poultry Science*, **88**, 1206-1215.

Rougière, N., and Carré, B. (2010). Comparison of gastrointestinal transit times between chickens from D+ and D- genetic lines selected for divergent digestion efficiency. *Animal*, **4**, 1861-1872.

Rougière, N., Malbert, C. H., Rideau, N., Cognie, J., and Carré, B. (2012). Comparison of gizzard activity between chickens from genetic D(+) and D(-) lines selected for divergent digestion efficiency. *Poultry Science*, **91**, 460-467.

Sakata, T., and Setoyam, H. (1995). Local stimulatory effect of short chain fatty acids on the mucus release from the hindgut mucosa of rats (Rattus norvegicus). *Comparative Biochemistry and Physiology. A. Physiology*, **111**, 429-432.

Saldeña, T. A., Saraví, F. D., Hwang, H. J., Cincunegui, L. M., and Carra, G. E. (2000). Oxygen diffusive barriers of rat distal colon: role of subepithelial tissue, mucosa, and mucus gel layer. *Digestive Diseases and Sciences*, **45**, 2108-2114.

Salter, D. N. (1973). The influence of gut micro-organisms on utilization of dietary ptotein. *Proceedings of the Nutrition Society*, **32**, 65-71.

Salter, D. N., and Fulford, R. J. (1974). The influence of the gut microflora on the digestion of dietary and endogenous proteins: studies of the amino acid composition of the excreta of germ-free and conventional chicks. *British Journal of Nutrition*, **32**, 625-637.

Salzman, N. H., Hung, K., Haribhai, D., Chu, H., Karlsson-Sjöberg, J., Amir, E., Teggatz, P., Barman, M., Hayward, M., Eastwood, D., Stoel, M., Zhou, Y., Sodergren, E., Weinstock, G. M., Bevins, C. L., Williams, C. B., and Bos, N. A. (2010). Enteric defensins are essential regulators of intestinal microbial ecology. *Nature Immunology*, **11**, 76-82.

Scheppach, W. (1994). Effects of short chain fatty acids on gut morphology and function. *Gut*, **35**, S35-S38.

Sharma, R., Young, C., and Neu, J. (2010). Molecular modulation of intestinal epithelial barrier: contribution of microbiota. *Journal of Biomedicine and Biotechnology*, doi:10.1155/2010/305879.

Shepherd, E. M., and Fairchild, B. D. (2010). Footpad dermatitis in poultry. *Poultry Science*, **89**, 2043-2051.

Shires, A., Thompson, J. R., Turner, B. V., Kennedy, P. M., and Goh, Y. K. (1987). Rate of passage of corn-canola meal and corn-soybean meal diets through the gastrointestinal tract of broiler and white leghorn chickens. *Poultry Science*, **66**, 289-298.

Snel, J., Heinen, P. P., Blok, H. J., Carman, R. J., Duncan, A. J., Allen, P. C., and Collins, M. D. (1995). Comparison of 16S rRNA sequences of segmented filamentous bacteria isolated from mice, rats, and chickens and proposal of "*Candidatus Arthromitus*". *International Journal of Systematic Bacteriology*, **45**, 780-782.

Souza, M. R., Moreira, J. L., Barbosa, F. H. F., Cerqueira, M., Nunes, A. C., and Nicoli, J. R. (2007). Influence of intensive and extensive breeding on lactic acid bacteria isolated from *Gallus gallus domesticus* ceca. *Veterinary Microbiology*, **120**, 142-150.

Stewart, J. A., Chadwick, V. S., and Murray, A. (2005). Investigations into the influence of host genetics on the predominant eubacteria in the faecal microflora of children. *Journal of Medical Microbiology*, **54**, 1239-1242.

Suzuki, K., Kodam, Y., and Mitsuoka, T. (1989). Stress and intestinal flora. *Bifidobacteria and microflora*, **8**, 23-38.

Svihus, B. (2011). The gizzard : function, influence of diet structure and effects on nutrient availability. *World's Poultry Science Journal*, **67**, 207-224.

Szylit, O., Champ, M., Aitabdelkader, N., and Raibaud, P. (1980). Role of 5 *Lactobacillus* strains on carbohydrate degradation in monoxenic chickens. *Reproduction Nutrition Development*, **20**, 1701-1706.

Taylor, R. D., and Jones, G. P. D. (2004). The influence of whole grain inclusion in pelleted broiler diets on proventricular dilatation and ascites mortality. *British Poultry Science*, **45**, 247-254.

Thomke, S., and Elwinger, K. (1998). Growth promotants in feeding pigs and poultry. I. Growth and feed efficiency responses to antibiotic growth promotants. *Annales de Zootechnie*, **47**, 85-91.

Timbermont, L., Haesebrouck, F., Ducatelle, R., and Van Immerseel, F. (2011). Necrotic enteritis in broilers: an updated review on the pathogenesis. *Avian Pathology*, **40**, 341-347.

Toivanen, P., Vaahtovuo, J., and Eerola, E. (2001). Influence of major histocompatibility complex on bacterial composition of fecal flora. *Infection and Immunity*, **69**, 2372-2377.

Torok, V. A., Hughes, R. J., Mikkelsen, L. L., Perez-Maldonado, R., Balding, K.,

MacAlpine, R., Percy, N. J., and Ophel-Keller, K. (2011). Identification and Characterization of Potential Performance-Related Gut Microbiotas in Broiler Chickens across Various Feeding Trials. *Applied and Environmental Microbiology*, **77**, 5868-5878.

Vispo, C., and Karasov, W. H. (1997). The interaction of avian gut microbes and their host : an elusive symbiosis. In *Gastrointestinal microbiology – 1997*, pp 116-155. Edited by R. I. Mackie and B. A. White. Vol. 1. Chapman Hall, Microbiology Series, New York (USA).

Williams, J., Mallet, S., Leconte, M., Lessire, M., and Gabriel, I. (2008). The effects of fructo-oligosaccharides or whole wheat on the performance and the digestive tract of broiler chickens. *British Poultry Science*, **49**, 329-339.

Yamauchi, K., Isshiki, Y., Zhou, Z. X., and Nakahiro, Y. (1990). Scanning and transmission electron microscopic observations of bacteria adhering to ileal epithelial cells in growing broilers and White Leghorn chickens. *British Poultry Science*, **31**, 129-137.

Yang, Y., Iji, P. A., and Choct, M. (2009). Dietary modulation of gut microflora in broiler chickens : a review of the role of six kinds of alternatives to in-feed antibiotics. *World's Poutry Science Journal*, **65**, 97-114.

Zhu, X. Y., Zhong, T., Pandya, Y., and Joerger, R. D. (2002). 16S rRNA-based analysis of microbiota from the caecum of broiler chickens. *Applied Environmental Microbiology*, **68**, 124-137.

Zoetendal, E. G., Collier, C. T., Koike, S., Mackie, R. I., and Gaskins, H. R. (2004). Molecular ecological analysis of the gastrointestinal microbiota: A review. *Journal of Nutrition*, **134**, 465-472.

Zschüttig, A., Zimmermann, K., Blom, J., Goesmann, A., Pöhlmann, C., and Gunzer, F. (2012). Identification and Characterization of Microcin S, a New Antibacterial Peptide Produced by Probiotic *Escherichia coli* G3/10. *PLoS One*, **7**, e33351.

12

PROGRESS ON THE ENGLISH PIG INDUSTRY ENVIRONMENT ROAD MAP

N. PENLINGTON AND A.E. DAVIS
BPEX, AHDB, Stoneleigh Park, Warwickshire.

Abstract

A definition for sustainability; *"Meeting the needs of the present generation without compromising the ability of future generations to meet their needs."*

The English Pig Industry launched its Roadmap; "Advancing Together" in May 2011 (BPEX, 2011a). This document is a clear statement of intent outlining how the industry will develop further improved sustainability and environmental responsibility. Delivery is taking place by improving performance throughout the whole industry from production to marketing of products. An integrated approach is taken, joining all the pieces of the jigsaw to make a complete picture, although there is no one simple solution. Producing pig meat sustainably in order to provide a growing world population with safe, affordable, highly desirable meat protein and other products of pig origin when faced with diminishing resources requires team effort.

Feed and nutrition are a crucial key piece of this jigsaw. Nutritionists are challenged by farmers to design rations which meet the production needs of their pigs at an affordable price, with high metabolic efficiencies that reduce emissions and pressures on the environment. Last, but not least, are the ethical questions addressed about the origin of ingredients, and even if we should feed some of them to animals at all?

As the World's population continues to increase, demand for pig products will continue to grow, especially as a source of low-carbon meat protein. A resource-efficient high yielding industry delivering what the market wants at a price it is willing to pay looks to be in a strong position.

Introduction

The Planet we inhabit is of finite size, with finite resources and many fragile ecosystems which play an important part in its stability. The impact of man on this planet is having a profound effect with many negative scenarios regularly appearing in scientific literature and the popular press. We are faced with a challenge to feed a growing population responsibly with fewer resources in terms of feed ingredients, water and energy whilst also minimising the effects of so-called Greenhouse Gases to limit the rate of climate change and environmental impact from food production. This is highlighted in many reports including "Livestock's Long Shadow, environmental issues and options" (FAO, 2006), which critically assessed livestock production.

The conclusion of many of our own leading scientists and Government advisors is that we need sustainable agriculture in order to meet the challenges. The UK Government Office for Science in its report; "Foresight, The Future of Food and Farming, challenges and choices for future sustainability" (Godfray et al., 2011) introduces the concept of "sustainable intensification" to deliver more affordable food for less impact, a challenge to agriculturalists.

The UK Department of Environment Food and Rural Affairs (Defra) introduced a Structural Reform Plan (SRP) in July 2011 that laid down three departmental priorities; i) support and develop British farming and encourage sustainable food production, ii) help to enhance the environment and biodiversity to improve quality of life, iii) support a strong and sustainable green economy, resilient to climate change. This not only gives the farming industry strong guidance but, most importantly, also sends a strong signal that food production is important. It provides the industry with a feeling of worth and a renewed sense of purpose. Within the SRP is the Department of Energy and Climate Change (DECC) and the Department for Business, Innovation and Skills (BIS) Roadmap which sets out to provide all of industry with a clear path to an eco-friendly economy.

The Climate Change Act of 2008 set in legislation for a reduction in green house gas emissions of 80% by 2050 from 1990 levels. An independent body - the Committee on Climate Change (CCC) - was established to advise Government on setting and meeting carbon budgets, and on preparing for the impacts of climate change. In its fourth carbon budget (http://www.theccc.org.uk/carbon-budgets/4th-carbon-budget-path-to-2030). English agriculture was set an annual emissions reduction target of 3 million tonnes CO_2-equivalent (Mt CO_2e), equating to an estimated 11%, with no sector differentiation in targets. Industry representatives agreed with Defra that they would work to encourage improvements in production efficiency focused on 15 key on-farm actions to deliver the targets in preference to a legislative approach and published; "Meeting the Challenge: agricultural industry GHG Action Plan" (GHGAP, 2011).

In parallel to this process, individual sectors have been developing their own Roadmaps for improved sustainability so that they can demonstrate responsibility to consumers and government, and to position themselves for the long term future. The English Pig Industry launched its Roadmap; "Advancing Together" in May

2011 (BPEX, 2011a), a clear statement of intent outlining how the industry will further develop improved sustainability and environmental responsibility in order to provide a growing world population with safe, affordable, highly desirable meat protein and other products of pig origin when faced with diminishing resources. Delivery is taking place by improving performance throughout the whole industry from production to marketing of products.

There are many definitions and interpretations of *"sustainability";* we elected to adopt; *"Meeting the needs of the present generation without compromising the ability of future generations to meet their needs."*

Parameters of the Roadmap

The English Pig Industry Roadmap is concerned with pig production from conception on the farm through to the production of pork and processing of pork products. We see the English pig industry as part of the UK and worldwide industries, and believe that our influence will extend beyond the geographical boundaries of our responsibility and remit through the export of goods and by continually working in co-operation with our counterparts overseas (for example in sourcing sustainable soya). We could simply export our industry, meet home targets for carbon reduction, and consume imported products. The responsible approach is to understand our strengths and weaknesses, provide leadership, and take control where this will deliver the best overall solution.

Our customers are essential to all that producers and processors do: their demand for products and goods drives the industry, provides the funds for investment and enthusiasm to go forward. The desires and aspirations of our customer base are recognised as paramount by the industry and throughout this document.

This Roadmap identifies the objectives for greater environmental sustainability in the English pig industry, objectively assesses where we are, current activity which will help achieve targets, recognises gaps and suggests how these may be addressed. Many Roadmaps and sustainability documents focus on carbon equivalents calculated from emissions of gases, principally nitrous oxide, methane and carbon dioxide bundled together and referred to as greenhouse gases. For the Pig Industry this is not the case; we look at a wider picture. Producers on the ground are facing challenges from the impacts of nitrogen-containing compounds, especially ammonia and nitrate, phosphate pollution of water bodies, and use of fossil fuel derived energy. These challenges are mediated through many pieces of legislation including, nitrates in water, habitats regulations, water framework directive, climate change levy. Pollution swapping, i.e. mitigating one type of pollution but allowing another to increase, is not a desirable outcome; thus we assess the four main measures of environmental consequences: climate change, eutrophication, acidification potentials, and abiotic resource depletion. Assessing these provides an understanding of the key drivers and their interactions so that we can aim for the best environmental solution with realistic and commercially viable targets. We are lucky in that often production efficiency will deliver reductions in environmental burdens, and better economic performance, the barrier often being the ability, and or decision making confidence to make the investments needed to deliver improvement.

Table 1. Assessment of environmental burdens of English pig meat production to farm gate.

Impact category	Unit	1 kg pork – 2001 average	1 kg pork – 2008 average	2001 – 2008 percentage improvement
Climate change	kg CO_2 eq	5.35	4.91	8%
Eutrophication	kg PO_4 eq	0.0510	0.0431	16%
Acidification	kg SO_2 eq	0.169	0.139	17%
Abiotic resource depletion	kg Sb eq	0.0286	0.0267	7%

Source; ERM Ltd for BPEX.

The success of the Roadmap - and ultimately of the English pig industry itself - will come only with engagement by industry and its people. Organisations such as the BPEX division of the Agricultural and Horticultural Development Board (AHDB), National Pig association (NPA), Pig Veterinary Society (PVS), British Meat Processors Association (BMPA), the Government and its agencies will put the mechanisms and tools in place. The active participation and commitment from pig producers to reduce the environmental impact of their activity is a prerequisite for recognition from the market place, consumers, regulators and policy makers. Producing pig meat sustainably requires team effort

To ensure such engagement, ambitious targets need also to be realistic and achievable. They need also to be communicated clearly so that producers are able to recognise that they can improve their businesses - both financially and operationally – while at the same time reducing their environmental footprint. There is no one simple formula to provide a quick route to our objectives; an integrated approach is required. Simply focusing on single issues, health, genetics, feed, will not be successful. We look at it as a jigsaw; all the pieces must be joined together in the right way to make a complete picture. **The Roadmap identifies three key areas of activity, i) using feed more efficiently, ii) improving productivity through the Two Tonne Sow (2TS) programme and iii) managing slurry/waste more effectively.**

A challenge for the Roadmap is to create a seamless transition for the changes and improvements to working practices, that producers can embrace and adapt to them without any feeling of distraction, or feeling that the changes are burdensome and unnecessarily onerous. Producers should have confidence that the industry as a whole is stimulated and motivated to deliver the long-term objectives that it has set itself.

Start of the journey

The Pig Industry has travelled a rough road since the late 1990s. "Advancing Together", is a continuation of the journey which commenced in 2002 when BPEX first launched its Road to Recovery strategy, Part 2 followed in 2006. Within this umbrella of activity came the BPEX Pig Health Scheme (BPHS), 2003, the Pig Industry Professional Register (PIPR), 2007, and the appointment of BPEX Knowledge Transfer Managers to empower farmers.

To lead the debate and industry, the Pig Environment Partnership (PEP) was developed in 2007. Unfortunately, this coincided with a period of rapidly falling farm gate pig prices. It was not seen as a priority by an industry fighting for economic survival, the background delivery work continued, but with a lower public profile. The Pigmeat Supply Chain Task Force, instigated in 2009 and chaired by UK Government Ministers, largely took over the function of PEP.

Table 2. Key performance targets for English pig producers

	2008	*2014*	*2020*	*2011 Update*
Pig performance				
Weight of pigs at weaning (kg)	7.7	7.9	8.0	7.6
Pigs weaned per sow per year	22.1	25.6	28.0	22.6
Finishing mortality (%)	3.3	2.0	1.8	2.9
Rearing Feed conversion ratio	1.7	1.5	1.5	1.71
Finishing Feed conversion ratio	2.87	2.40	2.30	2.82
Finishing daily live-weight gain (g)	766	835	875	784
Average live weight at slaughter (kg)	103	110	110.	103
Average dead weight (kg)	79.8	81.3	86.0	79.1
Killing out percentage (cold)	77.0	75.5	76.0	76.7
Sow feed (kg) per sow per year	1,456	1,560	1,360	1,169
Pigmeat (kg) per sow per year	1,608	2,000	2,200	1,680

Source; Advancing Together (BPEX, 2011a).

Despite implementation of the various schemes and strategies, the English industry continued to lag behind other European countries in terms of pig performance and cost of production. Thus in 2010, the simple concept of the Two Tonne Sow (2TS) was introduced. The aim being to focus on raising the industry average of 1.6 tonnes of pig meat per year to 2.0 tonnes by 2014, a substantial and theoretically achievable increase, but still behind the levels of production being achieved elsewhere in Europe, most notably Denmark. 2TS is a holistic strategy with six key focus areas, or pillars as they are referred to. The Pillars are; breeding, finishing, health, nutrition, buildings and training.

Two tonne sow and health

The Pillars are the front line activity with BPEX leading work on improving farm performance, concentrating on one at a time with the possible exception of health which is a parallel continuous work stream. Performance targets for 2TS are projected to exceed Government climate change reduction targets for the current period, providing a good platform for the next period when targets may be harder to achieve.

Table 3. Projected improvements in environmental burdens of English pig meat production.

Impact category	Unit	1 kg pork – 2008 average	2008 – 2020 forecast improvement
Climate change	kg CO_2 eq	4.91	17%
Eutrophication	kg PO_4 eq	0.0431	15%
Acidification	kg SO_2 eq	0.139	15%
Abiotic resource depletion	kg Sb eq	0.0267	16%

Source; ERM Ltd for BPEX.

The 2TS programme has become recognised throughout the industry as the main vehicle for knowledge transfer in the pig production industry. BPEX Knowledge Transfer (KT) Managers are engaging directly with producers through targeted and co-ordinated meetings, events, workshops and conferences backed up by a professional communications team. This approach means messages are disseminated effectively and by different means. The 2012 BPEX Annual Pig Meat Industry Survey (AHDB, 2012) results showed an increase in the last year in the use of BPEX services from 71% to 76% by respondents in the producer category.

Endemic disease has been a burden to our industry for too long, pulling down productivity and limiting advances perhaps most dramatically in nutrition and genetics where the UK is a recognised world leader and exporter. Thus investment in Health is a fundamental of success for the Roadmap.

In August 2011 a new strategy was launched; "20:20 Pig Health and Welfare, A Vision for 2020" (BPEX, 2011b) with cross industry support. The strategy is presented in a sister document to "Advancing Together", sharing a common holistic approach to solving problems and placing the industry in a better position to face challenges of the future. Health and welfare improvement targets covering disease elimination and impact reduction, welfare outcomes are listed which address both on-farm need and protecting consumer health and aspirations. There is also a pledge to continue working with the meat Supply Chain to improve food safety and to protect the Environment.

The Pig Health Improvement Programme (PHIP) is partnership working and has evolved from local to regional initiatives to become a national scheme soon to employ four co-ordinators. Focused cluster groups of farmers are working with veterinary practitioners and other specialists, utilising Defra grants to carry out on-farm activity to improve pig health status. Looking at disease and health is not enough, the housed environment is important, thus housing and ventilation are also receiving attention as often some small but critical changes can have a significant impact.

Feed and nutrition form one important pillar of 2TS and a crucial key piece of the Environmental Jigsaw. Besides the challenge of designing rations for farmers that meet the production needs of their pigs at an affordable price, high metabolic efficiencies are required to reduce emissions and pressures on the environment. Last, but not least, are the ethical questions about the origin of ingredients, and even if we should feed certain ingredients to animals at all?

Feed and the environment

Feed is the largest single component of the cost of pig production on the farm. It also is the largest contributor to the Carbon Footprint and environmental burdens of production. Co-product use is a good news story, but food manufacturers are under similar pressures to maximise returns from sales as well, so established products may change and new ones emerge. Feeding catering waste and processed animal protein is on the political radar, and is supported by some environmental non-governmental organisations (NGOs); will it become acceptable? Although the Industry may elect not to use these as a point of differentiation for marketing purposes, their use elsewhere may still provide an opportunity as we can supply product to other countries which do elect to use them. The more of the pig which can be utilised, the lower will be the burdens associated with production and use.

Genetically Modified Organisms (GMOs) are another topic of debate, the pig industry is participating and monitoring the science, but maintains that freedom of choice of the individual will remain an option for those who desire it.

BPEX Marketing and Environment Teams continue to work with Government departments, retailers, NGOs and consumer-facing media on these more contentious areas associated with the use and production of pig feeds. Soya is perhaps the most immediate of the issues on account of the quantities of Soyabean Meal used each year, although its use has decreased by one half in the last decade in favour of domestically grown proteins such as rape meal.

Promoting the use of sustainable soya remains an important issue. At present there is little RTRS (Round Table on Responsible Soy) certified soya on the market, but customer interest is increasing to the extent that FEMAS (Feed Materials Assurance Scheme used in the UK compound feed industry) and RTRS have recently launched a joint module for responsible soya supply. The module brings together the sustainability criteria of RTRS at farm level with the existing robust supply chain certification of the FEMAS scheme without adding significantly to auditing costs. The source of soya imports into the United Kingdom (UK) is reported to be mostly from Argentina (57%) with Brazil accounting for only 38% (Source AIC).

Land Use change (LUC) associated with the production of soya remains a hot topic of debate, there is an acceptance that the amount of soya grown in areas of cleared rainforest is relatively small (WWF, 2011) and the indications are that since the introduction in 2006 of a voluntary moratorium on the sourcing of soya, it has become less of a catalyst for deforestation (Union of Concerned Scientists, 2011). BPEX continues to play a leading role in the activities of the International Meat Secretariat (IMS) in pressing for greater availability and use of ethically produced soya in pig production. Life cycle assessment has been carried out as part of the Sustainable use of home grown proteins in livestock production (Green Pig project, Defra LINK LK0682) which highlights the importance of sourcing. This study reported that the LUC associated emissions in Brazil and Argentina are 7.69 and 0.93 kg CO_2-eq / kg soya, respectively. Also the Global Warming potential (GWP) of grower and finisher pig diets based on soyabean meal was calculated to be 1.69 kg CO_2-eq / kg pig without land use change included in the calculation and 2.37 kg CO_2-eq / kg pig (Topp et al. 2012).

Table 4. The environmental impact of pea, bean and soya based grower and finisher diets on pig production

	GWP (No LUC) (kg CO_2-eq / kg pig)	GWP (LUC) (kg CO_2-eq / kg pig)	Eutrophication (kg PO_4 / kg pig)	Acidifcation (kg SO_4 / kg pig)
Pea	1.61	1.85	0.130	0.012
Bean	1.66	1.86	0.140	0.015
Soya	1.69	2.37	0.131	0.018

Soya inclusion rates are reported to have reduced by a half in the last decade and now account for only 10% of the diet. There has been a corresponding increase in the use of home grown proteins.

As availability of RTRS and other certified sources of sustainable soya increases in the coming year, we will bring this to the attention of the industry. BPEX will also follow with interest the recently announced partnership agreement between the Brazilian Confederation of Agriculture and Livestock (CAN) and the British Embassy in Brazil on the programme aimed at spreading the use of sustainable agricultural practices.

Results from feeding trials of finishing pigs using peas and beans (Defra LINK project LK0682 "Green Pig") are being disseminated, and a total of five papers were accepted for the British Society of Animal Science conference in 2012. Commercial scale trials demonstrated that inclusion rates of up to 30% peas or beans can be fed successfully to pigs from 30 kg to slaughter weight (105 kg) without detriment to performance, as part of a diet specifically formulated to be nutritionally balanced. Inclusion levels of beans have to be higher than those of more protein dense soyabean meal, and there is a need for supplementary amino acids. Interest from farmers in the trial has been encouraging with renewed interest in growing and utilising beans especially. However achieving uptake is not without its challenges; beans are not very economical to grow due to variable yields, but can be a useful break crop for this particular system.

A wide range of co-products from the food and drinks industries continue to make a valuable contribution to pig diets continuing a long tradition of recycling. The effective utilisation of these products by our industry reduces the environmental burdens both of the source food or drink, and of the pig meat and pig carcase products; the well recognised green credentials of pig production. Furthermore, use of co-products reduces the industry's need for raw products such as cereal grains and pulses. The opportunities for improving co-products and identifying new potential supplies is something at which feed suppliers are very adept. The latest great hope comes from the UK and European fledgling bio-ethanol industry, wheat dried distillers grains with solubles (DDGS). At the present time there is no UK production taking place, however two feed mills are understood to be using French sourced wheat DDGS in pig rations. Experience with this and initial products from the ENSUS plant on Teeside is indicating that DDGS can be included successfully in finisher pig feed. Further studies within Defra LINK Project; The Environmental and Nutritional Benefits of Bio-ethanol Co-products (ENBBIO) are in the planning stages, but these will allow nutritionists to understand the full nutritional characteristics of this product.

Nutritional improvement is not confined to indoor herds, the "EcoPig" project led by pig production company British Quality Pigs (BQP) with Defra financial support, has successfully proved the benefits of feeding outdoor pigs in long troughs as opposed to the conventional floor method. Reduced feed and fuel use, carbon footprint, nitrate leaching and improved soil management are all positive outcomes. Results have given BQP the confidence to invest over £1M in trough feeding across all their outdoor production sites (around 25% of the English outdoor sow herd). Other production companies have visited the site and are looking to implement changes in their businesses.

One effect of improving health is improvement in feed utilisation and pig growth rate, but direct feed use improvement is still important, BPEX KT continues to raise the importance of management to reduce waste from spoilage and spillage to trough feeding of sows on outdoor units. The finishing stage of production accounts for 50% of feed volume and so small gains in productivity can make a significant impact. BPEX has launched the Finisher Challenge as the next stage of the Two Tonne Sow Programme (2TS). Knowledge Transfer Managers are helping to fine tune performance, identify lost potential and improve businesses by October through competitive spirit9.

In addition to its goal of utilising resources more effectively, the pig industry has to address ammonia emissions and their impact. The housing component of 2TS is looking at improving the atmosphere for the pigs themselves through design and management but possibly the biggest external pressures restricting potential development of new and replacement facilities is that of odour and ammonia emissions to the atmosphere and their effect on their locality. Through implementation of legislation to protect wildlife habitats, the impacts of ammonia from livestock farms is having to be assessed and computer simulation models used to demonstrate that the atmospheric concentrations or deposition is not going to cause damage, in some cases at a distance of up to 10 kilometres. This is bringing the composition of diets sharply into focus. Feed formulation and inclusion of ingredients which result in a reduction in protein levels whilst maintaining production can make the difference between whether a development can go ahead, or an environmental permit be issued or not. This is one area where the skills of nutritionists are going to be increasingly called upon to help deliver greater nutritional uptake and consequential reduced nitrogen excretion.

Managing excretion

Managing slurries and wastes and realising their full potential is an important part of a complex and interrelated series of activities promoted by BPEX, information for producers is available on the BPEX Environment Hub; www.bpex.org.uk/environment-hub/. Included are calculators to estimated volumes of manures and slurries produced on a farm together with the nitrogen excreted in order to fulfil statutory obligations. Further to this, help is provided to improve the understanding of the crop nutritional benefits of manures and slurries, how these may be best utilised and the financial opportunities available form reducing the use of manufactured fertilisers. The use of low emissions spreading equipment is increasing by farmers and contractors. This is in part driven by the need to comply with nitrate pollution prevention regulations which are driving a move to spreading on growing crops as opposed to bare land, but also the economics. The fertiliser savings by reducing ammonium nitrogen losses at spreading can be greater than the additional cost of using the high technology complex spreaders. Financial drivers such as this example are a very good way to drive improvements in performance both from the business and environmental perspectives.

One potential barrier to uptake of better practice, is confidence in the nutritional content of organic manures. This has partly been addressed by another Defra Link project; "Improving Analysis of Solid Manures and Slurries". The knowledge gained in this project has been commercialised offering producers an analysis service at lower cost and improved accuracy.

Significant amounts of ammonium nitrogen can be lost from stored slurry. In addition, slurry stores are often contentious sources of localised odour leading in complaints from neighbours and a poor image for the industry. Legally Environment Permitting Regulations (EPR) permitted farms have to cover their slurry stores, but increasingly other farmers are recognising the benefits of covers, less ammonia and odour loss, reduced volume of rainwater collected and increased storage period as a result. A number of pig producers have been early adopters of new Light Expanded Clay Aggregate (LECA) products with catalytic coatings applied to the granules which reduce ammonia and odour emissions. These products have been successful in overcoming local odour issues and offer a comparatively lower cost method of covering stores to comply with EPR requirements. Roadmap activity includes communicating the options and opportunities covering provides.

Energy and water

Energy used on farms has traditionally been of fossil fuel origin, the objective of controlling costs has driven many pig units to assess their energy demands and start installing more efficient equipment such as lights, motor drives and heaters as well as improving their control. New technologies, or manufacturing processes which reduce the cost of these mean we will see the introduction of different types of equipment, for example compact fluorescent lamps have rapidly replaced tungsten filament light bulbs in many piggeries. The next advance is a move to light emitting diode (LED) lamps, already in the poultry industry these are reducing lighting energy use by up to 90%, allowing behaviour control and simulation of day night transition. A BPEX study into the lighting needs of pigs (Taylor, 2010) concluded that these lights should not have negative consequences for pig health or welfare, guidance has been published (BPEX, 2010) and consequently a number of suppliers have entered the market.

Farms also offer many opportunities for renewable energy production including the recovery of heat from buildings and slurries besides the increasingly familiar site of solar panels and wind turbines as well as biogas production. Government incentives have encouraged a number of production sites to invest in these technologies as the returns on investment make this a sensible business decision, it also allows farmers to fix their energy costs for a number of years ahead providing a degree of security against inflation. BPEX continues to provide information to producers describing the systems on offer, benefits and incentives. New material has been added to the BPEX Website, including a case study featuring a £300k investment in solar PV technology on a midlands farm. We are also working with producers seeking to claim renewable heat incentive (RHI) payments from the use of biomass fuel to understand the system and assist others take advantage of this.

People and skills

Returning to the theme of a joined up approach, people and skills are the binder brining all the threads together. The Pig Sector has led agricultural industries from the front by developing formal skill training packages for all levels of staff, both on and off farm from stock people to owners and directors. Uptake has been good and continues to be driven by BPEX and the National Pig Association (NPA).

The BPEX website has been refreshed and improved to make our services more accessible to users. New material is constantly being published including photo stories and case studies. We have started to use webinars as another means of building engagement in the industry and reaching those who through location or for other reasons find it difficult to attend meetings and events but who still value interaction and participation even if it cannot be face to face.

Markets and utilisation

Besides producing animals efficiently, maximising use of the carcase and its components offers further opportunity to reduce the environmental impacts of production. The old saying of you can use "everything but the squeak" holds true today. Besides improving the yield of meat products through reducing carcase condemnations in the abattoir and adopting new cutting techniques world trade is important. Some components not favoured by the UK consumer can be highly valued in other parts of the world; for example trotters, heads and other parts can find ready markets in the Far East. Opening of export markets and exploiting these components increases their value from low to high, thus reducing the overall measure of Carbon Footprint for primary meat. Besides the edible parts, fats and oils can be converted to bio-fuels, and it is looking increasingly likely that bones and other elements will be able to be converted into processed animal protein (PAP) and marketed rather than being treated as a waste in rendering plants. Even if UK pig producers elect to maintain a point of differentiation for their product by not using PAP, export markets will become available adding financial yield.

Thus world trade is part of the solution and efforts of government, industry organisations and export companies continue to drive progress forward. The question of a "Green Premium" for home produced pig meat produced in low carbon systems is often suggested, at the present time there is little evidence from the market place that the majority of consumers are willing to pay a premium for a differentiated product like they do for animal welfare. Thus to add another layer of labelling and differentiation will add to confusion and deliver great benefits. Our approach continues to drive improvements in all production systems leaving the consumer with choice of product fitting their financial constraints and or aspirations.

Conclusions

The pig industry is engaged in a wide range of activity from conception to grave which is delivering lower environmental consequences making pig derived products more sustainable and improving the long-term prospects of the industry. The biggest barrier to progress being low or negative returns for producers and processers, the consequence of which is low confidence and unwillingness to invest in businesses and move forward. As the World's population continues to increase, demand for pig products will continue to grow, especially as a source of low carbon meat protein. A resource efficient high yielding industry delivering what the market wants at a price it is willing to pay looks to be in a strong position.

References

AHDB (2012) *2012 BPEX Annual Pig Meat Industry Survey.* Agricultural and Horticultural Development Board, Warwickshire, England.
BPEX (2011a) *Advancing Together, a Roadmap for the English Pig Industry.*

BPEX, Warwickshire, England.

BPEX (2011b) *20:20 Pig Health and Welfare, A Vision for 2020*. BPEX, Warwickshire, England.

BPEX (2010) *Research into Action 5; Lighting for pig units*. BPEX, Warwickshire, England.

FAO (2006) *Livestock's Long Shadow – environmental issues and options*. Food and Agriculture Organisation, Rome.

Godfray, H.C.J., et al. (2011) *Foresight. The Future of Food and Farming (2011)*. Final Project Report. The Government Office for Science, London.

Greenhouse Gas Action Plan (2011) *Meeting the Challenge: agricultural industry GHG Action Plan*. 2011.

Topp, C.F.E., Houdijk, J.G. M., Tarsitano, D., Tolkamp, B.J. and Kyriazakis, I. (2012) Quantifying the environmental benefits of using home grown protein sources as alternatives to soyabean meal in pig production through life cycle assessment. *Advances in Animal Biosciences*, **3**, 15.

Taylor, N. (2010) *Lighting for Pig Units*. BPEX, Warwickshire, England.

Union of Concerned Scientists (2011) *The Root of the Problem – what's driving tropical deforestation today*. Union of Concerned Scientists, Cambridge, MA, USA.

WWF (2011). *Soya and the Cerrado: Brazil's forgotten jewel*. WWF-UK, Goldaming, UK.

13

ASPECTS OF AMINO ACID DIGESTIBILITY IN FEED INGREDIENTS FED TO PIGS

F. N. ALMEIDA AND H. H. STEIN
Department of Animal Sciences, University of Illinois, Urbana, Illinois, USA

Introduction

Knowledge about the nutritional quality of feed ingredients is imperative for success in nutrition of pigs. For the protein fraction, it is generally agreed that the most accurate estimate of the quality of a feed ingredient is described by the digestibility of protein and amino acids in the ingredient. The objective of this chapter is to review digestion and absorption of protein and amino acids in pigs, to provide information about factors that influence protein and amino acid digestibilities in feed ingredients fed to pigs, and to discuss factors that may negatively impact protein and amino acid digestibility by pigs.

Digestion and absorption of protein and amino acids

Protein digestion in pigs starts in the stomach where pepsinogen, which is secreted by the Chief cells in the Fundic region, is activated to pepsin by H ions. In this stage, between 15 and 50% of all peptide bonds in proteins are hydrolyzed by pepsin, thus forming small oligopeptides. Activation of pepsinogen is best achieved at pH 2, and this may be a challenge for young pigs because HCl secretion is limited compared with that in older pigs. Therefore, activation of pepsinogen in young pigs may be limited and digestion of proteins may not be as effective as in older pigs, but there are limited data to demonstrate the extent to which protein digestion is impaired in young pigs. After gastric digestion, small and larger oligopeptides proceed to the small intestines where pancreatic enzymes (i.e., trypsin, chymotrypsin, elastase, and carboxypeptidase) and aminopeptidase, which is secreted from the small intestinal brush border, hydrolyze most of the peptide bonds in the oligopeptides. The resulting free amino acids, di-peptides, and tri-peptides are subsequently absorbed into the enterocytes using four different active transport systems. After absorption, di-peptides and tri-peptides are broken down to free amino acids in the enterocytes by the action of di-peptidases and tri-peptidases, respectively. The majority of the free amino acids then leave the enterocytes via the basolateral membrane and are subsequently taken up by the hepatic portal vein and transported to the liver. These amino acids are used for synthesis of proteins that may be used for maintenance or for production by the animal. Excess amino acids are not stored in the body. Instead, excess amino acids are deaminated and metabolized, and the N is excreted in the urine in the form of urea. The carbon skeletons are used for ketogenesis or gluconeogenesis and thus provide energy for the animal.

Amino acid digestibility

Absorption of amino acids takes place only in the small intestine. Amino acids that pass the last portion of the small intestine (the ileum) into the large intestine can no longer be absorbed by the animal and may be metabolized by microorganisms in the large intestine and subsequently excreted as microbial protein in the feces. Thus, determination of amino acid digestibility is believed to be more accurate if determined at the end of the ileum than in the faeces (Stein et al., 2007). Amino acid digestibility is generally expressed as apparent ileal digestibility (AID), true ileal digestibility (TID), or standardized ileal digestibility (SID; Stein et al., 2007; Urbaityte et al., 2009).

APPARENT ILEAL DIGESTIBILITY

Values for AID of amino acids are used to describe the net disappearance of protein and amino acids from the digestive tract proximal to the distal ileum (Stein et al., 2007). To determine AID values, pigs are surgically fitted with a T-cannula in the distal ileum from which ileal digesta are collected using standard procedures (Almeida et al., 2011). The concentration of protein and amino acids in the ileal digesta is then subtracted from the concentration of protein and amino acids in the diet, and the difference is divided by the concentration of protein and amino acids in the diet (Stein et al., 2007). Values for the AID of protein and amino acids, however, are not to be additive in mixed diets because they do not account for the endogenous losses of protein and amino acids, which is the main disadvantage of the use of values for AID (Stein et al., 2005). This issue, however, may be overcome by correction for endogenous protein and amino acids losses.

ENDOGENOUS PROTEIN AND AMINO ACID LOSSES

Endogenous protein and amino acid losses are composed of protein and amino acids resulting from mucoproteins, sloughed cells, digestive enzymes, microbial protein, amides, and ingested hair (Souffrant, 1991; Nyachoti et al., 1997). Endogenous protein and amino acid losses may be divided into 2 categories: 1) basal endogenous losses, which relates to the physical flow of feed dry matter through the gastrointestinal tract and represent the minimum amount of protein and amino acids inevitably lost by the pig; and 2) specific endogenous losses, which is stimulated by specific characteristics of feed ingredients such as fibre and antinutritional factors, and represent the losses above the basal endogenous losses (Schulze et al., 1995; Stein et al., 2007).

Methods used to determine basal endogenous losses of protein and amino acids include feeding a protein-free diet, the regression procedure, and the peptide alimentation procedure (Fuller, 1991; Jansman et al., 2002; Moughan, 2003). Use of the N-free diet is the simplest and easiest of these procedures and is, therefore, the most commonly used procedure. However, it is recognized that the N-free procedure may overestimate endogenous losses of proline and glycine (Stein et al., 2007).

Total endogenous losses of protein and amino acids, which include basal plus specific losses, may be estimated using the homoarginine method or the isotope tracer technique (Krawielitzki et al., 1977; Hagemeister and Ebersdobler, 1985). Both of these procedures are expensive and tedious to use and only estimate the loss of one or a few amino acids and they are, therefore, not commonly used in practical feed ingredient evaluation (Stein et al., 2007).

TRUE ILEAL DIGESTIBILITY

Values for the TID of amino acids are determined by correcting AID values for total endogenous losses of protein and amino acids. True ileal digestibility values, therefore, represent the amount of dietary protein and amino acids that disappear from the gastrointestinal tract proximal to the distal ileum (Stein et al., 2007). However, because of the difficulties in determining the total endogenous losses, values for TID of amino acids are not commonly determined for feed ingredients and these values are not used in practical feed formulation.

STANDARDIZED ILEAL DIGESTIBILITY

Values for the SID of amino acids represent the quantities of dietary protein and amino acids that disappear from the gastrointestinal tract proximal to the distal ileum but, in this case, AID values are corrected for the basal endogenous losses of protein and amino acids (Stein et al., 2007). For this reason, it is expected that values for the SID of protein and amino acids are greater than values for AID and less than values for the TID. Utilization of SID values may overcome some of the limitations of using AID and TID values as observed by Stein et al. (2005). Specifically, SID values are additive in mixed diets, which is of great practical importance for the feed industry because the SID of AA in mixed diets can be predicted from the SID of AA in the individual ingredients.

Factors affecting amino acid digestibility

Many factors may influence the digestibility of amino acids in feed ingredients. These include factors intrinsic to feed ingredients such as nutritional composition and antinutritional factors. Other factors relate to the physiological condition of the pig (i.e., weanling, growing, gestation, lactation), or to management practices, which include, but are not limited to, feed intake of animals. Processing of feed ingredients also may have a direct effect on amino acid digestibility.

PHYSIOLOGICAL ASPECTS

Body weight may influence the efficacy of pigs to digest protein and amino acids (Nitrayová et al., 2006). Little research, however, has been conducted to compare the digestibility of protein and amino acids among pigs at different physiological states.

Early studies revealed that the AID of protein and amino acids in growing pigs is less than the AID of protein and amino acids in lactating sows (Stein et al., 1999a). When compared with gestating sows, however, the AID of protein and amino acids in growing pigs is similar for most amino acids although the AID of histidine, lysine, threonine, and tryptophan are greater for gestation sows (Stein et al., 1999a). The assumptions for the differences observed were that the endogenous protein and amino acid losses may have been different among each group of pigs. Thus, pigs with less endogenous losses would have greater AID of amino acids (Stein et al., 1999a). This hypothesis was later confirmed by Leterme and Théwis (2004), and Presto and Lindberg (2010) who observed that endogenous losses of protein and amino acids are lower in growing pigs than in finishing pigs. The AID of protein and amino acids was greater for pigs at 61.7 kg than for pigs at 20.6 kg (Nitrayová et al., 2006). Similarly, the AID of protein and amino acids in piglets fed canola meal was lower than in growing pigs (Mariscal-Landín et al., 2008).

FEED INTAKE

Voluntary feed intake of pigs is associated with many factors, such as gender, group size, and lysine level in the diet (Hyun et al., 1997) and the level of feed intake affects the endogenous losses of protein and amino acids in growing pigs and gestating sows (Stein et al., 1999b; Moter and Stein, 2004). Consequently, values for the SID of protein and amino acids, which is calculated by correcting AID values for basal endogenous losses, are also affected by feed intake (Stein et al., 2001; Moter and Stein, 2004). Specifically, values for the AID of protein and some amino acids increases as the feed intake level increases, whereas the SID of protein and most amino acids decreases with increasing levels of feed intake (Moter and Stein, 2004). These observations were later confirmed for weanling pigs, where SID of protein and amino acids decrease if the level of feed intake increases above 2 times the maintenance requirement for energy (Goerke et al., 2012). However, values for SID of protein and amino acids are identical if pigs arc fcd 3 times the level of maintenance energy or if they are allowed ad libitum access to feed (Chastanet et al., 2007). It is, therefore, recommended that pigs are fed at a level of at least 3 times the energy requirement for maintenance when experiments to determine protein and amino acid digestibility are conducted.

FIBRE

The concentration of fibre in diets fed to pigs is negatively correlated with the digestibility of some amino acids (Lehnen et al., 2011). Specifically, crude fibre decreases the AID of phenylalanine, lysine, leucine, proline, and serine. Neutral detergent fibre also reduces the AID of arginine, histidine, isoleucine, lysine, and methionine, and acid detergent fibre reduces the AID of aspartate, glutamate, alanine, phenylalanine, and proline. Lignin was also negatively correlated with the AID of glutamate, alanine, and phenylalanine (Lehnen et al., 2011).

Some of the reduction in the AID of amino acids by dietary fibre may be attributed to an increase in N excretion from endogenous origin (Huang et al., 2001). Dietary fibre may increase sloughing of cell in the small intestines, in addition to increased mucus production (Huang et al., 2001). Dietary fibre also affect gelling and viscosity properties that may decrease the mixing of intestinal contents, and therefore, impair interactions between proteins and enzymes, thereby reducing digestibility (Huang et al., 2001). In addition, an unstirred water layer may form as a result of increased concentration of dietary fibre, thus reducing absorption and consequently reducing the AID of amino acids (Huang et al., 2001).

ANTINUTRITIONAL FACTORS

Antinutritional factors are defined as natural occurring plant metabolites or compounds formed as a result of processing of feed ingredients that may negatively affect utilization of nutrients by the animal, and consequently reduce productive performance (Gilani et al., 2005). Among the natural occurring metabolites that directly affect protein and amino acid digestibility are gossypol, phytic acid, and trypsin inhibitors.

Gossypol, a naturally occurring polyphenolic compound in cotton seeds, is present in the plant in the forms of bound gossypol or free gossypol (Martin, 1990). Bound gossypol is non-toxic to pigs, but free gossypol is associated with growth depression and reduced lysine digestibility in pigs (Martin, 1990). Free gossypol is believed to bind lysine, thus reducing its availability. Increasing levels of cottonseed meal from 25 to 50, and to 75% in diets fed to pigs caused a reduction on the digestibility of amino acids (Li et al., 2000). The detrimental effects of free gossypol on pig performance, however, may be reduced if ferrous sulfate is added to diets in a 1:1 ratio (Martin, 1990).

The majority of phosphorus in plant feed ingredients such as maize and maize co-products is bound to phytic acid (Eeckhout and de Paepe, 1994; Selle and Ravindran, 2008; Almeida and Stein, 2012). Because of the negative charges of phosphate groups in phytic acid, complexes between phytic acid and proteins may be formed in feed ingredients (Lehnen et al., 2011). Phytic acid may also form complex molecules with free amino acids in the gastro intestinal tract (Kies et al., 2001). For these reasons, the digestibility of amino acids may be reduced as a result of high concentrations of phytic acid in some feed ingredients. Phytases are enzymes commonly added to pig diets to hydrolyze phytic acid and release phosphorus to be used by the pig (Almeida and Stein, 2012). Thus, it has been hypothesized that phytases may also reduce the binding of phytic acid to proteins and, therefore, increase the digestibility of amino acids (Mroz et al., 1994). Results from a meta-analysis indicate that addition of phytase to diets increased the digestibility of arginine by 2%, but did not increase the digestibility of other amino acids (Lehnen et al., 2011). However, results of some experiments have indicated that phytase improves amino acid digestibility (Sands et al., 2007; Nortey et al., 2007; and Kiarie et al., 2010), whereas results of other experiments indicate that addition of phytase to diets fed to pigs does not improve amino acid digestibility (Cervantes et al., 2011; Yanez et al., 2011). Based on these observations, it is not clear if microbial phytase can improve the digestibility of amino acids in feed ingredients.

Trypsin inhibitors are present in many commonly fed feed ingredients such as soybean meal, peas, triticale, and rye (van Heugten, 2001), and they impair digestion and metabolism of protein, therefore, causing reduction in pig performance (van Heugten, 2001). The negative effects of trypsin inhibitors on protein digestibility in pigs are a result of the negative impact of these inhibitors on the activity of trypsin, chymotrypsin, and other pancreatic enzymes (Yen et al., 1977). Because of their proteic nature, however, trypsin inhibitors may be inactivated by heat processing, and therefore, soybean meal is usually heat processed before it is used in diets for pigs (Gilani et al., 2005; Goebel and Stein, 2011). Heat treatment of full fat soybeans also improves the AID and SID of amino acids (Goebel and Stein, 2011).

Glucosinolates are sulfur-containing plant metabolites present in Brassica that have been associated with reduced performance of pigs, when fed at high dietary levels (Tripathi and Mishra, 2007). It is recommended that dietary levels of glucosinolates are kept below 2μmol/g of diet (Tripathi and Mishra, 2007). Iodine deficiency, increased thyroid hormone levels, and thyroid hypertrophy have been observed in pigs when dietary concentration of glucosinolates exceeded the recommended maximum concentration (Bourdon and Aumaitre, 1990; Corino et al., 1991). Thyroid hormones play important role in metabolism and hyperthyroidism in humans and have been associated with increased oxidation of protein, loss of muscle mass, and increased protein catabolism (Martin et al., 1991; Møller et al., 1996; Riis et al., 2002). It has been show in humans that hypothyroidism causes both an increase in protein catabolism and anabolism, although the rate of protein catabolism is greater than that of anabolism (Riis et al., 2005). To our knowledge, the secondary detrimental effects of glucosinolates leading to hyperthyroidism and consequent effects on protein metabolism in pigs have not been demonstrated. Nevertheless, it is likely that reduced performance of pigs fed diets containing high levels of glucosinolates is a result of both reduced feed intake due to reduced palatability and also due to an increase in protein catabolism as observed in humans.

Heat damage of amino acids

The nutritional value of feed ingredients may be reduced during storage and processing (Friedman, 1996). This is probably a consequence of a combination of heat and humidity that leads to the Maillard reaction, which starts with the condensation between an amino group of an amino acid or protein and a carbonyl group of a reducing sugar. Lysine is an essential amino acid that has an -amino group that easily condenses with the carbonyl group of a reducing sugar (Nursten, 2005). In the initial stage of the reactions, Amadori products are formed. These products go through subsequently reactions called Strecker degradation, which later lead to the formation of pre-melanoidins and melanoidins at the final stage of the reactions (Nursten, 2005). Melanoidins are heterocyclic brown polymers that are responsible for color formation during heat processing of feed ingredients.

Distillers dried grains with solubles (DDGS) that were oven-dried at 50, 75, or 100°C had reduced concentration of reactive lysine (Pahm et al., 2008). When autoclaving DDGS for 45 min at 120°C, the digestibility of amino acids was reduced, especially that of lysine (Martinez-Amezcua et al., 2007), and it was suggested that the reduction in the digestibility of amino acids other than lysine was a result of the formation of Maillard reaction products that interfered with the absorption of other amino acids. Heat treatment of whey protein in the presence of lactose at temperatures that ranged from 75 to 121°C also caused a decrease in the availability of lysine from 75 to 45% (Desrosiers et al., 1989). González-Vega et al. (2011) reported that the SID of lysine by pigs was reduced from 93% (non-heated soybean meal) to 89.3 and 84.2% when soybean meal was autoclaved for 15 and 30 min, respectively, at a temperature of 125°C. In another experiment, Cozannet et al. (2010) observed that the SID of lysine in wheat DDGS was highly variable and that the samples with the least values for SID were darker and contained less lysine as a percent of crude protein, thus suggesting that color and lysine:crude protein ratio may be used as indicators of heat damage in wheat DDGS. As observed by Stein and Shurson (2009) and confirmed by Cozannet et al. (2010), when feed ingredients are heat damaged the concentration of lysine is reduced whereas the concentration of crude protein remains relatively constant. Therefore, the concentration of SID lysine in wheat DDGS fed to pigs may accurately be predicted ($R^2 = 0.86$) from the lysine:crude protein ratio (Cozannet et al., 2010). Kim et al. (2012) determined the SID of crude protein and amino acids in 21 sources of corn DDGS and observed that there is a positive correlation between the SID of lysine and the lysine:crude protein ratio, which further confirms the above theory. Cysteine and arginine also participate in the Maillard reactions (Ledl and Schleicher, 1990). Heat processing may cause oxidation of unsaturated lipids leading to formation of hydroperoxides (Meade et al., 2005).

Hydroperoxidases may oxidize cysteine, thus, limiting its utilization by the animal. In feed ingredients that have been heat damaged to a higher degree, pre-melanoidins may also react with cysteine and arginine (Finot, 1990). Cysteine may also go through Strecker degradation reactions producing hydrogen sulfide, ammonia, and acetaldehyde (Mottram and Mottram, 2002). The products of these reactions serve as intermediates to the formation of aroma compounds, such as thiazoles and disulphides, which are associated with the Maillard reactions (Mottram and Mottram, 2002). The participation of arginine in the Maillard reactions resulting from heat processing is associated with the formation of cross-links with lysine through imidazopyridinium bridges (Ledl and Schleicher, 1990).

There is, therefore, ample evidence that heat damage to feed ingredients may reduce the nutritional value of feed ingredients, specifically the concentration and digestibility of most amino acids and crude protein. Because many feed ingredients are heated during manufacturing or preparation, it is necessary to evaluate the nutritional quality of these feed ingredients in a quick and reliable manner to accurately use them in feeding programs.

Conclusions

Amino acids are indispensable nutrients that need to be available for pigs to synthesize protein. Most feed ingredients used in practical feed formulation contain protein that is digested in the stomach and small intestine with a subsequent absorption of amino acids. Absorption takes place only in the small intestine and amino acids that are not absorbed by the end of the small intestine will enter the large intestine and be used for the synthesis of microbial protein, which is excreted in the feces. Digestibility of amino acids, therefore, needs to be determined by the end of the small intestine. However, values for AID of amino acids are not always additive in mixed diets fed to pigs because of the influence of endogenous losses of amino acids on AID values. In contrast, values for SID of amino acids, which are calculated by correcting AID values for the basal endogenous losses, are additive in mixed diets and are, therefore, used in practical feed formulation.

Several anti-nutritional factors including gossypol, phytate, trypsin inhibitors, and glucosinolates may negatively impact protein and amino acid digestibility. However, heat treatment will reduce the concentration of trypsin inhibitors in feed ingredients and use of low-glucosinolate varieties will reduce the impact of glucosinolates on amino acid metabolism.

Processing of feed ingredients involving heat will often result in Maillard reactions, which involves the condensation between the amino group of Lys or other AA, and the carbonyl group of reducing sugars. Consequently, Lys becomes unavailable to pigs, thus reducing the digestibility of this AA. The Maillard reactions are a series of complex reactions that remain to be fully understood, although much is known about the initial and intermediate stages. For several feed ingredients it has been shown that calculation of the lysine to crude protein ratio provides a reasonable estimate for heat damage in the ingredient.

References

Almeida, F. N. and Stein, H. H. (2012). *Journal of Animal Science*, **90**, 1262-1269

Almeida, F. N., Petersen, G. I. and Stein, H. H. (2011). *Journal of Animal Science*, **89**, 4109-4115

Bourdon, D., and Aumaitre, A. (1990). *Animal Feed Science and Technology*, **30**:175-190.

Cervantes, M., Gómez, R., Fierro, S., Barrera, M. A., Morales, A., Araiza, B. A., Zijlstra, R. T., Sánchez, J. E. and Sauer, W. C. (2011). *Journal of Animal Physiology and Animal Nutrition*, **95**, 179-186

Chastanet, F., Pahm, A. A., Pedersen, C. and Stein, H. H. (2007). *Animal Feed Science and Technology*, **132**, 94-102

Corino, C., Baldi, A, and Bontempo, V. (1991). *Animal Feed Science and Technology*. **35**:321-331

Cozannet, P., Primot, Y., Gady, C., Métayer, J. P., Callu, P., Lessire, M., Skiba, F. and Noblet, J. (2010). *Animal Feed Science and Technology*, **158**, 177-186

Desrosiers, T., Savoie, L., Bergeron, G. and Parent, G. (1989). *Journal of Agriculture and Food Chemistry*, **37**, 1385-1391

Eeckhout, W. and de Paepe, M. (1994). *Animal Feed Science and Technology*. **47**, 19-29

Finot, P. A. (1990). In *The Maillard Reaction in Food Processing, Human Nutrition and* Physiology, pp. 259-272. Ed. Finot, P. A., Aeschbacher, H. U., Hurrel, R. F. and Liardon, R. Birkhaüser Verlag, Berlin, Germany

Friedman, M. (1996). *Journal of Agriculture and Food Chemistry*, **44,** 631-653

Fuller, M. (1991). In *Digestive Physiology in pigs, Proceedings of the Fifth International Symposium*, pp. 273-288. Ed. Vestergen, M. W. A., Huisman, J. and den Hartog, L. A. Wageningen Academic Publishers, Wageningen, the Netherlands

Gilani, G. S., Cockell, K. A. and Sepehr, E. (2005). *Journal of AOAC International*, **88**, 967-987

Goebel, K. P. and Stein, H. H. (2011). *Asian-Australasian Journal of Animal Science*, **24**, 88-95

Goerke, M., Eklund, M., Sauer, N., Rademacher, M., Piepho, H-P., Börner, C.

and Mosenthin, R. (2012). *Journal of Science and Food Agriculture*, **92**, 1261-1266

González-Vega, J. C., Kim, B. G., Htoo, J. K. and Stein, H. H. (2011). *Journal of Animal Science*, **89**, 3617-3625

Hagemeister, H. and Ebersdobler, H. (1985). *Proceedings of the Nutrition Society*, **44**, 133A

Huang, S. X., Sauer, W. C. and Marty, B. (2001). *Journal of Animal Science*, **79**, 2388-2396

Hyun, Y., Ellis, M., McKeith, F. K. and Wilson, E. R. (1997). *Journal of Animal Science*, **75**, 1443-1451

Jansman, A. J. M., Smink, W., van Leeuwen, P. Rademacher, M. (2002). *Animal Feed Science and Technology*, **98**, 49-60

Kiarie, E., Owusu-Asiedu, A., Simmins, P. H. and Nyachoti, C. M. (2010). *Livestock Science*, **134**, 85-87

Kies, A. K., van Hemert, K. H. F. and Sauer, W. C. (2001). *World`s Poultry Science Journal*, **57**, 110-126

Kim, B. G., Kil, D. Y., Zhang, Y, and Stein, H. H. 2012. *Journal of Animal Science,* **90**, doi:10.2527/jas.2011-4103

Krawielitzki, R., Volker, R., Smulikowska, S., Bock, H. D. and Wuensche, J. (1977). *Archives of Animal Nutrition*, **27**, 609-621

Ledl, F. and Schleicher, E. (1990). *Angewandte Chemie International Edition in English*, **29**, 565-594

Lehnen, C. R., Lovatto, P. A., Andretta, I., Kipper, M., Hauschild, L. and Rossi, C. A. (2011). *Pesquisa Agropecuária Brasileira*, **46**, 438-445

Leterme, P. and Théwis, A. (2004). *Reproduction Nutrition Development*, **44**, 407-417

Li, D., Xu, X. X., Qiao, S. Y., Zheng, C. T., Chen, Y., Piao, X. S., Han, In K. and Thacker, P. (2000). *Journal of Animal Science*, **13**, 521-527

Mariscal-Landín, G., Reis de Souza, T. C., Parra S, J. E., Aguilera B, A. and Mar B, B. (2008). *Livestock Science*, **116**, 53-62

Martin, S. D. (1990). *Feedstuffs*, **62**, 14-17

Martin, W. H., Spina, R. J., Korte, E. Yarasheski, K. E., Angelopoulos, T. J., Nemeth, P. M. and Saffitz, J. E. (1991). *Journal of Clinical Investigations.* **88**, 2047-2053

Martinez-Amezcua, C., Parsons, C. M., Singh, V., Srinivasan, R. and Murthy, G. S. (2007). *Poultry Science*, **86**, 2624-2630

Meade, S. J., Reid, E. A. and Gerrard, J. A. (2005). *Journal of AOAC International*, **88**, 904-922

Moter, V. and Stein, H. H. (2004). *Journal of Animal Science*, **82**, 3518-3525

Mottram, D. S. and Mottram, H. R. (2002). In *Heteroatomic Coumpounds,* pp. 73-92. Ed. Reineccius, G. A. and Reineccius, T. A. American Chemical

Society, Washington, DC

Moughan, P. J. (2003). In *Digestive Physiology in pigs, Proceedings of the Ninth International Symposium*, pp. 199-221. Ed. Ball, R. O. University of Alberta, Alberta, Canada

Mroz, Z., Jongbloed, A.. W. and Kemme, P. A. (1994). *Journal of Animal Science*, **72**, 126-132

Møller, N., Nielsen, S., Nyholm, B., Pørksen, N., Alberti, K. G., and Weeke, J. (1996). *Clinical Endocrinology, Oxford.* **44**, 453-459.

Nitrayová, S., Hger, J., Patráš, P. and Brestenský. (2006). *Slovakian Journal of Animal Science*, **39**, 65-68

Nortey, T. N., Patience, J. F., Simmins, P. H., Trottier, N. L. and Zijlstra, R. T. (2007). *Journal of Animal Sciences*, **85**, 1432-1443

Nursten, H. (2005). In *The Maillard Reaction. Chemistry, biochemistry, and implications.* Royal Society of Chemistry, Cambridge, UK.

Nyachoti, C. M., de Lange, C. F. M., McBride, B. W. and Schulze, H. (1997). *Canadian Journal of Animal Science*, **77**, 149-163

Pahm, A. A., Pedersen, C. and Stein, H. H. (2008). *Journal of Agriculture and Food Chemistry*, **56**, 9441-9446

Presto, M. H., Lyberg, K. and Lindberg, J. E. (2010). *Livestock Science*, **134**, 18-20

Riis, A. L. D., Jørgensen, J. O. L. Gjedde, S., Nørrelund, H., Jurik, A. G., Nair, K. S., Ivarsen, P., Weeke, J., and Møller, N. (2005). *American Journal of Physiology, Endocrinology and Metabolism.* **288**:E1067-E1073

Riis, A. L. D., Gravholt, C. H, Djurhuus, C. B., Nørrelund, H., Jørgensen, J. O. L., Weeke, J. and Møller, N. (2002). *Journal of Clinical Endocrinology and Metabolism.* **87**:4747-4753

Sands, J. S., Dilger, R. N., Ragland, D. and Adeola, O. (2007). *Livestock Science*, **109**, 208-211

Schulze, H., van Leeuwen, P., Verstegen, M. W. A. van den Berg, J. W. O. (1995). *Journal of Animal Science*, **73**, 441-448

Selle, P. H. and Ravindran, V. (2008). *Livestock Science*, **113**:99-122

Souffrant, W. B. (1991). In *Digestive Physiology in pigs, Proceedings of the Fifth International Symposium*, pp. 147-166. Ed. Vestergen, M. W. A., Huisman, J. and den Hartog, L. A. Wageningen Academic Publishers, Wageningen, the Netherlands

Stein, H. H., Aref, S. and Easter, R. A. (1999a). *Journal of Animal Science*, **77**, 1169-1179

Stein, H. H., Kim, S. W., Nielsen, T. T. and Easter, R. A. (2001). *Journal of Animal Science*, **79**, 2113-2122

Stein, H. H., Pedersen, C., Wirt, A. R. Bolke, R. A. (2005). *Journal of Animal Science*, **83**, 2387-2395

Stein, H. H., Sève, B., Fuller, M. F., Moughan, P. J. and de Lange, C. F. M. (2007). *Journal of Animal Science*, **85**,172-180

Stein, H. H. and Shurson, G. C. (2009). *Journal of Animal Science*, **87**, 1292-1303

Stein, H. H., Trottier, N. L., Bellaver, C., and Easter, R. A. (1999b). *Journal of Animal Science*, **77**, 1180-1187

Tripathi, M. K., and Mishra, A. S. (2007). *Animal Feed Science and Technology.* **132**, 1-27

Urbaityte, R., Mosenthin, R. and Eklund, M. (2009). *Asian-Australasian Journal of Animal Science*, **22**, 1209-1223

van Heugten, E. (2001). In *Swine Nutrition*, pp. 563-584. Ed. Lewis, A. J. and Southern, L. L. CRC Press, Boca Raton, Florida

Yáñez, J. L., Beltranena, E., Cervantes, M. and Zijlstra, R. T. (2011). *Journal of Animal Science*, **89**, 113-123

Yen, J. T., Jensen, A. H. and Simon, J. (1974). *Journal of Nutrition*, **107**, 156-165.

14

SOW NUTRITION: HORMONAL MANIPULATION VIA NUTRITION

R. GERRITSEN AND P.J. VAN DER AAR

Schothorst Feed Research, PO Box 533, 8200 AM Lelystad, The Netherlands

Introduction

Due to genetic selection for increased litter size in modern sow lines, the number of piglets weaned per sow per year has increased. For example, the number of piglets weaned per sow per year for sows in the Schothorst Feed Research (SFR) pig herd has increased from 24.9 in 2005 to 30.6 in 2011. This increase is mainly the result of an increase in number of piglets born alive (from 11.6 to 13.7). As uterine capacity is limiting (Foxcroft et al., 2006), the increase in litter size has reduced individual birth weight from 1456 g on average in 2005 to 1247 g on average in 2011. Additionally variation within birth weight between litter mates has increased, thus reducing the homogeneity of the litter.

Furthermore, genetic selection for lean meat content and average daily gain (ADG) in growing-finishing pigs has resulted in a higher ADG potential in young sows (Foxcroft and Aherne, 2001) and more meatier-type sows. These two developments in pig genetics have resulted in great challenges for the sow feed industry: 1. how to feed modern genotype sows with high reproductive performance according to their requirements and 2. how to feed modern genotype sows to improve piglet survival, birth weight and homogeneity of the litter. The first challenge can be faced by re-evaluating the energy and amino acid requirements of gestating and lactating sows as well as amino acid ratios, as has been described by several scientific groups (e.g. Kim et al., 2009; Samuel et al., 2011). The second challenge can be seen as the fine tuning of gestating and lactating sow diets. In the past, when wanting to improve birth weight, the focus was on fine tuning of nutrition of the sow during the last trimester of gestation. Recently, studies have also shown that fine tuning during the end of lactation and during the weaning to oestrus interval can affect birth weight and homogeneity of the litter. In both cases the nutritional measures taken in order to improve piglet quality have their effect via hormones. Thus, there is fine-tuning of sow performance and performance of offspring via manipulation of hormones. The hormone playing the most important role (based on current knowledge) is insulin. How insulin is affected by feeding strategy such as feeding level and diet composition as well as how insulin affects birth weight and homogeneity of the litter will be discussed in this paper.

Role of insulin in sow performance

INSULIN AND SOW REPRODUCTIVE HORMONES

It is commonly known that in order for follicle development and oestrus to occur within 5 days post-weaning, the luteinising hormone (LH) pulsatility pattern of high amplitude, low frequency observed during lactation needs to shift to a pattern of low amplitude, high frequency immediately at weaning (Shaw and Foxcroft, 1985). During lactation, LH pulsatility is low as it is being suppressed by the suckling frequency of the piglets (e.g. Stevenson et al., 1981; De Rensis et al., 1999) and the metabolic state of the sow (for review see Prunier et al., 2003). As lactation progresses, suckling frequency decreases and inhibition of LH is less pronounced (Edwards and Foxcroft, 1983), resulting in a gradual increase in LH pulsatility towards the end of lactation (Quesnel and Prunier, 1995). Under normal conditions this increase in LH pulsatility will not result in the growth of follicles up to pre-ovulatory size. Nevertheless, the gradual increase in LH pulsatility during lactation is important for post-weaning follicle development. Quesnel et al. (2007) have shown that follicular development at day 3 post-weaning is highly correlated to LH characteristics during mid-lactation. Thus, LH pulsatility is very important for adequate commencement of follicle development and consequently the weaning to oestrus interval (WOI) in sows. When LH pulsatility is inhibited or reduced, this also affects follicle development and oestrus.

Insulin is one of the factors known to affect LH secretion. For example, Tokach et al. (1992) found that serum insulin concentrations during lactation are related to the number of LH peaks at days 14, 21 and 28 during lactation. A recent study in multiparous sows has shown that insulin levels during the WOI are also related to LH secretion (Wientjes et al., 2012a). Not only LH secretion but also follicle development/quality have been found to be stimulated by insulin levels. Whitley et al. (1998) found that administration of exogenous insulin (0.4 IU/kg BW) once per day around feeding in primiparous sows during the first 5 days post-weaning did not affect the total number of follicles or follicle diameter at day 5 post-weaning but did affect the level of steroid hormones (oestradiol, testosterone) in the follicular fluid of the medium and large sized follicles. These higher levels of steroid hormones indicate a better development of the follicle and oocyte. In this study no effects of exogenous insulin administration on hormone levels were found in small sized follicles (Whitley et al., 1998). Insulin therefore, seems to affect oocyte development in medium to larger size follicles. Wientjes et al. (2012a) found a positive relation between basal insulin levels and follicle diameter at ovulation. Ramirez et al. (1997) found an increased farrowing rate (92.3% vs. 76.7%) when primiparous sows were administered with exogenous insulin (0.4 IU/kg body weight) for four days post-weaning compared to control (saline) and greater litter size (+1 piglet) when insulin was administered for two days post-weaning. Improved farrowing rate and embryo survival may be related to higher progesterone levels during the first 10 days of gestation, which were related to mean insulin during the WOI during the first 10 days of gestation (Wientjes et al., 2012b). Possibly, the better developed follicle will also result in a better developed corpus luteum (CL). These results indicate that by stimulating the development of the medium to larger size follicles, this can lead to improved sow performance. This theory is also supported by Van den Brand et al. (2009) who state that the stimulating effect of insulin of LH secretion will positively affect development of the larger follicles as these have LH receptors which the smaller follicles do not. As a result, the small follicles will not grow and the larger follicles will, resulting in a more homogenous follicle pool. This may finally lead to a more homogenous litter.

Not only insulin but insulin growth factor I (IGF-1) also has been put forward as metabolic hormone affecting sow reproductive performance. In pigs IGF-1 has been found also to be present in granulosa cells of 2-8 mm follicles and interacts with follicle stimulating hormone (FSH) to stimulate oestradiol production by granulosa cells (Webb et al., 2007). Wientjes et al. (2012a) found a positive relationship between basal LH levels and IGF-1 levels during days 3-5 post-weaning. Furthermore not only insulin but also IGF-1 has been related to progesterone production as IGF-1 has been found to play an important role in the early development of the corpus luteum (CL) and stimulates progesterone secretion (Miller et al., 2003).

In summary, both insulin and IGF-1 play a role in follicle development and oocyte quality. The effects of insulin seem to work via interactions with LH and on medium and large sized follicles via higher concentrations of steroid hormones in the follicular fluid. A better quality oocyte may also have beneficial effects on birth weight and homogeneity of the litter. Nutritional measures affecting insulin secretion may therefore also affect sow reproductive performance which will be discussed subsequently.

THE ROLE OF INSULIN DURING THE LAST TRIMESTER OF GESTATION

For optimal foetal growth, which is highest during the last part of gestation, foetuses mainly depend on glucose and lactate as energy sources. As described earlier, birth weight has decreased as a result of the increase in litter size. Additionally variation in birth weight has increased and is already apparent after day 45 of gestation (Kim et al., 2009). In order to increase birth weight and reduce variation it is important to study the last trimester of gestation as the sow naturally already has a system to optimize the flow of glucose to the foetuses. To facilitate an optimal flow of glucose from the sow to the foetuses, the glucose blood level of the sow is 2.5 times higher than of the foetus (Pere, 1995). Within the placenta, glucose is converted to lactate which is used by the foetus as an energy source. To optimize the flow of glucose to the foetuses even more the sow develops a reversible type of insulin resistance which delays insulin secretion, reduces the sensitivity of the sow to insulin and thereby increases the time of high glucose blood levels (Pere et al., 2000). The longer the period of high blood glucose, the more glucose can be transported to the foetuses. In some species, insulin resistance remains present during lactation in order to stimulate the transport of glucose to the udder (Pere and Etienne, 2007). In sows, insulin resistance seems to reduce gradually as lactation progresses (Quesnel et al., 2007; Pere and Etienne, 2007). This process, however, seems to be dependent on the metabolic status of the animal. Compared to other species the period of insulin resistance in the sow is not only short, but the level of resistance is also relatively mild. This may explain the low energy reserves of piglets at birth even though the sows become insulin resistant. Piglets store energy in the form of glycogen in the liver and muscles mainly during days 60 and 110 of gestation (Randall and L'Ecuyer, 1976; Okai et al., 1978). By finding measures to increase the amount of glucose that is transported to the foetuses, glycogen storage also can be increased. Increasing the energy storage of piglets at birth may also improve piglet survival. There are nutritional measures that can be taken during the gestation period to improve glycogen storage in the sow via insulin. These possibilities will be discussed further subsequently.

Hormonal manipulation via nutrition: weaning to oestrus interval

FEEDING MANAGEMENT

Management of feeding is important in order to realize an optimal feed intake during lactation but is also of importance during the WOI. It is striking that not many sow farmers know how much feed a sows eats during the WOI. When wanting to fine-tune sow performance by hormonal manipulation via nutrition, it is important that the feed management is optimized as well. This includes parameters as how many meals do sows receive during the WOI, what is the feeding level and how much of the feed supplied do the sows actually eat? Baidoo et al. (1992) fed second parity sows diets containing 160g CP/kg and 9.14 MJ NE/kg at either a low feeding level of 3 kg/day or a high feeding level of 6 kg. Sows fed at 3 kg/d ate all of the feed supplied, whilst sows fed the high feeding level ate on average 4.7 kg/day which is only 0.78 of the feed supplied. In a more recent study in multiparous sows, sows achieved feed intakes of 0.73 and 0.63 of the supplied 3.8 and 3.6 kg/day of a feed containing 136g CP/kg and 8.86 MJ NE/kg (Wientjes et al., 2012a). Thus during the WOI sows do not by definition consume all the feed that is supplied, which needs to be taken into account when wanting to manipulate sow performance.

The number of studies examining feed intake and feeding level during the WOI is very limited as is the effects of these factors on insulin parameters. It is commonly known that a low feed intake during lactation has a negative effect on sow reproductive performance post-weaning. Particularly with the large litters, it is therefore important to stimulate lactational feed intake. When this is achieved, it is possible to fine-tune feeding management and diet composition during the WOI via insulin.

In gilts, several studies have been published in which the effects of feeding level on reproductive performance have been examined (e.g. Almeida et al., 2001; Hazeleger et al., 2005). Hazeleger et al. (2005) fed gilts during the last week of altrenogest treatment either 2.8 M (high) or 1.5 M (low) and found that gilts fed the high feeding level had a greater follicle size during the first three days after the end of the altrenogest treatments. Furthermore, an increase in the number of follicles with a diameter of 4.5 mm or greater was observed at the high feeding level. Even though insulin was not measured in this study, the greater number of follicles larger than 4.5 mm indicates that the higher feeding level does affect insulin and LH secretion. As described earlier, insulin will stimulate LH secretion, resulting in the outgrowth of larger follicles with LH receptors. Thus in gilts, feeding level may affect insulin secretion and consequently reproductive performance.

In multiparous sows, not many studies have been performed in which the feeding level during the WOI was studied. Wientjes et al. (2012a) fed sows either two times per day (12 h intervals) of a control diet or six times per day (4 h intervals) a diet containing lactose/dextrose during the WOI. Insulin levels recorded in sows after feeding were higher in sows fed two times per day up to 240 min post-feeding. Feeding sows six times per day did not result in higher insulin levels or a longer period of insulin secretion. It seems that when sows are fed more often per day and thus the meals are smaller, the effects on insulin are also smaller. Therefore, when studying the effects of diet composition on hormone levels, the number of feedings and feed amounts are of importance.

As insulin (and IGF-1) are related to reproductive hormones (LH and progesterone) it may be that a high feeding level during early pregnancy positively affects embryo survival rate. Hoving et al. (2012) fed primiparous sows either 2.5 kg/d or 3.25 kg/d of a gestation diet (130g CP/kg, 8.8 MJ NE/kg) from day 3 post-insemination until day 35 of gestation. Sows on the high feeding level achieved higher insulin levels and also recorded the peak level later post-feeding (48 vs. 24 min post-feeding). No correlations between insulin and LH or embryo survival were found. The authors concluded that feeding level during early gestation does not affect metabolic parameters or sow reproduction. It is thus not clear if a higher feed intake during early gestation can stimulate sow performance via insulin. It must be noted, however, that a high feeding level during early gestation has a positive effect on recovery of body condition.

In summary, feeding management is important when wanting to improve sow reproductive performance via insulin and reproductive hormones. There seem to be effects of feeding level on insulin levels which may lead to improved reproductive performance. Furthermore, the number of feedings is of importance. Feeding small portions at several times per day reduces the effect of insulin compared with feeding only two times per day.

DIET COMPOSITION

A number of studies have been performed in which the effects of diets containing insulin-stimulating ingredients on sow reproductive performance have been studied (Table 1).

In all studies diet changes were made using different carbohydrate sources. In many of the studies dextrose had been used alone or in combination with for example lactose. Sugars such as dextrose and sucrose are easily absorbed and when fed result in a high and quick response of insulin (Wientjes et al., 2012d). Other carbohydrates such as lactose or those found in sugar beet pulp are not digested in the small intestine but are fermented by the microflora of the large intestine and are called fermentable non starch polysaccharides (NSP). These ingredients result in a slower but longer release of insulin. In a comparative study, Wientjes et al. (2012d) fed multiparous sows seven different diets and measured the glucose, insulin and IGF-1 response. Sows were fed the following diets: 1. control; 2. dextrose (54 g/kg); 3. sucrose (50 g/kg); 4. lactose (50 g/kg); 5. dextrose and lactose; 6. sucrose and lactose; 7. dextrose and sugar beet pulp (400 g/kg). The other diets also contained sugar beet pulp but in a much lower quantity (120 g/

Table 1. Effects of insulin stimulating diets on sow reproductive performance

Reference[1]	Diet composition[2]			Feeding level (kg/d)	Number of meals[3]	Main results
	Insulin stimulating ingredient	Crude protein (g/kg)	Energy level (MJ NE/kg)			
Van den Brand et al., 2001	Starch (178 g maize starch / kg; 60 g/ dextrose /kg)	200	8.8	2xM	2x/day	higher insulin pre- and post-ovulation higher percentage of oestrus within 9 days
Van den Brand et al., 2006	150 g dextrose /kg	156	9.4	3.5	2x/day	reduction in CV birth weight
Ferguson et al., 2007	500g unmolassed sugar beet pulp/kg	140	8.38	2.8	-	higher frequency LH pulsatility at D18 more oocytes in Metaphase II after 46 h culture higher ESR D27-29
Van den Brand et al., 2009	L: 25 g dextrose/kg 25 g lactose/kg WOI: 150g dextrose/d 150 g lactose/d	L: 165 WOI: 136	L: 9.5 WOI: 9.3	L: voluntary WOI: 3.6	-	tendency for lower CV birth weight tendency higher birth weight
Wientjes et al., 2012a	150 g dextrose /d 150glactose/d	136	8.86	3.8	6x/day	lower insulin levels higher basal LH level greater follicle diameter at ovulation
Wientjes et al., 2012b	150 g dextrose /d 150 g lactose /d	136	8.86	3.8	6x/day	higher progesterone during 1st 10 days gestation
Wientjes et al., 2012c	L + WOI 150g sucrose/d 150 g lactose/d	L: 163 WOI: 68	9.1	L: max 7.5 WOI: 3.0	L: 2x/day WOI: 1x/ day	-

[1] all studies were performed with multiparous sows, except Ferguson et al. who used gilts; [2] diets with insulin stimulating ingredients were compared with control diets without the ingredients, except van den Brand et al. (2001) who compared high starch with a high fat diet; In all studies diets were fed isocaloric; [3] not all studies mentioned the number of meals per day

kg). The highest insulin response was observed when dextrose and sucrose were fed in combination with lactose, when compared with the control and lactose diet. Insulin response of the other treatments was intermediate. It must be noted, however, that the sows used in this study were not in the WOI and not catabolic.

Even though in the study of Wientjes et al. (2012d) no clear effect of sugar beet pulp on insulin was observed, Ferguson et al. (2007) did find an effect of high fibre from sugar beet pulp on oocyte development and embryo survival in gilts. As by European legislation it is required that gestation diets contain a certain amount of fibre, it is interesting to investigate further the effect of sugar beet pulp on insulin secretion and follicle development in sows during the WOI.

In the other studies presented in Table 1, insulin-stimulating diets were produced by the inclusion or top dressing with dextrose and/or lactose. A reduction in the variation in birth weight was found when using dextrose and the combination of dextrose and lactose (Van den Brand et al., 2006; 2009). This effect was not found by Wientjes et al. (2012c) but a possible explanation is the fact that organic sows were used with a longer lactation length. Sows lost a small amount of body weight during lactation and were no longer in a catabolic state. In the other studies of Wientjes (2012a; 2012b) sows were slaughtered and thus birth weight could not be measured. In these studies a greater follicle diameter at ovulation (Wientjes et al., 2012a) and a higher progesterone concentration (Wientjes et al., 2012b) were found. No other effects or even negative effects on insulin were found compared to the control diet. This can be explained by the fact that sows were fed six times per day whilst the control animals were fed two times per day, resulting in lower feed amounts and thus lower insulin peaks.

In summary, the inclusion of sugars such as dextrose and sucrose alone or in combination with carbohydrates that are fermented in the large intestine can affect insulin secretion in sows during the WOI. Higher insulin peaks in combination with longer insulin secretion can affect follicle development (more homogenous pool by selection of only the larger follicles) finally resulting in a more homogenous but not larger litter at birth. Best results are obtained when feeding management is also adjusted (feeding level, number of feedings) and sows are in a catabolic state at the end of lactation.

Hormonal manipulation via nutrition: end of gestation

Piglets have very low energy reserves at birth compared to other species. Furthermore, it has been shown that the level of glycogen is depended on the size of the piglet. Larger piglets at birth have greater total glycogen levels without having more liver or muscle glycogen (Theil et al., 2011). A large variation in birth weight, therefore, also results in large variation in glycogen reserves. If via nutritional measures in gestating sows diets the naturally occurring form of insulin resistance can be influenced to increase the amount of glucose transported to the foetuses, piglet birth weight and survival may be affected.

Several studies have been performed which investigated the effects of diet composition in gestating (and lactating) sows on glycogen levels and piglet survival (Table 2). In these studies, whether possible effects on piglet parameters can be explained by the effect of diet composition on insulin and glucose levels in the sow was also measured. Fat is the main component studied as Storlien et al. (2000) described in a review that saturated (S) fats increase insulin resistance and polyunsaturated (U) fats decrease insulin resistance. In several of the studies effects of saturated fatty acids such as medium chain triglycerides (MCT), coconut oil and palm oil on piglet survival were found. Both Azain (1993) and Jean and Chiang (1999) found a higher piglet survival when sows were fed MCT at day 3 post-farrowing compared to the control (93% vs. 84% (Azain, 1993); 99% vs. 88% (Jean and Chiang, 1999). In both studies the greatest effects on survival were found in piglets with low birth weights. Azain (1993) for example found that survival in piglets with a birth weigh < 900 g was 68% when sows were fed MCT compared with only 32% when fed the control diet. Piglets with a birth weight lower than 1100 g also had a higher survival in the study of Jean and Chiang (1999) and not only MCT but also coconut oil improved survival in this category. This higher survival rate may be related to higher blood glucose levels found at birth (Azain, 1993) or higher glycogen in liver and muscles (Jean and Chiang, 1999). Inclusion of palm oil also positively affected litter size and birth weight, especially when it was fed during the first 60 days of gestation (Corson et al., 2008). When examining the period before farrowing, the highest birth weight was achieved when sows were fed palm oil and the lowest birth weights were found when sows were fed unsaturated fats such as sunflower oil and olive oil. In contrast to these positive findings, Theil et al. (2011) did not find any effects of inclusion of different fats on piglet glycogen levels; the diets were only fed the last week before farrowing, which may have been too short to affect glycogen levels in the piglet.

The question is whether these positive effects of saturated fats on piglet parameters can be explained by effects on glucose and insulin parameters in the sow. Bikker et al. (2007) performed a glucose tolerance test on days 7, 84 and 112 of gestation and no differences were found in glucose and insulin levels between a diet with a high or low U:S ratio. On day 84, glucose and insulin levels of sows fed the low U:S ratio diet (diets containing high levels of saturated fats) remained higher for a longer period of time than levels of sows fed a high fat diet composed of saturated and short chain unsaturated fatty acids (see Figure 1). On day 84 of gestation sows on the low U:S ratio diet were switched to a high starch

Table 2. Effects of diet composition on insulin resistance and piglet performance

Reference	Diet composition[123]	Period	Results sow (glucose/insulin)	Results piglet
Azain, 1993	1. Control 2. LCT 120g soybean oil/kg 3. MCT 100g MCT, 20g soybean oil/kg	D91-D7 lactation	Tendency decreased blood glucose sows fed MCT	Higher survival piglets when sows fed MCT Especially piglets with birth weight <900 g Piglets higher blood glucose at birth
Jean and Chiang, 1999	1. Soybean oil 2. Coconut oil 3. MCT	D84-D28 lactation D84-farrowing	- -	Higher survival first 3 days post-farrowing for piglets of birth weight <1100 g on MCT and coconut oil Higher liver and muscle glycogen in piglets of sows fed MCT or coconut oil
Van der Peet et al., 2004	1. NSP 2. NSP + 360 g starch (wheat starch) 3. NSP + 164 g fat (soybean oil)	D85-farrowing	High fat diet resulted in less glucose tolerant sows	NSP diet higher number live born No effect on birth weight or piglet survival
Bikker et al., 2007	1. High unsaturated fat (U:S ratio 6.1) 2. Low U:S ratio (1.6) 3. High starch (179 g maize starch/kg; U:S ratio 4.9)	1. D1-D115 2. D1-D84 3. D84-D115	D84: low U:S ratio diet resulted in longer period of high glucose and insulin levels D112: high starch resulted in lower glucose and insulin levels	Lower liver glycogen in piglets at birth when sows fed high starch Higher piglet survival when sows fed high starch diet
Corson et al., 2008	1. Control 2. extra energy 3. palm oil 4. olive oil 5. sunflower oil 6. fish oil	G1. 1st 60 days G2. 60 days before farrowing	No effects on glucose and insulin levels sows	G1 greater litter size and birth weight mainly when using palm oil compared with sunflower oil G2 no effect on birth weight Lowest birth weight with olive and sunflower oil; highest birth weight with energy and palm oil
Theil et al., 2011	1 3g animal fat/kg 2 1. + 2.5 g/d hb 3 8 g coconut oil/kg 4 8 g fish oil/kg 5 4 g octanoic acid + 40 g fish oil/kg	D108-farrowing		No effect of diet on glycogen contents in piglets No effect on piglets survival rate

[1] NSP: non starch polysaccharides; [2] U:S ratio: ratio between unsaturated and saturated fatty acids; [3] hb: hydroxyl-methyl butyrate

diet to improve glucose supply to the foetuses. As shown in Figure 1, the high starch diet did not increase but reduced the glucose and insulin levels of the sows. These results indicate that a diet containing a high level of saturated fatty acids (low U:S ratio) can affect glucose and insulin levels. Furthermore, a diet high in both saturated and unsaturated fats is better able to influence glucose and insulin levels than a high starch diet.

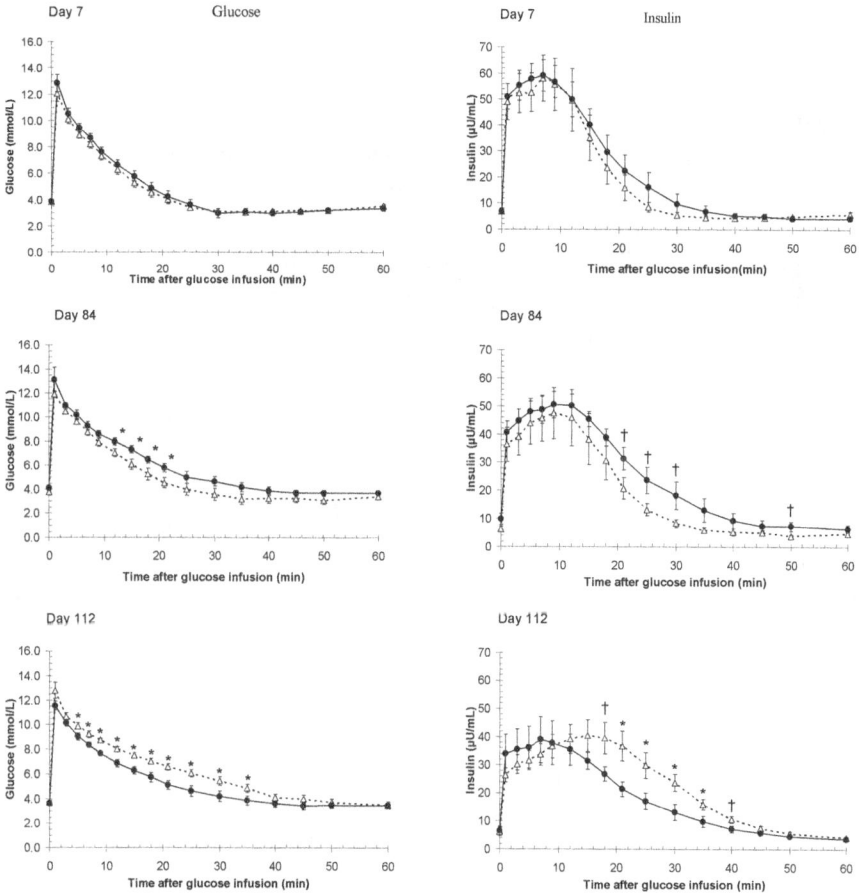

Figure 1. Plasma glucose and insulin levels of sows in response to glucose infusion at days 7, 84 and 112 of gestation fed either a control diet with an U/S ratio of 6.1 containing a high percentage of saturated fat and short chain unsaturated fatty acids (--△---) until lactation or a diet with a low U/S ratio of 1.5 containing 60 g palm oil/kg (—•—) until day 84 of gestation and a high starch diet (340 g/kg starch) from day 85 onwards.

* indicates a significant (P<0.05) difference between the diets; † indicates a tendency (P<0.10) towards a significant difference between the diets (Courtesy of Gerritsen et al., 2010)

A high starch diet may increase the supply of glucose to the piglets but was shown not to increase glucose levels in blood of the sow. Additionally Van der Peet et al. (2004) did not find a positive effect of high starch levels. Bikker et al. (2007) even found lower glycogen levels in piglets of which the sows were fed the high starch diet compared with the high fat diet. Nevertheless, the high fat diet was associated with a higher mortality which according to Kemp et al. (1996) can be explained by the occurrence of hypoglycaemic shock after birth after having been exposed to high levels of glucose during gestation. Another possibility for higher survival when fed high starch diets (low insulin resistance) is that piglets are used to low glucose levels and are better able to cope with low glucose levels at birth.

In summary, it is possible to improve piglet survival by including saturated fatty acids in gestating sow diets. It remains unclear whether this higher survival is the result of a higher insulin resistance as a high insulin resistance has also been related to a lower survival. Possibly the positive effects of e.g. MCT on survival are not mediated via insulin resistance but via more nutrients that become available to the piglet. Inclusion of saturated fatty acids in gestating sow diets can positively affect piglet performance but manipulating the hormone insulin via nutrition may not be the most successful method.

Conclusion

Sow reproductive performance can be influenced by hormonal manipulation via nutrition. Insulin is the most investigated hormone which can be affected by nutrition during different stages of the sow's cycle. Current practical problems such as low birth weights and a large variation in birth weight within litters can be reduced by manipulating the sow's diet during the WOI. Sugars such as dextrose and sucrose as well as fermentable NSPs (e.g. sugar beet pulp) affect insulin levels and duration of secretion, stimulating secretion of reproductive hormones and consequently follicle development. Additionally during the end of gestation, insulin seemed to be promising as sows develop a reversible form of insulin resistance to increase glucose transport to the foetuses. Manipulating this insulin resistance may improve piglet survival. Saturated fats have been found to affect insulin resistance but results on piglet performance have been variable. MCT seem promising in improving survival of smaller piglets but most likely not via the insulin mechanism.

In conclusion, sow reproductive performance can be affected by manipulating metabolic hormones via nutrition. Most interesting is manipulating during the WOI, but this fine-tuning is only effective when other factors on the farm such as feed management are functioning properly.

References

Almeida, F.R.C.L., Kirkwood, R.N., Aherne, F.X., Foxcroft, G.R. (2001) Consequences of different patterns of feed intake during the oestrous cycle in gilts on subsequent fertility. *Journal of Animal Science*, **78**, 1556-1563.

Azain, M.J. (1993) Effects of adding medium-chain triglycerides to sow diets during late gestation and early lactation on litter performance. *Journal of Animal Science*, **71**, 3011-3019.

Baidoo, S.K., Aherne, F.X., Kirkwood, R.N., Foxcroft, G.R. (1992) Effect of feed intake during lactation and after weaning on sow reproductive performance. *Canadian Journal of Animal Science*, **72**, 911-917.

Bikker, P., Kluess J., Fledderus J., Geelen M.J.H. (2007) Invloed van voeding van dragende zeugen op vitaliteit en glycogeenreserves van pasgeboren biggen. Schothorst Feed Research report 801.

Corson, A.M., Laws, J., Litten, J.C., Dodds, P.F., Lean I.J., Clarke L. (2008) Effect of dietary supplementation of different oils during the first or second half of pregnancy on the glucose tolerance of the sow. *Animal*, **2**, 1045-1054.

De Rensis, F., Cosgrove, J.R., Willis, H.J., Hofacker, S., Foxcroft, G.R. (1999) Ontogeny of the opioidergic regulation of LH and prolactin secretion in lactating sows II: interaction between suckling and morphine administration. *Journal of Reproduction and Fertility*, **116**, 243-251.

Edwards, S.A, and Foxcroft, G.R. (1983). Endocrine changes in sows weaned at two stages of lactation. *Journal of Reproduction and Fertility*, **67**, 161-172.

Ferguson, E.M., Slevin, J., Hunter, M.G., Edwards, S.A., Ashworth, C.J. (2007) Beneficial effects of a high fibre diet on oocyte maturity and embryo survival in gilts. *Reproduction*, **133**, 433-439.

Foxcroft, G.R. and Aherne F. (2001) Rethinking management of the replacement gilt. In: *Advances in Pork Production*, volume 12, pp. 197-210. Proc. Banff Pork Seminar, Banff, Alberta, Canada.

Foxcroft, G.R., Dixon, W.T., Novak, S., Putman, C.T., Town, S.C., Vinsky, M.D.A. (2006) The biological basis for prenatal programming of postnatal performance in pigs. *Journal of Animal Science*, **84**, E105-E112.

Gerritsen, R., Bikker, P., Van der Aar, P.J. (2010). Glucose metabolism in reproductive sows. In: *Dynamics in Animal Nutrition* – 2010, pp 99-112. Edited by: J. Doppenberg and P.J. Van der Aar. Wageningen Academic Publishers, Wageningen, The Netherlands.

Hazeleger, W., Soede, N.M., Kemp, B. (2005) The effect of feeding strategy during the pre-follicular phase on subseuqent follicular development in the pig. *Domestic Animal Endocrinology*, **29**, 362-370.

Hoving, L.L., Soede, N.M., Feitsma, H., Kemp, B. (2012) Embryo survival, progesterone profiles and metabolic responses to an increased feeding level during second gstation in sows. *Theriogenology*, **77**, 1557-1569.

Kemp, B., Soede, N.M., Vesseur, P.C., Helmond, F.A., Spoorenberg, K.H., Frankena, K. (1996). Glucose tolerance of pregnant sows is related to postnatal pig mortality. *Journal of Animal Science*, **74**, 879-885.

Kemp, B., Soede, N.M., Helmond, F.A., Bosch, M.W. (1995) Effects of energy source in the diet on reproductive hormones and insulin during lactation and subsequent estrus in multiparous sows. *Journal of Animal Science*, **73**, 3022-3029.

Kim, S.W., Hurley, W.L., Wu, G., Ji, F. (2009). Ideal amino acid balance for sows during gestation and lactation. *Journal of Animal Science*, **87**, E123-E132.

Miller, E.A., Ge, Z., Hedgpeth, V., Gadsby, J.E. (2003). Steriodogenic responses of pig corpora lutea to insulin-like growth factor I (IGF-1) throughout the oestrous cycle. *Reproduction*, **125**, 241-249.

Okai, D.B., Wyllie, D., Aherne, F.X., Ewan, R.C. (1978) Glycogen reserves in the fetal and newborn pig. *Journal of Animal Science*, **46**, 171-187.

Pere, M.-C. (1995). Maternal and fetal blood levels of glucose, lactate, fructose, and insulin in the conscious pig. *Journal of Animal Science*, **73**, 2994-2999.

Pere, M.-C., Etienne, M. (2007) Insulin sensitivity during pregnancy, lactation, and postweaning in primiparous gilts. *Journal of Animal Science*, **85**, 101-110.

Pere, M.-C., Etienne, M., Dourmad, J.Y. (2000) Adaptations of glucose metabolism in multiparous sows: effects of pregnancy and feeding level. *Journal of Animal Science,* **78**, 2933-2941.

Prunier, A., Soede, N.M., Quesnel, H., Kemp, B. (2003) Productivity and longevity of weaned sows. In *Weaning the pig: concepts and consequences* – 2000, pp 385-419. Edited by: J.R. Pluske, J. Le Dividich, M.W.A. Verstegen. Wageningen Academic Publishers, Wageningen, The Netherlands.

Quesnel, H., and Prunier, A. (1995) Endocrine basis of lactational anoestrus in the sow. *Reproduction nutrition development*, **35**, 395-414.

Quesnel, H., Etienne, M., Pere, M.-C. (2007) Influence of litter size on metabolic status and reproductive axis in primiparous sows. *Journal of Animal Science*, **85**, 118-128.

Ramirez, J.L., Cox, N.M., Moore, A.B. (1997) Influence of exogenous insulin before breeding on conception rate and litter size of sows. *Journal of Animal Science*, **75**, 1893-1898.

Randall, G.C.B., L' Ecuyer, C.L. (1976) Tissue glycogen and blood glucose and fructose levels in the pig fetus during the second half of gestation. *Biology of the Neonate*, **28**, 74-82.

Shaw, H.J., and Foxcroft G.R. (1985) Relationships between LH, FSH and prolactin secretion and reproductive activity in the weaned sow. *Journal of Reproduction and Fertility*, **75**, 17-28.

Stevenson, J.S., Cox, N.M., Britt, J.H. (1981) Role of the ovary controlling Luteinising Hormone, Follicle Stimulating Hormone, and prolactin secretion during and after lactation in pigs. *Biology of Reproduction*, **24**, 341-353.

Storlien, L.H., Higgins, J.A., Thomas, T.C., Brown, M.A., Wang, H.Q., Huang, X.F., Else, P.L. (2000) Diet composition and insulin action in animal models. *British Journal of Nutrition*, **83**, Suppl. 1, S85-S90.

Theil, P.K., Cordero, G., Henckel, P., Puggaard, L., Oksbjerg, N., Sorensen, M.T. (2011) Effects of gestation and transition diets, piglet birth weight, and fasting time on depletion of glycogen pools in liver and 3 muscles of newborn piglets. *Journal of Animal Science*, **89**, 1805-1816.

Tokach, M.D., Pettigrew, J.E., Dial, G.D., Wheaton, J.E., Crooker, B.A., Johnston, L.J. (1992) Characterization of luteinizing hormone secretion in the primiparous, lactating sow: relationship to blood metabolites and return-to-estrus interval. *Journal of Animal Science*, **70**, 2195-2201.

Van den Brand, H., Soede, N.M., Kemp, B. (2006) Supplementation of dextrose to the diet during the weaning to oestrus interval affects subsequent variation in within-litter piglet birth weight. *Animal Reproduction Science*, **91**, 353-358.

Van den Brand, H., Van Enckevort, L.C.M., Van der Hoeven, E.M., Kemp, B. (2009) Effects of dextrose plus lactose in the sows diet on subsequent reproductive performance and within litter birth weight variation. *Reproduction in Domestic Animals*, **44**, 884-888.

Van der Peet, C.M.C., Kemp, B., Binnendijk, G.P., Den Hartog, L.A., Vereijkens, P.F.G., Verstegen, M.W.A. (2004). Effects of additional starch or fat in late-gestating high non starch polysaccharide diets on litter performance and glucose tolerance in sows. *Journal of Animal Science*, **82**, 2964-2971.

Webb, R., Garnsworthy, P.C., Campbell, B.K., Hunter, M.G. (2007). Intra-ovarian regulation of follicular development and oocyte competence in farm animals. *Theriogenology*, **68S**, S22-S29.

Whitley, N.C., Moore, A.B., Cox, N.M. (1998). Comparative effects of insulin and porcine somatotropin on postweaning follicular development in primiparous sows. *Journal of Animal Science*, **76**, 1455-1462.

Wientjes, J.G.M., Soede, N.M., van den Brand, H., Kemp, B. (2012a). Nutritionally induced relationships between insulin levels during the weaning-to-ovulation interval and reproductive characteristics in multiparous sows: I. luteinizing hormone, follicle development, oestrus and ovulation. *Reproduction in Domestic Animals*, **47**, 53-61.

Wientjes, J.G.M., Soede, N.M., van den Brand, H., Kemp, B. (2012b) Nutritionally induced relationships between insulin levels during the weaning-to-ovulation interval and reproductive characteristics in multiparous sows:

II. Luteal development, progesterone and conceptus development and uniformity. *Reproduction in Domestic Animals*, **47**, 62-68.

Wientjes, J.G.M., Soede, N.M., van der Peet-Schwering, C.M.C., van den Brand, H., Kemp, B. (2012c) Piglet uniformity and mortality in large organic litters: effects of parity and pre-mating diet composition. *Livestock Science*, **144**, 218-229.

Wientjes, J.G.M., Soede, N.M., Aarsse, F., Laurenssen, B.F.A., Koopmanschap, R.E., van den Brand, H., Kemp, B. (2012d) Effects of dietary carbohydrate sources on plasma glucose, insulin and IGF-1 levels in multiparous sows. *Journal of Animal Physiology and Animal Nutrition,* **96**, 494-505.

15

EXTRA-PHOSPHORIC EFFECTS OF PHYTASE – LOW PHYTATE NUTRITION IN NON-RUMINANTS

M.R. BEDFORD AND C.L. WALK
AB Vista Feed Ingredients Ltd., Marlborough, Wiltshire, UK SN8 4AN

Summary

The vast majority of phytase use to date has been with reduced supplementation of inorganic phosphates in poultry and swine rations in mind. Such an application saves considerable costs whilst at the same time providing a benefit to the environment with regards to reduced phosphorus (P) pollution. Phytases deliver the P of interest through de-phosphorylation of phytic acid, and it is the destruction of the phytic acid *per se*, not the provision of phosphate which is the focus of this paper. Considerable quantities of P are delivered at commercial phytase dosage rates, but such dosages are insufficient to consistently destroy more than 60% of the phytic acid in the diet. Phytic acid has several anti-nutritive properties, not least the ability to chelate minerals (Adeola et al., 1995; Kies et al., 2006), rendering them unavailable, which in some cases may precipitate deficiency. However such effects are well understood and circumvented by supplementation with the appropriate mineral premixes. Indeed current mineral requirements for monogastrics more than likely have taken this anti-nutritive phytate effect into account so the advent of phytase may justify a review of all mineral requirements. However, recent work has suggested a more profound anti-nutritive effect of phytic acid (Cowieson et al., 2004; Cowieson and Ravindran, 2007; Onyango et al., 2004), and that more complete destruction of phytic acid *per se* can yield benefits which are unrelated to P release. Whereas the mechanism has been well described as to how phytic acid may detract from energetic efficiency of the animal, there is little information on the potential scale of response attainable if the target for phytase use was specifically phytic acid destruction rather than P release. This is because the vast majority of work where very high dosages of phytases have been used has employed diets which are deficient in P (Augspurger and Baker, 2004; Cowieson et al., 2006; Pirgozliev et al., 2011). As a result, it is not possible to ascertain when the response to incremental phytase dosage switches from meeting the P requirement to phytic acid destruction, if indeed phytic acid is involved at all in the work reported. However, recently several trials have been conducted which do indeed suggest that benefits beyond P release are attainable. This effect however, requires use of phytase dosages which are well in excess of current practice. If such an effect proves to be consistent then it may profoundly alter the way this enzyme is used in the future.

Current usage

The approximate cost of inorganic phosphates at time of press was £450 per tonne which results in a gross savings of approximately £2-3 per tonne of feed if 1g/kg P is replaced with a given dose of phytase. Since phytases cost considerably less than this (the return on investment is approx. 5 to 1), it is clear why most monogastric feeds contain a phytase. Indeed usage of the enzyme has increased over the years as compounders have attempted to save more money by taking out even more inorganic phosphate. However, two problems need addressing in this regard:

1. The relationship between dosage of phytase and P release is log-linear (Kornegay et al., 1996; Rosen, 2002). As a result, to double the P spared by this enzyme requires a 10 fold increase in dose. Thus least cost formulation packages must be adapted to account for this non-linear relationship if errors are to be avoided. Nevertheless significant savings continue to be realised at doses which are several multiples above that currently used commercially.

2. The P that a phytase can release relates to how much phytate P is in the diet. Most phytase research from which matrix values were constructed has been conducted in corn–soy based diets, which likely contain 2.4 g/kg phytic acid P or greater. If a diet rich in animal protein meal is employed then the phytic acid P content could be as low as 1.5g/kg. In such a case the P release from any given dosage will likely be less than expected and thus the matrix should be adjusted accordingly. In no case, for obvious reasons, should a matrix be applied to a very high dosage of phytase which exceeds the dietary phytic acid P content, and thus it is important for feed manufacturers to be aware of the approximate phytic acid P content of the diets they are using.

Provided the two conditions listed above are considered, then the P replacement benefits of phytase addition should be realised. Usage of phytase in this manner has been commercially undertaken in some parts of the world for many years, with dosages of 1000 FTU/kg and greater being employed on a regular basis. The purpose of such an approach is simply to return performance of a low P diet to that of a P adequate diet at lower cost, with no intention to exceed the performance of the P adequate diet. Such a concept has been amply researched and is nicely demonstrated with body weight gain in the work by Kornegay et al. (1996; Figure 1).

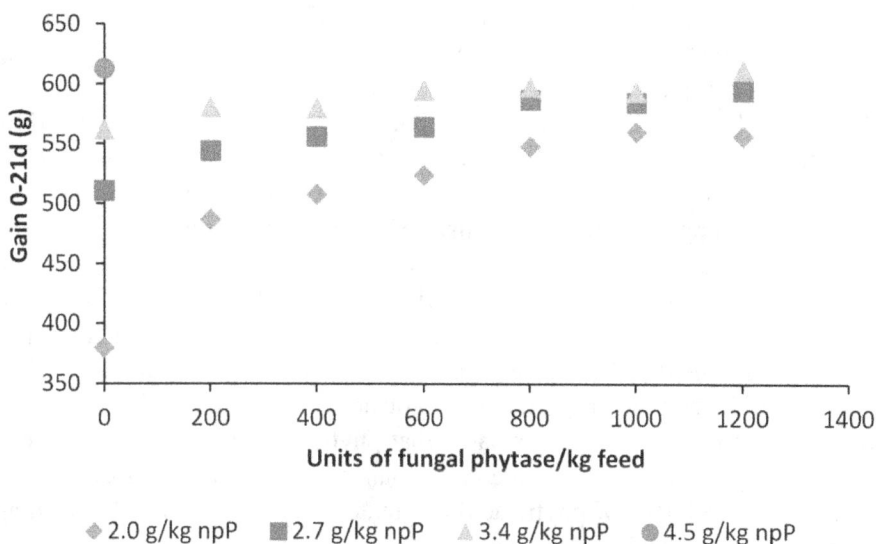

Figure 1. Effects of increasing doses of phytase on weight gain of male broilers to 21 d of age in diets varying in non-phytate P content. (Adapted from Kornegay et al., 1996)

However such high dosages do not necessarily constitute "superdosing" as subsequently defined in this paper since the dosages employed are largely insufficient to elicit the desired degree of phytate destruction. Furthermore, in most cases the diets employed are P deficient and thus growth rate is mostly limited by the digestible P content of the diet rather than the anti-nutritive effect of phytate. Successful superdosing requires use of phytase dosages that result in far greater rates of phytate destruction than currently practiced and in diets which are clearly not limited by digestible P content.

Another factor which clouds interpretation of superdosing in the literature is the fact that the response per FTU (or phytase unit) varies considerably between phytases. Unfortunately whilst the current assay is perfectly adequate for quality control of phytases, the conditions used for analysis (Engelen et al., 2001) bears little resemblance to those in the GIT where the enzyme operates. The biological value of phytases from different sources, therefore, differ substantially per assayed

FTU (Bedford, 2012). Part of this difference relates to the fact that the pH of the AOAC assay is set at 5.5 whereas it is largely accepted that the majority of phytase activity takes place in the stomach (Blaaberg, 2011; Igbasan, 2002; Kemme et al., 1999; Kemme et al., 2006; Pagano et al., 2005; Schlemmer et al., 2001), which is considerably lower in pH. Indeed recent work has suggested that the biological efficacy of all commercial phytases in use today is reasonably well described by shifting the pH of the assay to 3.0 (Bedford, 2012). Since the pH profile of the different phytase sources differs considerably (Igbasan et al., 2000; Simon and Igbasan, 2002), some displaying more activity at pH 3.0 than 5.5 and some far less, it is clear that some enzymes will need far fewer AOAC units than others to release a given quantity of P and succeed in superdosing through destruction of phytate. Indeed Table 1 illustrates this point from the P matrices declared by the manufacturers of the different phytases available on the market. If 500 FTU (measured as per the AOAC assay) of each phytase is employed in a broiler ration, then depending upon the source organism of the phytase, it will spare anything from 0.67 to 1.5 g of P/kg. As suggested above, the enzymes with the lowest P matrix have least activity at pH 3.0 and vice versa for those with the highest P matrix. If a simple assumption is made that this relates proportionately to phytic acid hydrolysis, and that the average vegetable protein-source diet contains 2.4 g/kg phytic acid P, then the proportion of phytic acid hydrolysed ranges from 0.28 to 0.63 g/kg. It is proposed in this paper that phytic acid P needs to be reduced below 0.4 g/kg for realisation of the performance benefits of superdosing. Thus approximately 850 g/kg of phytic acid or greater needs to be hydrolysed in an average vegetable protein source diet in order to benefit from superdosing.

Table 1. Assumed proportion of phytic acid destruction from P matrix values of selected phytases

Source	P matrix (g/kg) for 500 FTU/kg feed	Proportion of phytic acid hydrolysed
Peniophora lycii	0.67	0.28
Aspergillus niger	1.00	0.42
Eschericia coli	1.20	0.50
Enhanced E coli	1.30	0.54
2nd generation enhanced E coli	1.50	0.63

Thus, given the log-linear dose response relationship for all phytases, to achieve benefits of superdosing slightly more than 1000 FTU/kg feed of the 2nd generation enhanced E coli would be required and upwards of 5000 FTU/kg feed of the Aspergillus phytase and significantly more of the Peniophora phytase would be needed. Due to the shape of the curves, if a greater proportion of phytate needed to be hydrolysed to achieve superdosing effects, then the differential between enzymes becomes larger as shown in Figure 2. However, it must be borne in mind that two significant errors exist in such an assumption:

Substrate limitations will start to influence the results once phytic acid is largely removed from the digesta. This effect influences the efficacy of some enzymes more than others and as a result, there will be a reduction in phytase efficacy as proportionately more phytic acid is hydrolysed.

Substrate availability. It is likely that not all phytic acid is released during transit through the stomach and that the proportion of "susceptible" phytic acid may vary considerably from diet to diet. As a result, it is highly unlikely that total phytic acid hydrolysis will take place and indeed it may not exceed 90% of total phytate content.

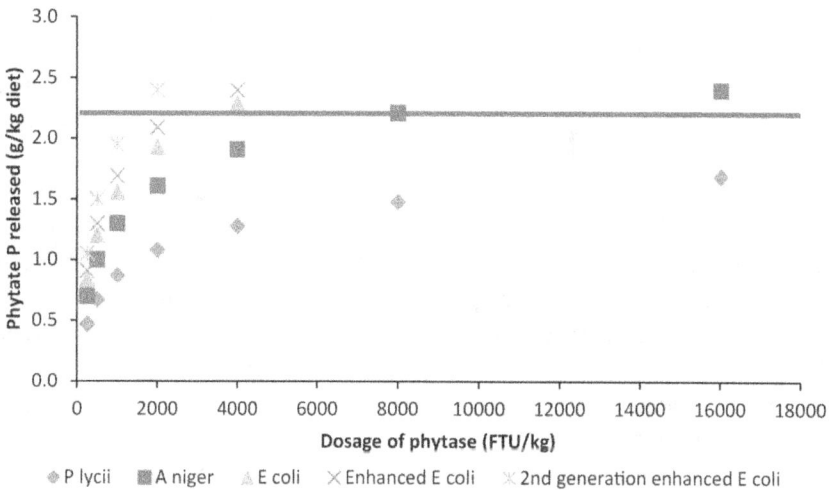

Figure 2. Relationship between source of phytase and amount of phytic acid P released from a broiler diet containing 2.4g phytic acid P provided substrate limitation were not a consideration. Horizontal line depicts proposed phytic acid P hydrolysis required to consistently achieve a superdosing effect

It is clear, therefore, that if the term superdosing is to be relevant, reference to a fixed FTU/kg feed is to be avoided as this bears no relationship to the biological value when phytases from different sources are compared.

Why should phytate destruction be beneficial?

It is likely that any "extra-phosphoric" effect of superdosing of phytases may rely on more than one mechanism at any one time. To date, four possible mechanisms are suggested and any or all may be relevant depending upon the circumstances of the animal concerned. These hypotheses are listed:

1. Considerable data have emerged recently which have identified phytic acid as a potent anti-nutrient (Cowieson et al., 2004; Cowieson et al., 2009; Cowieson and Ravindran, 2007; Onyango et al., 2004). The proposed mechanism is that it interferes with gastric digestion, either by direct association with dietary proteins and/or digestive enzymes, or by reducing the available water content in a kosmotropic manner (Selle and Ravindran, 2007; Selle et al., 2006; Selle et al., 2000). Regardless of which mechanism dominates, the animal responds to impaired gastric protein digestion by secretion of more pepsin and more hydrochloric acid, the latter in particular necessitating increased secretion of mucin in the stomach to protect against the reduction in pH. Much of this mucin is voided due to its particularly indigestible nature. All of the above responses reduce the efficiency of utilisation of digested and absorbed nutrients with an end result of reduced feed efficiency. Research has indicated an increase in gastric pH with use of phytase (Walk et al., 2012b) and reduced mucin production (Cowieson et al., 2004), the latter being sufficiently quantitative to be reflected in the composition of amino acids spared (Cowieson and Ravindran, 2007; Onyango et al., 2009). Indeed the pattern of amino acids spared as a result of reduced mucin secretion (threonine, glycine, serine and cysteine dominating) may be of benefit in animal protein free diets as these tend to contain much lower and possibly deficient levels of glycine plus serine. It is noteworthy that the metabolic cost of manufacture of mucin, acid and digestive enzyme is captured not in AME or TME studies, but in NE studies since this benefit relates to partitioning of AME into NE_m and NE_g. Indeed work has shown that whilst large benefits of superdosing of phytase can be measured in an NE assay, the effects on dietary AME are muted and not always significant (Pirgozliev et al., 2011).

2. The continued destruction of phytic acid inescapably results in incremental release of bound minerals as well as phosphate. It has been well documented that the mineral binding capacity of phytic acid (IP6) is proportionately greater than that of IP5, which in turn is greater than that of IP4 and so on (Luttrell, 1992; Persson et al., 1998). As a result, the release of bound cations is initially extremely rapid but then slows with each successive P release from the inositol ring. With specific regard to Ca and P, such an effect results in the initial activity of phytase resulting in significantly more Ca release relative to P (the initial ratio perhaps being as high as 3:1), and as more phytase is added or more time is allowed, proportionately more P is released compared with Ca

until the final ratio of 1.5 Ca:1 P is achieved (Walk et al., 2012a). Ironically, one of the potential reasons of the "extra-phosphoric" effects of phytase may actually therefore relate to the balancing of the Ca:P ratio. Such an effect is noted in some trials with regards to reduced litter moisture on higher phytase diets as a result of a better Ca:P balance. Care is thus needed in designing trials to test the extra-phosphoric effects of phytase, to ensure that the effect is not related to balancing of the Ca:P ratio.

3. Complete dephosphorylation of phytic acid and co-ordination with endogenous alkaline phosphatases yields an inositol ring which is known to be involved in fat metabolism and transport (Holub, 1986). Some work has suggested that inositol per se may be of benefit in broiler performance and thus may play a role in the extra-phosphoric effect. Once absorbed inositol can be reconstituted to phytate which is thought to play a role in the anti-oxidant status of the animal, thus potentially preserving other anti-oxidants. Indeed, very high doses of an enhanced E coli phytase were shown to increase hepatic stores of fat soluble vitamins and Coenzyme Q10, which may indicate improved fat metabolism and reduced oxidative pressure (Karadas et al., 2009). Further evidence of superdosing benefits in a high metabolic environment is given by the fact that motility and concentration of sperm from male broiler breeders was improved in a dose dependent manner (Al-Sa'aidi et al., 2009). High dosages of phytase may therefore, ironically, increase phytate stores in the body thus sparing other anti-oxidant sources (Karadas et al., 2009; Liu et al., 2010). Such a mechanism would rely on sufficient stores of phosphorus to re-phosphorylate the inositol ring which may explain the lack of superdosing effects noted in low P diets.

4. Despite the fact that the pathway of IP6 degradation down to IP1 by the various phytases on the market has been determined in vitro, and such work suggests bioactive intermediates are not generated, it cannot be ruled out that such intermediates are indeed generated in concert with phosphatase activity from endogenous and microbial origin. Such effects may or may not prove to be beneficial, depending upon the status of the animal at the time of generation of the intermediates.

Thus there are at least four possible reasons why significant, if not complete de-phytinisation, of the ration may prove beneficial, the relevance of each is clearly dependent upon the circumstances of the diet and the animal under test. Nevertheless empirical data suggests that the benefits derived from de-phytinisation of the diet can be substantial as discussed below.

Empirical evidence

One of the first studies in which phytase was used at higher doses was described by Nelson et al. in 1971. In this work there was clearly a significant benefit from feeding large quantities of phytase in a P deficient diet with the response being best described as log-linear: logarithmic increases in phytase dosage required to maintain linear increments in performance. Although all of the growth responses obtained were likely driven by P release rather than phytate destruction, this work established an important relationship between dose and response which was later confirmed by the definitive review of Rosen in 2002, where the continued improvement in performance required a logarithmic increment in phytase dose. Many papers even up to the present day still make the mistake of claiming an asymptote has been achieved in experimental designs where the dosages are linearly spaced. Such claims are clearly not properly tested as the highest dose employed is well below that required to establish or refute such a claim. As a result the debate with regards to the existence or not of superdosing continues. Logarithmic increments in phytase dosage have been employed in several papers where it has been almost unequivocally shown that at extremely high dosages (>10,000 FTU/kg of E coli or better), performance continues to improve and often exceeds that of the positive control (Shirley and Edwards, 2003; Augspurger and Baker, 2004; Cowieson et al 2006; Pirgozliev et al., 2007) although it is never clear whether the improvement in performance beyond that of the P adequate diet is due to the P adequate diet in fact being marginally deficient in P. Augspurger and Baker (2004) employed 500 and 10,000 FTU of an E coli phytase in a semi-synthetic diet which was sufficient in P and Ca and observed no benefit in performance which suggests there was no superdosing effect from phytase supplementation. However, it should be noted that there was less than 0.09% phytate P in these diets which limits not only the anti-nutritive effect of phytate but also the expected benefit of superdosing a phytase.

More recent work with turkeys has indicated that performance beyond that of the marginally P deficient diet was achieved with increasing doses of an evolved E coli phytase to the point that, at 2,000 FTU/kg feed, body weight gain was approximately 10% superior to that of the P adequate diet and FCR approximately 15 points improved. Given the P adequate diet was designed to meet the Ca and P requirements of the birds it is unlikely that all of the benefits noted were related to P nutrition, although without a high P control this cannot be ruled out of course. This work was subsequently repeated with substantially similar results, i.e. the 2,000 FTU/kg diet significantly outperformed the P adequate diet, and such results have been replicated in large scale field tests (no statistics, but >5,000 birds were tested on 2,000 FTU of a 2nd generation evolved E coli phytase vs. a standard phytase diet with "requirement P and Ca" levels).

Recent work by Persia (2010) has indicated that broilers fed P deficient diets supplemented with as much as 5,000 FTU/kg feed of an enhanced E coli phytase resulted in growth rates and in some cases FCR that was significantly improved over a P adequate control. Use of equivalent dosages of phytase in a semi-synthetic diet which did not contain appreciable levels of phytic acid did not result in improved performance, indicating that phytic acid *per se* was the anti-nutrient (Persia, 2010). A further trial, where the positive control contained copious amounts of nPP in the starter, grower and finisher diets (5.4 and 4 g/kg, respectively) was compared with a negative control (nPP levels reduced by 2 g/kg) supplemented with up to 146,000 FTU /kg feed revealed significant benefits of the higher doses over the P adequate control (FCR was 1.63; Figure 3). These data are instructive in that they clearly show increasing benefits in FCR when up to 65,000 FTU/kg of either an E coli or Aspergillus phytase are fed (with the former tending to be more effective than the latter). The apparent loss in efficacy at the highest dosage may relate to changes in macronutrient content of the diet since at this level as much as 30 g/kg of the diet would be supplied by the phytase premix. The fact that growth and feed efficiency continue to respond at such high phytase dosages suggests that rate of phytate hydrolysis in the stomach is not fast enough at commercial dosages. This partly relates to the efficacy of the enzyme in surviving and functioning in the conditions of the gastric environment, but may also be a consequence of the rapid rate of phytic acid evacuation from the stomach (Blaaberg, 2011), which severely limits the time available for a phytase to act before a significant fraction of the phytic acid escapes to the small intestine.

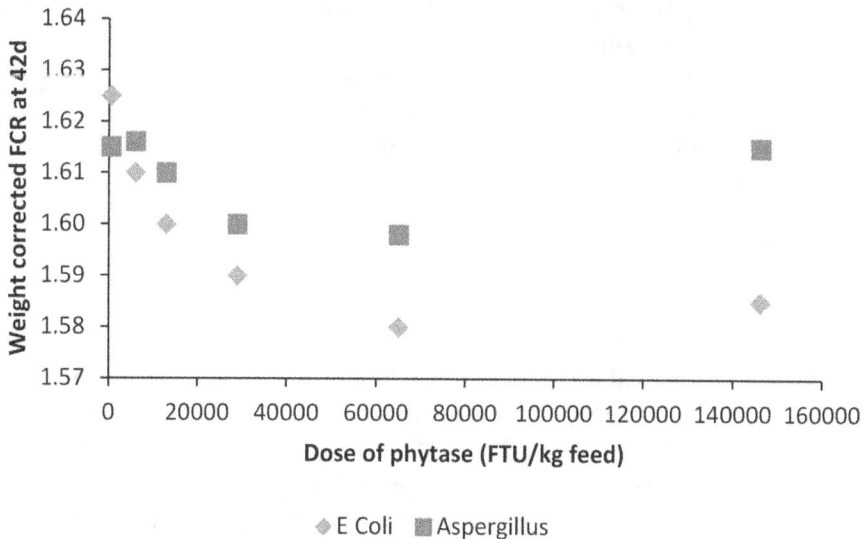

Figure 3. Influence of incremental dosages of phytases from E coli or A niger sources on weight corrected FCR of 42d old male broilers when applied in a low P diet (Persia, 2010) (weight corrected FCR of the P adequate control was 1.63).

More definitive work has recently been completed in 4 identical broiler trials (d 0 to 42). Birds were fed either a positive control (PC) corn-soy based diet which contained recommended levels of P and Ca, or a further PC supplemented with an additional 0.10% P and Ca to determine whether there was any response to further increments of P. The PC was then reduced moderately in P and Ca (0.15 and 0.165%, respectively) to generate a negative control (NC) which was then supplemented with 500, 1000 or 1500 FTU/kg of a 2nd generation evolved E coli phytase. The 500 FTU/kg dose was designed to replenish the down-specification with the subsequent dosages being in excess (superdose). All 4 trials gave similar responses and when analysed together it was apparent that the birds on the PC did not respond to additional P indicating that the PC was indeed adequate in P and thus any improvement in performance over this diet was likely not related to P nutrition. The addition of the phytase to the NC resulted in dose-dependent improvements in weight corrected FCR to the point that at the 1000 FTU/kg dose birds performed significantly better than the positive control by 2 points and those fed the 1500 FTU/kg dose were 4 points ahead. These data suggest a P independent effect of high dosages of phytase more-so than any other data to date. Further work is needed to determine the extent to which this effect can be exploited and whether it is dependent upon phytate source and concentration, dietary P and Ca concentration and vitamin D concentration, in addition to enzyme source and dose. Nevertheless the evidence for extra-phosphoric effects of phytase is becoming more secure and opens the door to a completely new way of using this enzyme commercially. It may well be that value and environmental benefits created by sparing P is secondary to that of the performance enhancement obtained with superdosing.

One final point of observation is that when phytases are replenishing a P deficiency, their performance benefit is seen mostly as a feed intake and weight gain response, with FCR rarely responding, whereas with superdosing the benefit is most often observed as an FCR benefit.

Conclusion

Phytases have been used in commercial feed for over 20 years. The pattern of use had remained largely unchanged during this period as the focus has been on P provision with moderate dosage levels of phytase rather than phytate hydrolysis through superdosages. Recent work suggests that the latter, either directly or indirectly is of great benefit to the animal and as a result may provide even greater nutritional and performance benefits than P provision. Applying the superdose concept to facilitate the extra-phosphoric effect of phytate destruction requires knowledge of the phytate content of the diet and the cost-effective phytase dose required to achieve maximal phytate destruction. Additionally, the extra-phosphoric benefits from superdoses of phytase may extend beyond simply ridding the digesta of phytic acid for example, to inositol production and antioxidant sparing capabilities in the blood. It is rare that an additive is introduced and used in the market for one activity for a long period of time but then an alternate use is adopted through a different approach with the same product. This rare event, due to falling phytase costs coupled with increasing prices of raw materials, may well be happening with the use of phytase.

References

Adeola, O., Lawrence, B.V., Sutton, A.L., Cline, T.R., 1995. Phytase induced changes in mineral utilisation in zinc supplemented diets for pigs. Journal of Animal Science. 73: 3384-3391.

Al-Sa'aidi, J.A.A., Ali, S.H., Al-Se'eide, M.J.A., 2009. Role of dietary supplementation of microbial phytase in roosters reproductive system efficiency of broiler breeder (Hubbard flex). Iraqi Journal of Veterinary Sciences. 23:Ar511-Ar520.

Augspurger, N.R., Baker, D.H., 2004. High dietary phytase levels maximize phytate-phosphorus utilization but do not affect protein utilization in chicks fed phosphorus- or amino acid-deficient diets. Journal of Animal Science. 82: 1100-1107.

Bedford, M.R., 2012. Alternate uses of phytases - superdosing. Asian Poultry, June, 8-11.

Blaaberg, K., Jorgensen, H., Tauson, A.H., Poulsen, H.D., 2011. The presence of Inositol phosphates in gastric pig digesta is affected by time after feeding a nonfermented or fermented liquid wheat- and barley-based diet. Journal of Animal Science. 89:3153-3162.

Cowieson, A.J., Acamovic, T., Bedford, M.R., 2004. The effects of phytase and phytic acid on the loss of endogenous amino acids and minerals from broiler chickens. British Poultry Science. 45:101-108.

Cowieson, A.J., Acamovic, T., Bedford, M.R., 2006. Supplementation of corn-soy based diets with an Eschericia coli-derived phytase: Effects on broiler chick performance and the digestibility of amino acids and metabolizability of minerals and energy. Poultry Science. 85: 1389-1397.

Cowieson, A.J., Bedford, M.R., Selle, P.H., Ravindran, V., 2009. Phytate and microbial phytase: Implications for endogenous nitrogen losses and nutrien availability. World's Poultry Science 65: 401-417.

Cowieson, A.J., Ravindran, V., 2007. Effect of phytic acid and microbial phytase on the flow and amino acid composition of endogenous protein at the terminal ileum of growing broiler chickens. British Journal of Nutrition. 98: 745-752.

Engelen, A.J., van der Heeft, F.C., Randsdorp, P.H.G., Somers, W.A.C., Schaefer, J., van der Vat, B.J.C., 2001. Determination of phytase activity in feed by a colorimetric enzymatic method: Collaborative interlaboratory study. Journal of AOAC International. 84: 629-633.

Holub, B.J., 1986. Metabolism and function of myo-inositol and inositol phospholipids. Annual Review of Nutrition. 6: 563-597.

Igbasan, F.A., 2002. A comparative study of the stability of microbial phytases and phytate phosphorus hydrolysis in the gastrointestinal tract of chickens. Tagung Schweine-Une Geflugelernahrung. 6:71-74.

Igbasan, F.A., Manner, K., Miksch, G., Borriss, R., Farouk, A., Simon, O., 2000. Comparative studies on the in vitro properties of phytases from various microbial origins. Archives of Animal Nutrition-Archiv fur Tierernahrung. 53: 353-373.

Karadas, F., Pirgozliev, V., Pappas, A.C., Acamovic, T., Bedford, M.R., 2009. Effects of different levels of dietary phytase activities on the concentration of antioxidants in the liver of growing broilers. Journal of Animal Physiology and Animal Nutrition. 94: 519-526.

Kemme, P.A., Jongbloed, A.W., Mroz, Z., Kogut, J., Beynen, A.C., 1999. Digestibility of nutrients in growing-finishing pig is affected by Aspergillus niger phytase, phytate and lactic acid levels 2. Apparent total tract digestibility of phosphorus, calcium and magnesium and ileal degradation of phytic acid. Livestock Production Science. 58: 119-127.

Kemme, P.A., Schlemmer, U., Mroz, Z., Jongbloed, A.W., 2006. Monitoring the stepwise phytate degradation in the upper gastrointestinal tract of pigs. Journal of the Science of Food and Agriculture. 86:612-622.

Kies, A.K., Kemme, P.A., Sebek, L.B., van Diepen, J.T., Jongbloed, A.W., 2006. Effect of graded doses and a high dose of microbial phytase on the digestibility of various minerals in weaner pigs. Journal of Animal Science. 84:169-1175.

Kornegay, E.T., Denbow, D.M., Yi, Z., Ravindran, V., 1996. Response of broilers to graded levels of microbial phytase added to maize-soyabean-meal-based diets containing three levels of non- phytate phosphorus. British Journal of Nutrition. 75: 839-852.

Liu, N., Ru, Y.J., Li, F.D., 2010. Effect of dietary phytate and phytase on metabolic change of blood and intestinal mucosa in chickens. Journal of Animal Physiology and Animal Nutrition. 94: 368-374.

Luttrell, B.M., 1992. The biological relevance of the binding of calcium ions by inositol phosphates. The Journal of Biological Chemistry. 268: 1521-1524.

Nelson, T.S., Shieh, T.R., Wodzinski, R.J., Ware, J.H., 1971. Effect of supplemental phytase on the utilization of phytate phosphorus by chicks. Journal of Nutrition. 101: 1289-1294.

Onyango, E.M., Asem, E.K., Adeola, O., 2009. Phytic acid increases mucin and endogenous amino acid losses from the gastrointestinal tract of chickens. British Journal of Nutrition. 101:836-842.

Onyango, E.M., Asem, E.K., Sands, J., Adeola, O., 2004. Dietary phytates increase endogenous losses in ducks and chickens. Poultry Science. 83: 149-150.

Pagano, A.R., Roneker, K.R., Lei, X.G., 2005. Fate of supplemental Escherichia coli phytase in the digestive tract of young pigs. Jounal of Animal Science. 83: 388-389.

Persia, M.E., 2010. An enzymatic approach to dealing with the negative consequences of phytate. Multi-State Poultry Meeting, May 25-27, pp. 1-9.

Persson, H., Turk, M., Nyman, M., Sandberg, A.-S., 1998. Binding of Cu^{2+}, Zn^{2+} and Cd^{2+} to inositol tri-, tetra-, penta- and hexa-phosphates. Journal of Agricultural and Food Chemistry. 46: 3194-3200.

Pirgozliev, V.R., Bedford, M.R., Acamovic, T., Mares, P., Allymehr, M., 2011. The effects of supplementary bacterial phytase on dietary energy and total tract amino acid digestibility when fed to young chickens. British Poultry Science. 52: 245-254.

Pirgozliev, V.R., Oduguwa, O., Acamovic, T., Bedford, M.R., 2007. Diets containing Escherichia coli-derived phytase on young chickens and turkeys: effects on performance, metabolizable energy, endogenous secretions, and intestinal morphology. Poultry Science. 86:705-713.

Rosen, G.D., 2002. Microbial phytase in broiler nutrition. In: Garnsworthy, P.C., Wiseman, J. (eds.), Recent Advances in Animal Nutrition 2002, Nottingham University Press, Nottingham, pp. 105-118.

Schlemmer, U., Jany, K.-D., Berk, A., Schulz, E., Rechkemmer, G., 2001. Degradation of phytate in the gut of pigs - pathway of gastro-intestinal inositol phosphate hydrolysis and enzymes involved. Archives of Animal Nutrition. 55: 255-280.

Selle, P.H., Ravindran, V., 2007. Microbial phytase in poultry nutrition. Animal Feed Science and Technology. 135: 1-41.

Selle, P.H., Ravindran, V., Bryden, W.L., Scott, T.A., 2006. Influence of dietary phytate and exogenous phytase on amino acid digestibility poultry: A review. Journal of Poultry Science. 43: 89-103.

Selle, P.H., Ravindran, V., Caldwell, R.A., Bryden, W.L., 2000. Phytate and phytase: Consequences for protein utilisation. Nutrition Research Reviews. 13: 255-278.

Simon, O., Igbasan, F., 2002. In vitro properties of phytases from various microbial origins. International Journal of Food Science and Technology. 37: 813-822.

Walk, C.L., Bedford, M.R., McElroy, A.P., 2012a. Influence of diet, phytase and incubation time on calcium and phosphorus solubility in the gastric and small intestinal phase of an in vitro digestion assay. Journal of Animal Science. In Press.

Walk, C.L., Bedford, M.R., McElroy, A.P., 2012b. Influence of limestone and phytase on broiler performance, gastrointestinal pH and apparent ileal nutrien digestibility. Poultry Science. 91: 1371-1378.

LIST OF PARTICIPANTS

The forty-fourth University of Nottingham Feed Conference was organised by the following committee:

MR M. HAZZLEDINE (*Premier Nutrition*)
MR R. KIRKLAND *(Volac International)*
MR W. MORRIS (*BOCM PAULS Lt*d)
DR D. PARKER (*Novus International*)
DR M.A. VARLEY (*Provimi Ltd*)
DR P. WILCOCK (*ABVista USA*)

DR J.M. BRAMELD
PROF P.C. GARNSWORTHY (*Secretary*)
DR T. PARR   *University of Nottingham*
PROF A.M. SALTER
DR K.D. SINCLAIR
PROF J. WISEMAN (*Chairman*)

The conference was held at the University of Nottingham Sutton Bonington Campus, 27-28 June 2012. The following persons registered for the meeting:

Armbruster, Mr D	Deutscher Fachverlag GMBh, Mainzer Landstrasse 251, Frankfurt Main 60326, Germany
Armstrong, Mr A	Kemin UK, Tudor House, Hampton Road, Southport PR8 6QD, UK
Armstrong, Mr N	University of Nottingham, Sutton Bonington Campus, Loughborough, Leics, LE12 5RD, UK
Auroy, Ms V	CCPA, ZA du Bois de Teillay, Quartier du Haut Bois, Rennes 35150, France
Beaumont, Mr D	Lohmann Animal Health, Maple Lodge, Ryknield Hill, Denby DE5 8NW, UK
Bedford, Dr M	A B Vista, 3 Woodstock Court, Marlborough Business Park, Marlborough SN8 4AN, UK
Brameld, Dr J M	University of Nottingham, Sutton Bonington Campus, Loughborough, Leics, LE12 5RD, UK
Brand, Dr T	University of Stellenbosch, P O Box 80, Elsenburg 7607, South Africa
Butler, Mr D	Freelance Journalist, 11 Meikle St, Meeniyan 3956, Australia
Carlsson, Ms C	A B Vista, 3 Woodstock Court, Marlborough Bus Park, Marlborough SN8 4AN, UK
Davies, Mr T	Kite Consulting, The Crown Buildings, Watling St, Brewood, Staffs ST19 9LL, UK
Down, Mr P	University of Nottingham, Sutton Bonington Campus, Loughborough, Leics, LE12 5RD, UK
Elve, Mr B E	Felleskjopet Rogaland Agder, Postboks 208, Stavanger 4001, Norway
Erregger, Ms E	Stapeley Veterinary Practice, The Gatehouse, Lordstone Lane, Minsterley, Shropshire SY5 0EU, UK
Evans, Mr B R	Hartpury College, Hartpury House, Hartpury, Gloucs GL19 3BE, UK

Ewing, Dr W	Context Products Ltd, 53 Mill St, Packingston, Leics LE65 1WN, UK
Fowers, Miss R	Nutreco, Veerstraat 38, Boxmeer 5831 JN, The Netherlands
Gabriel, Dr I	INRA, Avian Poultry Research, Nouzilly 37380, France
Garnsworthy, Prof P C	University of Nottingham, Sutton Bonington Campus, Loughborough, Leics, LE12 5RD, UK
Gentle, Miss C	Cargill plc, Witham St Hughes, Lincoln LN6 9TN, UK
Gerritsen, Dr R	Schothorst Feed Research (SFR), Meerkoetenweg 26, Lelystad 8218 NA, The Netherlands
Gibbons, Dr J	DairyCo, Stoneleigh Park, Kenilworth CV8 2TL, UK
Gill, Prof M	University of Aberdeen, 14B/10 Riversdale Cresc, Edinburgh EH12 5QT, UK
Golds, Mrs S	University of Nottingham, Sutton Bonington Campus, Loughborough, Leics, LE12 5RD, UK
Graham, Mr M R	Five F Agri LLP, 4 Breidden Avenue, Arddleen, Llannymynech SY22 6SP, UK
Hancox, Miss L	University of Nottingham, Sutton Bonington Campus, Loughborough, Leics, LE12 5RD, UK
Hansen, Dr P	University of Florida, P O Box 110910, Gainesville FL 32611-0910, USA
Harison, Miss E R	B.A.T.A. Ltd, Main St, Amotherby, Malton, North Yorkshire YO17 6TA, UK
Heed, Miss N	University of Nottingham, Sutton Bonington Campus, Loughborough, Leics, LE12 5RD, UK
Houseman, Dr R	MCS Nutrition, 18 Melrose Rd, Bishop Monkton, Harrogate HG3 3RH, UK
Hume, Prof D	The Roslin Institute & R(D)SVS, University of Edinburgh, Easter Bush, Roslin, EH25 9RG, UK
Husband, Mr J	Evidence Based Veterinary Consultancy Ltd, Redhills Rural Enterprise, Penrith CA11 0DT, UK
Jagger, Dr S	AB Agri, 64 Innovation Way, Lynchwood Business Park, Peterborough, P12 6FL, UK
Johnson, Miss S G	Premier Nutrition, The Levels, Rugeley WS15 1RD, UK
Johnston, Miss C	5M Publishing, Benchmark House, 8 Smithy Wood Drive, Chapeltown, Sheffield S35 1QN, UK
Kendal, Mr R	Alltech, Larchwood, Hawksdale, Dalston, Carlisle, Cumbria CA5 7BX, UK
Kirkland, Dr R	Volac, 50 Fishers Lane, Royston SG8 5QX, UK
Kirwan, Dr S	Dr Eckel GmbH, Im Stiefelfeld 10, Niederzissen 56651, Germany
Lander, Miss R	NWF Agriculture Ltd, Wardle, Nantwich, Cheshire CWS 6AQ, UK
Lavrencic, Dr A	University of Ljubljana, Jamnikarjeva 101, Ljublhana 1000 , Slovenija
Lawson, Mrs K	University of Nottingham, Sutton Bonington Campus, Loughborough, Leics, LE12 5RD, UK

Le Bon, Miss M	University of Nottingham, Sutton Bonington Campus, Loughborough, Leics, LE12 5RD, UK
Massey O'Neill, Dr H V	A B Vista, 3 Woodstock Court, Marlborough Business Park, Marlborough SN8 4AN, UK
May, Ms K	University of Nottingham, Sutton Bonington Campus, Loughborough, Leics, LE12 5RD, UK
McCartney, Dr E	Pen & Tec Consulting S.L., Pl. D'Ausias March, 1, 4th Floor DO1, Sant Cugat, del Valles 08195, Spain
Mellits, Dr K	University of Nottingham, Sutton Bonington Campus, Loughborough, Leics, LE12 5RD, UK
Morris, Mr W	BOCM Pauls Ltd, Unit 15A (First Floor), Gelders Hall Road, Shepshed LE12 6NH, UK
Neal, Miss H	AB Agri, 64 Innovation Way, Lynch Wood, Peterborough PE2 6FZ, UK
Newbold, Prof J	IBERS, Aberystwyth University, Penglais Campus, Aberystwyth SY23 3DA, UK
Nordang, Dr L	Felleskjopet Forutvikling, Bromstadvegen 57, Trondheim N-7005, Norway
Northover, Mrs S	University of Nottingham, Sutton Bonington Campus, Loughborough, Leics, LE12 5RD, UK
Parr, Dr T	University of Nottingham, Sutton Bonington Campus, Loughborough, Leics, LE12 5RD, UK
Pedersen, Dr C	Livestock Feed Consultancy, 6 Randalls Croft Road, Salisbury SP2 0EX, UK
Penlington, Mr N	BPEX, Agriculture & Horticulture Development Board, Stoneleigh Park, Kenilworth, Warks CV8 2TL, UK
Pinas-Fernandez, Dr A	Biosciences Knowledge Transfer Network, The Roslin Institute, Easter Bush, Midlothian EH25 9RH, UK
Pope, Mr B	BASF plc, P O Box 4, Earl Rd, Cheadle Hulme, Cheadle, Cheshire SK8 6QG, UK
Raj, Dr J	Micron Bio-Systems Ltd, BFF Business Park, Bath Rd, Bridgwater TA6 4NZ, UK
Retter, Dr W	Heygate & Sons, Bugbrooke Mill, Northampton NN73 3QH, UK
Richards, Dr S	HST Feeds, 4th Avenue, Weston Road, Crewe CW1 6BN, UK
Robinson, Mr M G	Sciantec Analyrical Services Ltd, Stockbridge Technology Centre, Cawood, York YO8 3SD, UK
Salter, Prof A	University of Nottingham, Sutton Bonington Campus, Loughborough, Leics, LE12 5RD, UK
Sartori, Mrs	c/o University of Sao Paulo, Brazil
Sartori, R	University of Sao Paulo, Av. Padua Dias, 11, Piracicaba SP. 13.418-900, Brazil
Saunders, Mr N	University of Nottingham, Sutton Bonington Campus, Loughborough, Leics, LE12 5RD, UK

Shingfield, Dr K	MTT Agrifood Research Finland, Animal Production Research, Jokioinen Fl, 31600, Finland
Sinclair, Dr K	University of Nottingham, Sutton Bonington Campus, Loughborough, Leics, LE12 5RD, UK
Sivam, Mr K	Westpoint Veterinary Group, Unit 1 Trevornick Business Park, Winnard's Perch, St Columb TR9 6DT, UK
Speelman, Mr R	A B Vista, 3 Woodstock Court, Marlborough Business Park, Marlborough SN8 4AN, UK
Springer, Mr B	Feed Magazine/Kraftfutter, Mainzer Landstrasse 251, Frankfurt (M) 63571, 63571, Germany
Stainsby, Mr A	B.A.T.A Ltd, Main St, Amotherby, Malton, North Yorkshire YO17 6TA, UK
Stein, Dr H	University of Illinois, 1207 West Gregory Drive, Urbana 61801, USA
Sullivan, Miss K	AB Agri, 64 Innovation Way, Lynchwood, Peterborough PE2 6FL, UK
Tan, Mr M Y	AB Vista, 3 Woodstock Court, Marlborough Business Park, Marlborough SN8 4AN, UK
Taylor, Mr D	Farmvets Southwest Ltd, Unit 8, Sedgemoor Auction Centre, Market Way, North Petherton TA6 6DF, UK
Ten Doeschate, Dr R H M	A B Vista, 3 Woodstock Court, Marlborough Business Park, Marlborough SN8 4AN, UK
Thornley, Mr B	Harper Adams University College, Newport, Shropshire TF10 8NB, UK
Van Adrichem, Mr P	Cargill Animal Nutrition, Veilingweg 23, Velddriel 5334LD, Netherlands
Vandaele, Mrs L	ILVO, Scheldeweg 68, MELLE 9090, Belgium
Velasquez-Estay, Mr H	Pen & Tec Consulting, SL, Pl. D'Ausias March, 1, 4th Floor DO1, Sant Cugat del Valles 08195, Spain
Vitit, Mr K	United Feeding Company Limited, 199/49-51 Vibhavadi Rangsit Road, Samsen Nai, Phaya Thai, Bangkok 10400, Thailand
Walk, Dr C L	A B Vista, 3 Woodstock Court, Marlborough Business Park, Marlborough SN8 4AN, UK
Walker, Dr N D	A B Vista, 3 Woodstock Court, Marlborough Business Park, Marlborough SN8 4AN, UK
Walton, Miss H	Provimi, Provimi Mill, Dalton Ind Estate, Thirsk Y07 3HE, UK
Wilcock, Dr P	A B Vista, 3 Woodstock Court, Marlborough Business Park, Marlborough SN8 4AN, UK
Wilkinson, Prof JM	2 Kirklington Close, Southwell, Notts NG25 OFA, UK
Wischer, Mr G	BASF SE, G-ENL/ED, F 31 Chemiestrasse 22, Lampertheim 68623, Germany
Wiseman, Prof J	University of Nottingham, Sutton Bonington Campus, Loughborough LE12 5RD, UK

Wonnacott, Dr K	BOCM Pauls Ltd, Unit 15A (First Floor), Gelders Hall Road, Shepshed LE12 6NH, UK
Woolf, Mr N	AB Agri, 64 Innovation Way, Lynchwood, Peterborough PE2 6FL, UK
Wynn, Dr R	AB Agri Ltd (KW Alternative Feeds), Bishopdyke Road, Sherburn in Elmet, LS25 6JZ, UK

INDEX

www.ingramcontent.com/pod-product-compliance
Lightning Source LLC
Chambersburg PA
CBHW052119230326
41598CB00080B/3890